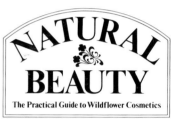

NATURAL BEAUTY

The Practical Guide to Wildflower Cosmetics

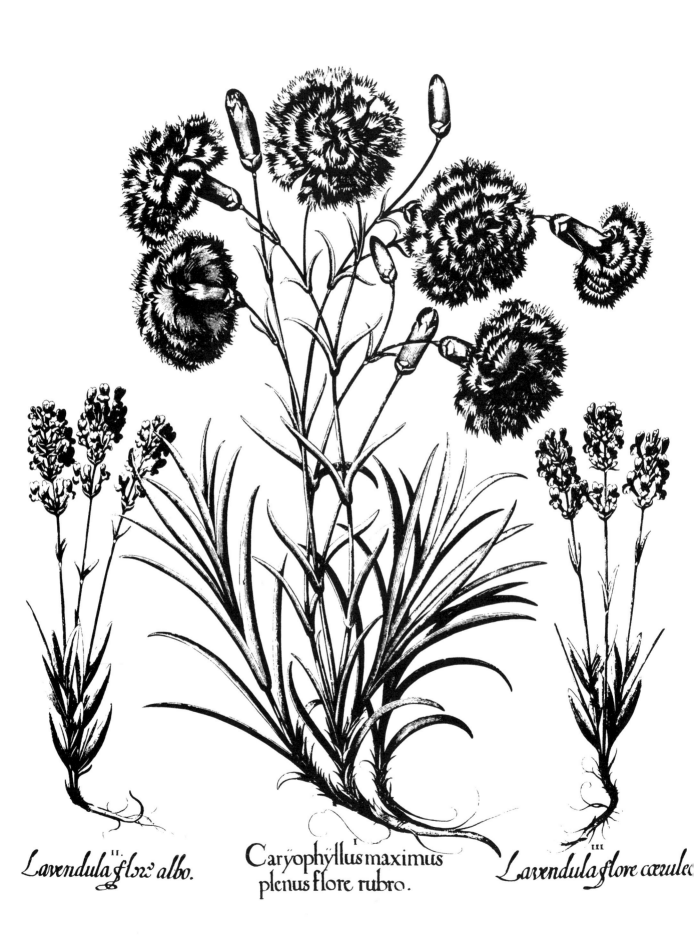

Lavendula II. *flo: albo.*

Caryophyllus maximus plenus flore rubro.

III. *Lavendula flore cœrulec*

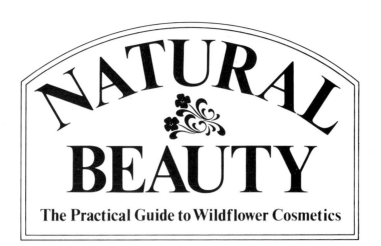

NATURAL BEAUTY

The Practical Guide to Wildflower Cosmetics

Roy Genders

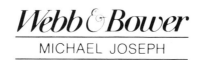

Webb & Bower

MICHAEL JOSEPH

A BDV Basilius Verlag Co-Publication
Copyright © 1985 by BDV Basilius Verlag AG,
CH-Basel
Copyright © UK edition Webb & Bower (Publishers) Ltd

This edition published 1986 by
Webb & Bower (Publishers) Limited
9 Colleton Crescent, Exeter, Devon EX2 4BY
in association with
Michael Joseph Limited
27 Wright's Lane, London W8 5SL

**British Library Cataloguing in
Publication Data**
Genders, Roy
  Wild flower beauty.
  1. Herbal cosmetics
  I. Title
  646.7'2   RA778

  ISBN 0 86350 078 1

Original Concept and Design by
EMIL M. BUHRER
Editor
MASSIMO GIACOMETTI
Captions and Copy Editor
DORIE BAKER
Picture Procuration
ROSARIA PASQUARIELLO
Printed by
G. CANALE & C. S.p.A. - TURIN, ITALY
Bound by
MAURICE BUSENHART, LAUSANNE, SWITZERLAND
Typeset in Great Britain by
KEYSPOOLS LIMITED, GOLBORNE,
WARRINGTON, LANCASHIRE
Photolithography by
BUFOT GMBH, BASEL, SWITZERLAND

Printed in Italy

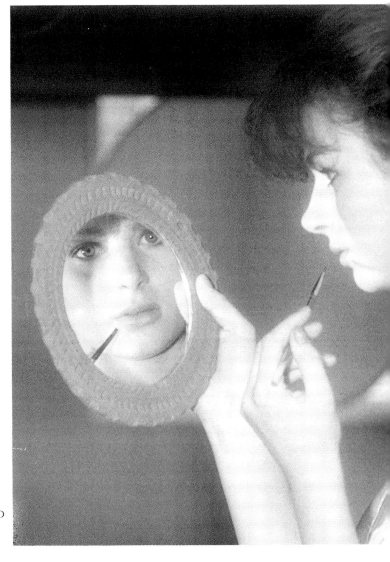

Contents

Plants have provided man's mate with all that is needed to beautify the body, to maintain its attractions for the opposite sex for the reproduction of the species just as flowers depend upon scent and colour to attract insects for their pollination and reproduction.

There are plants for all parts of the body, to give sparkle to the eyes, to add lustre to the hair,

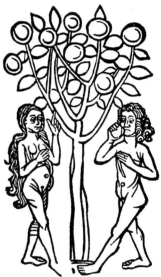

colour to the cheeks and lips, and also provide a sense of comfort and well being to every part of the human frame. Many of today's most respected beauty preparations contain flowers and fruits, vegetables and herbs as their principal ingredients and man is becoming ever more conscious of their goodness.

Then took Mary a pound
of ointment of spikenard,
very costly, and anointed
the feet of Jesus,
and wiped his feet
with her hair: and the house
was filled with the odour
of the ointment ...

John 12:3

On the basis of tradition
supported by the gospel text
Mary Magdalene is
worshipped as the patron
saint of perfume makers. In
this painting by the Master
of Moulins, she is shown
bearing the alabaster box
containing the very precious
ointment with which she
anointed Christ. Spikenard
is just one of the very valued
herbal plants whose oil has
figured in the legend and
lore of Western civilization.

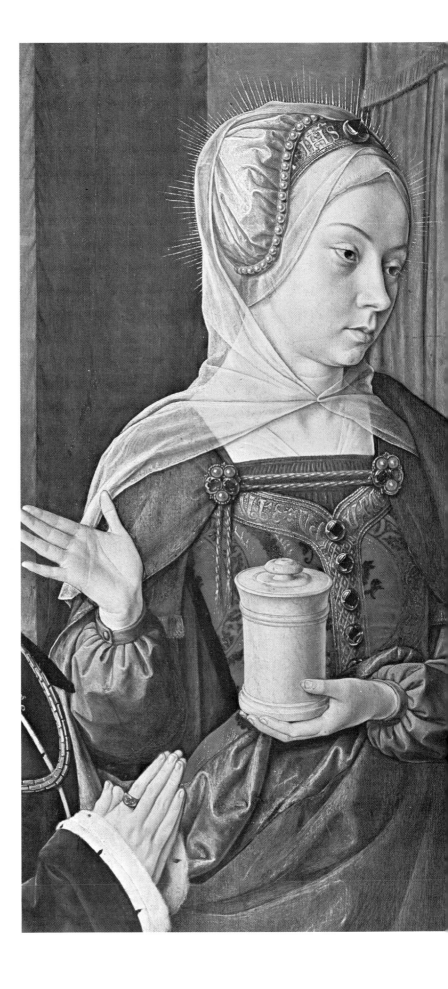

Introduction

Among the manifold creatures of God . . .
none have provoked men's studies more or satisfied their desires
so much as plants have done, and that upon just and worthy causes.
For if delight may provoke men's labour,
what greater delight is there than to behold the earth apparalled with plants,
as with a robe of embroidered work, set with pearls of the Orient,
and garnished with great diversitie of rare and costly jewels? . . .
If odours or if taste may work satisfaction,
they are both so common in plants and so comfortable
that no confection of apothecaries can equal their excellent virtues.

John Gerard in the Dedication to the Herbal, 1597

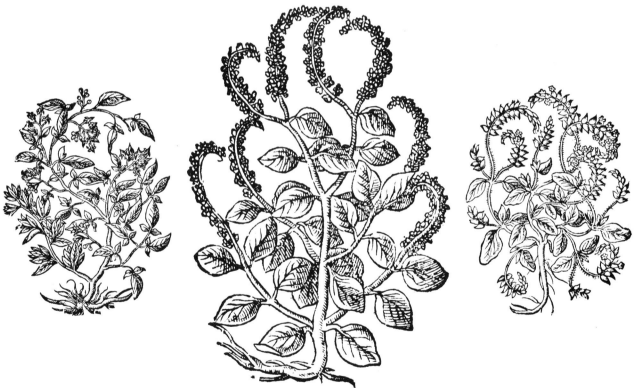

From the beginning of time, plants have provided man with all his needs, cures in time of sickness and disease, and foods to maintain the body in health and vitality by providing it with vitamins and mineral salts to meet the body's total requirements. Plants have also provided man's mate with all that is needed to beautify the body, to maintain its attractions for the opposite sex for the reproduction of the species just as flowers depend upon scent and colour to attract insects for their pollination and reproduction.

There are plants for all parts of the body, to give sparkle to the eyes, to add lustre to the hair, colour to the cheeks and lips, and also provide a sense of comfort and well being to every part of the human frame. Many of todays most respected beauty preparations contain flowers and fruits, vegetables and herbs as their principle ingredients and man is becoming ever more conscious of their goodness.

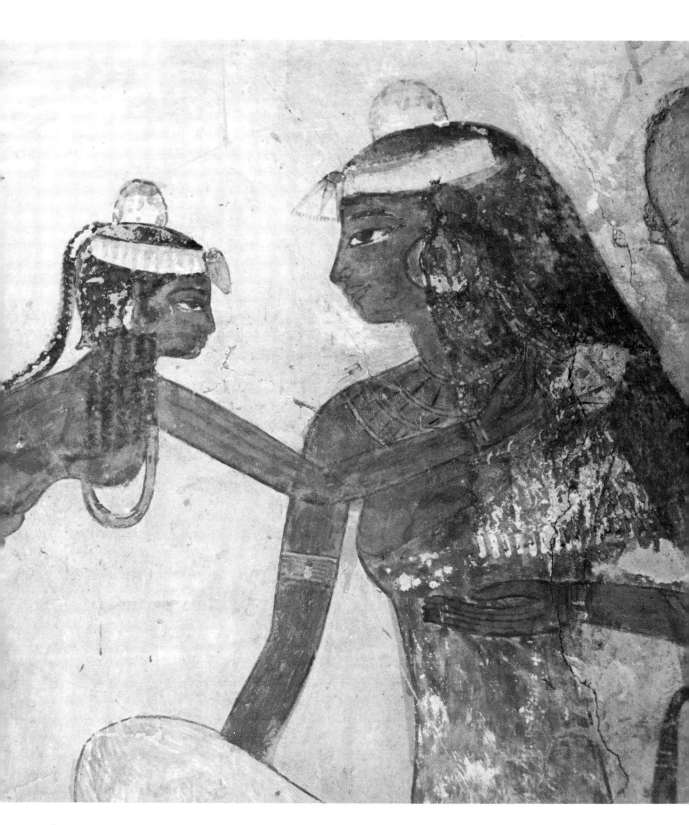

The cosmos of cosmetics

Since mankind first appeared on earth, those plants which contributed to his well being, to the pleasures rather than the necessities of life, have played as large a part in everyday life as the food bearing plants and those of economic value.

The first Book of the Bible, written some 6000 years ago, shortly before the building of the Sphinx and the great pyramid of Cheops, tells that "the Lord God planted a garden eastward in Eden in which grew every tree that is pleasant to the sight and good for food ... and a river went out of Eden to water the garden".

Gold, frankincense and myrrh were then recognised as the most valuable of man's possessions. Both frankincense and myrrh are plants of the same family Burseraceae and are closely related to the citrus family. They are shrubs of twiggy habit, whose small leaves keep transpiration to a minimum in the hot and arid conditions in which they grow. The plants are found in ravines and on barren hillsides, usually growing amongst rocks and boulders. The gummy exhudations appear throughout the year and are collected by Arab people today exactly as in ancient times: from the beards and fleeces of goats and sheep which nibble at the evergreen leaves for nourishment.

The gum is made into cakes and sold in the markets of Arabia and East Africa, eventually reaching all parts of the world.

Another of the important gum-resins of the ancient world was labdanum, the Rock or Cretan rose (in no way connected to the Damask rose used in perfumery). It is *Cistus ladaniferus*, found on hillsides throughout Syria and Palestine, as well as on the islands of Cyprus and Crete where the purest labdanum is obtained. It is collected from the plants with a special instrument known as a ladanisteron, rather than from the beards of goats as in the Holy Land. When used as incense, pure labdanum, which is reddish-black, burns with a clear flame and gives off a pleasing balsamic perfume, free of the noticeable smell of ammonia encountered from burning animal hairs. Like myrrh, labdanum was one of the bases of all ancient perfumes, as it is still today.

The sweet cinnamon known to the peoples of the Near East would be the bark of the species *Cinnamomum glanduliferum*, like spikenard, present in remote valleys of the Himalayas and known in perfumery as Nepal Sassafras. Its bark is brown and is readily peeled from the tree without harming it.

From another species of *Cinnamomum*, the "cassia" oil of the Scriptures was obtained. Again it is the bark that is used, whilst from the young bud-stalks and leaves, a fragrant oil is obtained and used in perfumery. In biblical times, this precious oil was mixed with oil from the fruit of the olive which abounded in Palestine. It was rubbed onto the feet and legs and massaged into the body to keep the skin soft and supple. The scented barks, and the dried roots of many plants including sweet calamus and spikenard, were ground to a fine powder and used to sprinkle amongst bedding and over the body after bathing, exactly as talcum powder is used today.

Opposite, the woman in this detail from a Theban tomb painting is being prepared by her servants for a feast. This is one of many illustrations depicting the ritual cosmetic process that preceded celebrations and life passages, including death.

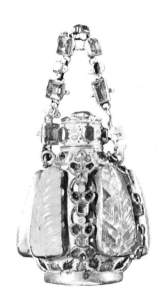

The expense lavished on this English gold and enamel perfume container set with chalcedony panels and mounted with rubies and diamonds, indicates the value placed on the scent contained.

The most precious of all the aromatics was spikenard, only obtainable from the most remote valleys of the Himalayas and collected and transported with extreme difficulty. Hence it was the most costly of all aromatics, to be used only on special occasions. The roots were either dried and ground down or an oil was extracted from them and made into an ointment (with olive or almond oil) to rub onto the feet and shoulders. The heavy and lasting perfume of the plant made it as precious to the Egyptians and the peoples of the Near East as it was in later years to the Greeks and Romans.

Saffron was included in most unguents. It is the product of the dried stigmata of *crocus sativus* which covers mountainous slopes throughout the Near East and in Kashmir and N India. It is the Karkom of the Song of Solomon and from this became "crocum", Linnaeus using the name *crocus* for the corm-bearing plants he grouped under this genus.

The "balm" of Genesis is thought to be the gummy exhudation of *Pistacia lentiscus*, a fragrant terebinthine which appears from the stems of the plant as pale yellow transparent drops. It was and still is chewed by the peoples of the Near East as it is believed to strengthen the teeth and gums. It is known as "mastick" and is an ingredient of modern tooth pastes. Arabia and the Near East abound in gum resins as nowhere else and their uses have been appreciated from earliest times. Gradually they reached Southern Europe, where the ancient civilisation of Greece and Rome made the maximum use of their many qualities.

From the petals or the whole flower of many plants, numerous beauty preparations are obtained. Astringents and "after shave" lotions are made from elder, centaury, lily of the valley and privet; complexion milks and washing waters from Solomon's seal, red clover, lime tree blossom and cowslips; body lotions from mignonette and mullein; hair tonics and restorers (though mostly from leaves) are made from cassia and chamomile; skin creams from marigold and marshmallow; and to soothe the eyes there is cornflower and clary.

Leaves are commonly used to treat balding and to colour hair; to soothe the eyes and to give them a sparkle; to make body powder when dried and ground; and to provide a relaxing bath. Sometimes only leaves are used or sometimes they are used in combination with the entire plant.

Leaves most used in perfumery and for cosmetics are those containing glands in the form of pellucid dots in which the fragrant oil is stored as a waste product. The fragrance is released when the leaves are pressed between the fingers. With certain plants, e.g. carnauba wax and balsam poplar, the leaf buds are covered with resin which is removed with spirits of wine and has the scent of storax.

In Pinnate the leaflets are arranged on either side of a central stalk as with agrimony, a decoction of which is used to soothe the eyes, and Jacob's ladder from which a black hair dye is obtained.

Lobed leaves have parts of the leaf edge protruding, as with feverfew, whose leaves are divided into several lobed segments. Boiled in milk, they remove soreness when applied cold to the face.

Lanceolate leaves are long, tapering to the apex as with patchouli, the principal ingredient (when dry) of Eastern talcum powders; and golden rod, whose leaves, when boiled in milk, are soothing to the skin.

The stems of certain plants yield gum – resin and bark.
Resin is collected by incisions made in the stem or trunk and allowed to solidify before being transported for use as a fixative for cosmetics.
Labdanum is the best known of gum-resins. It is exuded by the stems and leaves in the intense heat where it grows and is collected from the fleece and beard of goats which browse amongst the bushes as in biblical times. Balsam of Peru and oil of ben (Benzoin), which is colourless and tasteless and does not turn rancid with age, is collected from tree trunks and is used to make hair oils and sun-tan lotions. The exudations of pistacia and elemi are used in perfumery.
The Bark of certain trees has important uses in perfumery, chiefly for talcum powder, as elemi and canella, being finely ground after drying. The bark of red elm provides mucilage which is soothing to the skin and to the lining of the stomach when taken internally.

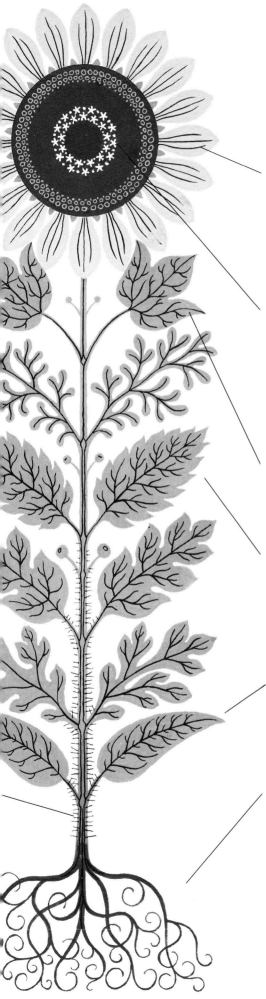

Certain plants provide their dried seeds for many beauty aids, most important being cereals, oats and barley, used for face packs or masks since Cleopatra's time. Sesame seed is used in sun-tan oils and to protect the skin from excessive ultra-violet light. Coriander and caraway seeds make soothing toilet waters and the sunflower provides seeds which make a softening skin cream. The seeds of ambrette and tonquin are ground to make talcum powders, and walnuts provide an oil to dye the hair black.

The fruits of several plants have similar uses. The fruit may take the form of nuts or berries. A berry is a fruit containing seeds embedded in its juice or pulp, whilst a nut is a hard, one-seeded fruit. Nuts may vary in size from almonds to coconuts and both yield valuable skin healing oils which protect and soothe the skin when used in creams and soaps. The avocado and quince, apple and olive are fruits whose pulp yields nourishment for the skin; tomatoes make ideal face packs. Lemons are good astringents and hair tonics; oranges are used in perfumes and toilet waters.

In Palmate the leaves are usually 5- or 7-lobed, divided like the fingers of a hand. This leaf is represented by the wax palm of Brazil, from which carnauba wax is obtained for use in mascara and soaps.

Ovate leaves are amongst the most common of the plant kingdom. They are broadest below the middle, being almost egg-shaped, as with those of the box which are smooth and glossy and provide a valuable hair tonic, and sage which are deeply channeled and rough to the touch.

Elliptic leaves are broadest at the middle, narrowing at both ends. Those of the henna plant are an example, the leaves being used since earliest times to colour the hair.

Roots take several forms and have many uses. From those of the alkanet, a dye is extracted to colour the cheeks red and from arnica, to colour the hair and act as a tonic. The root of marshmallow provides a soothing skin preparation and carrot, mashed and mixed with a little olive oil, a face mask or pack which will cleanse the skin of blemishes. From the rhizomatous root of orris and sassafras, after drying and grounding, perfumed talcum powder is made, whilst the bulbous roots of the madonna lily and garlic (also of the lily family) yield juices which when mixed with oil or lard, make an effective ointment to clear the skin of soreness and blemishes. The edible tuberous root of the potato acts as an astringent, and when peeled and placed raw on the neck, it will help to remove wrinkles and sagginess by tightening the skin.

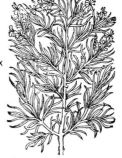

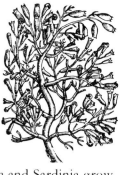

The five illustrations from the 17th century herbal of Adamo Lonicero depict plants that have been prized for their medicinal and cosmetic properties from ancient times to the present. From left to right rosemary, cloves, coriander, cisthus, stirax benzoin.

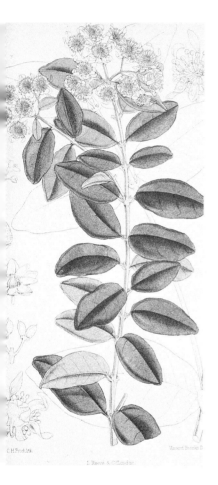

Boldoa fragrans, a native shrub of the Chilean Andes mountains is used by the natives of the area for many medicinal and cosmetic purposes. The leaves have a highly scented essential oil which is used commercially to make perfume and soap. The bark and twigs of this aromatic plant are ground to make dusting powders.

Among other plants native of the Near East was the very much valued Red Rose whose natural habitat is believed to be Persia and the land between the Black and Caspian Seas.

A hybrid of the red rose, possibly from a crossing with the Damask rose, which abounds in Syria (*suri* means "land of roses") and which provides its essential oil for perfumes, is depicted on a wall of the excavated Palace of Knossos in Crete, believed to be more than 4000 years old. It has been identified as the Holy Rose, the *Rosa Sancta* of Arabia and Abyssinia (Ethiopia) and which has been found, still fragrant, in Egyptian tombs of 4000 years ago.

One of the most beautiful of all plants indigenous to the Holy Land and Near East is the Camphire of the song of Solomon. It is thought to have been planted for hedges in the Hanging Gardens of Babylon, for the scent of its flowers exceeds that of all others. It was one of the poet Milton's "odorous shrubs" which grew in the Garden of Eden and is today planted throughout the Near East to protect vineyards from prevailing winds. The small white flowers are borne along the twiggy stems and are woven into chaplets by maidens. Until quite recent times, sprigs of blossom were sold in the streets of Cairo, with the cry of "oh odours of Paradise; of flowers of henna". Since earliest times the dried leaves, made into a paste, have proved the best of all colouring agents for the hair. Southern Europe itself, was the habitat of many plants famed for their scented flowers and more especially, their leaves. Along the coast of France and Italy and on the

islands of Corsica and Sardinia grow rosemary and lavender, marjoram, the thymes and plants that have been used in perfumery and cosmetics since earliest times. They were probably introduced into Britain with the Roman invasion, where, ever since, they have been cultivated to meet their many uses. They are amongst the most effective of all plants for conditioning the hair, whilst their dried and ground leaves add strength to sachet and talcum powders. From the flowers of lavender, a popular handkerchief perfume is made and a brilliantine to set the hair.

For centuries, olive and almond trees have been established in southern Europe, on the rocky ground with which they are familiar in their native lands. Greece and Italy abound with the small trees which are found as far west as the Spanish peninsula. The citrus fruits grow with them and all are now cultivated in large plantations to supply the leading perfumers with the essential oils of their fruits for there are few perfumes which do not include at least one of them.

Several of those plants with fragrant roots, which when dried and ground down are used in talcum powders, are native of southern Europe and the Near East. These include orris root (*Iris florentina*) and (*Iris pallida*) and further east, in India, Burma and Malaysia, are found zedoary and spikenard, kuchoora and kapur-kadri, each increasing in strength with keeping. They mostly have the violet perfume, present also in the Indian violet grass, *Andropogon muricatus*. Those eastern plants with scented roots are mostly of the ginger

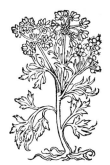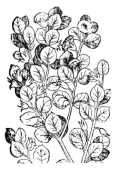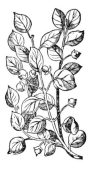

family, their culture now extending to SE Asia. When ground they are often mixed with cloves and with fragrant woods such as cedar and sandalwood which have a similar "flowery" fragrance. From the deep yellow roots of *Curcuma aromatica*, a fragrant oil is extracted which Eastern women rub onto the body, imparting a delicious perfume and from the dried roots of *C. zedoaria*, along with powdered cloves and scented woods, Hindu women make a talcum powder called zedoary.

Plants of SE Asia, tropical Australia and islands of the Pacific include the coconut palm, famed for its oil, used in many beauty preparations, especially bath oils and shampoos, and sandalwood, its essential oil used as a fixative and in the "green and woody" perfumes known as "bouquets". Usually included with them is vetivert, the violet-scented rhizomatous roots of the Indian violet grass.

In the hot and rain drenched forests of Queensland grows the evergreen *Melaleuca linarifolia* and from its fresh leaves yellow oil of cajaput is obtained; also in Queensland the Gum acacia or cassie tree is found. Here too, grows the elemi, native also to the Philippine Islands, from which is obtained a fragrant gum much used in perfumery. It has a sharp lemony scent.

In the Indonesian islands grows *Styrax benzoin*, gum styrax or storax, whose fragrant gum enables perfumers to give permanence to those flowery odours obtained by maceration. The closely related *Styrax officinale* grows in Asia Minor and is used in the same way. By stuffing its

collected bark into horsehair bags and pressing the contents with a wooden lever, a resin is extracted with an odour similar to that of musk and ambergris. Although unpleasant when in bulk, in small amounts it has the delicious smell of jonquil and tuberose.

Where it is not quite so warm, in China and Japan, flowers figure prominently in perfumes and cosmetics, and include the lilac and gardenia, white jasmine and orange blossom. Here too, grows *Cinnamomum camphora*, as it does in Sri Lanka and Malaysia and on many of the islands of SE Asia, its bark being widely used in cooking and in perfumery. It has the delicious scent of orange and bergamot and when ground down is included in talcum powders. *Cinnamomum cassia* and *Cinnamomum glanduliferum* are confined to north India and west China. From the young bud-stalks and its leaves, cassia (not to be confused with cassie) oil is obtained and also from the bark by distillation.

The forests of N America abound with trees and shrubs useful in many cosmetics. In the eastern states, *Hamamelis virginiana* grows in dense coppices and from its bark the finest of all skin astringents is obtained. It is a clear liquid known as witch hazel and is used in every beauty parlour in the West.

From the bark of the birch, *Betula lenta*, an aromatic oil identical to oil of wintergreen, which often grows with it, is obtained and used in medicated soaps to treat skin infections and blemishes. From its leaves an astringent lotion is obtained.

The Balsam poplar yields from the

Of those plants common to most parts the cereal crops must take pride of place. Barley, wheat and oats were used for food and for bodily care before the quest for beauty emerged as a force in daily life. As Cleopatra was to discover, barley is the best of all face masks.

The elder grows in many places and has many uses, particularly among northern peoples: its hollow stems were used for kindling, its fruit for preserves, its flowers to bring relief and to impart a sparkle to sore eyes and to use as an astringent and body lotion. It continues to be in great demand. Of other plants enjoying a wide distribution there is horsetail and horseradish, sowthistle and eyebright, the loosestrifes, watercress and succory, each having food value in addition to its uses in the care of the body. They are "green" plants, mostly distributed across N. Europe and Asia, and are used fresh from the countryside.

No place produces more plants for beauty and allurement than the Mediterranean, for on its shores or in close proximity, grow lavender and rosemary, marjoram and thyme, woody aromatic plants that can be used fresh or dry. They have been used in the making of sweet waters, to include in washing waters and pot pourris and sweet bags since earliest times. Of even greater importance to the world of beauty is the fruit of the lemon and orange, which have many uses in perfumery, and the softening oils of almond and olive, which have been used to give lustre to the hair and to maintain the elasticity of the skin since the time of ancient Egypt.

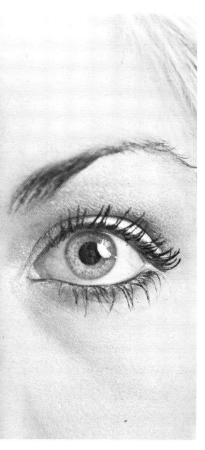

The window of the soul is the eye, and there is perhaps no facial feature more alluring to the opposite sex than bright receptive appealing eyes. The art of making them up properly is one well worth developing. Two herbs associated with the enhancement of ocular beauty are eyebright and belladonna.

scales of its leaf buds, a balsamic resin which, when extracted by spirits of wine, yields a substance with the scent of storax used as a fixative in perfumes. Another of the balsams of the New World is the Balsam of Peru. It has no connections with the country of that name and is found only in dense coastal forests of El Salvador along a strip of land known as the Balsam Coast and with it grows the only other species of the genus, Balsam of Tolu. The resins of the New World match those of the Old in their many medicinal and cosmetic uses. And there are plants whose barks replace the cinnamon and cassia of the Old World which are ground down to make sweet-scented talcum powders. In Chile grows *Boldoa fragrans* whose smooth brown bark yields the scented powder known as Boldo and whose leaves yield an essential oil used in perfumery and soap making.

In the tropical forests of Florida, the Bahamas and Cuba grows *Canella alba*, its white bark having the aroma of cloves, for it contains eugenol, which gives the clove its unique fragrance.

North America abounds in plants famed for the fragrance of their bark, being used in perfumery and cosmetics as "sassafras". They are trees or shrubs of the Laurel order, common in woodlands from eastern Canada to Missouri where, in the warmer climate of the south it will attain a height of 100 feet (30 m). *Laurus sassafras* has deeply furrowed bark which is extremely fragrant and so are the roots of young plants which have a shrub-like habit. They are usually present on wooded slopes and with them grows the closely

related *Magnolia grandiflora* with its glossy laurel-like leaves and fragrant cup-shaped flowers which the early French settlers in Louisiana made into garlands to decorate their homes. Safrol is present in the bark or outer skin of the roots and from safrol heliotropin is obtained synthetically and reproduces the scent of heliotrope in perfumery.

The early settlers of Carolina made use of the bark of the "Sweet-scented shrub" or *Calycanthus* whose bark has a cinnamon smell, whilst its roots smell of camphor, but it was the bark that was most in demand as a substitute for cinnamon though the settlers burnt the dried roots to fumigate their homes.

The Sweet Fern of North America also yields a fragrant oil and is used in perfumery and cosmetics, often with oil of wintergreen obtained from the evergreen *Gaultheria procumbens* whose heath-like leaves when dry are used as a substitute for tea. The plant is especially prevalent in New Jersey and North Carolina. Otto of wintergreen is the principal ingredient of Iceland Wintergreen, a popular handkerchief perfume a century ago and which has remained so. It is prepared from esprit de rose; essence of lavender and extract of cassie, neroli and vanilla. It has much of the refreshing fragrance of eau de Cologne but in which the vanilla essence is absent.

Used the world over in cooking and in cosmetics and perfumery, to which it imparts its own subtle flavour, is the vanilla, an epiphytic plant of the forests of Mexico and Brazil. It is the pods or beans (like pole or runner beans) that are used for so many purposes. The perfumer

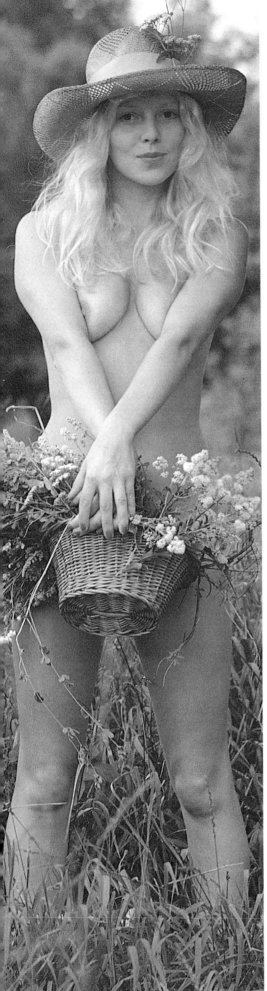

Hair

The hair is one's crowning glory and reflects the health of one's body. For a natural shampoo which will impart a gloss to the hair and feed the roots, those preparations containing bay rum, chamomile, caraway and marjoram (with beer) are recommended. To use as a tonic, there is bay rum, chamomile and rosemary, sage and box, marjoram and thyme, southernwood and wormwood, all promoting new hair growth if used persistently.

Eyes

There are plants to sooth the eyes, to take away soreness caused by long hours of close work or by strong sunlight or cold winds and amongst these are elder flowers and clary, fennel, marigold, cornflower and melilot. To brighten the eyes, to give them a sparkle, agrimony, vervain and eyebright are recommended.

Face or Complexion

For a face pack or mask that will leave the skin clean and soft, there are barley and oats, tomato and red elm, which have been used since earliest times. Amongst the best natural ingredients to include in face creams is the avocado (present in the most expensive creams) and cucumber, which is almost as good, marigold and marshmallow, almond, olive and coconut oil, quince seed mucilage, oil of Balanos and carnauba wax.

Mouth (lips and teeth)

To maintain the teeth in condition and to keep them white and clear of tartar, regular brushing with the juice of strawberry or sloes, the fruit of the blackthorn, will be effective.

Neck

It is in the neck that the first signs of age appear with wrinkling and flabbiness of the skin. Elderflower water (with glycerine and borax) or witch hazel (with almond oil and lanolin) should be massaged into the neck at bedtime. Or peel a large tomato and cut into slices and place over the neck for an hour at a time.

Breasts and Body

To keep the breasts firm, cloths soaked in an infusion of lady's mantle whilst warm and placed on the breasts will bring about firmness. Extract of arnica massaged into the breasts will give similar results.

Arnica (with witch hazel) or rosemary is a reliable deodorant and a refreshing toilet soap can be made with bay laurel, myrrh, caraway, lavender, pine or wintergreen as ingredients.

Hands and Nails

To keep the hands clean and free from stains, place the juice of half a lemon in a basin of warm water and soak them for several minutes. Then scrub them in warm water with soap. To prevent the nails becoming brittle and the hands chapped, massage olive oil or almond oil into the hands at bedtime. White iodine from sea kelp is the best of nail "varnishes".

Legs and Feet

Once a week at bedtime, soak the feet and ankles for 15 minutes in a footbath of warm water into which rosemary, mint or wild thyme has been placed. Then massage olive oil into the feet and legs and wear long stockings over night.

To prevent callouses forming on the feet, upon rising, rub into the soles lemon juice or witch hazel.

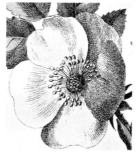

Above, the wild rose or dog rose (the root of which was supposed to cure mad dogs' bites), ancestor of the infinite array of roses enjoyed today.

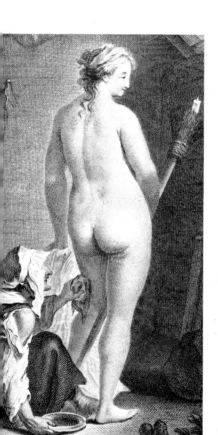

Witches were supposed to be expert in filters and other herbal concoctions leading them to wildly erotic encounters with the devil on sabbath nights. A renewed knowledge of the power of plants to enhance beauty may help today's "witches" in the game of allurement.

uses it in the "green" and "woody" perfumes – the "bouquets" – usually with extract of Tonquin.

The tomato and strawberry are native of Chile and Peru and are amongst the most efficient of nature's products to use as a face pack, as they leave the skin soft and smooth and clear of blemishes. Chile and Peru are also the original home of the potato, now a staple food the world over. To improve the neckline, to take away wrinkles and to firm the flesh, the juice of a potato has no equal.

In the islands of the West Indies and in the Bahamas, in Cuba and Haiti grows the West Indian Bay, a plant of the myrtle family whose leaves and pea-sized fruits yield an aromatic oil which when mixed with Jamaica rum, yields the best of all hair tonics, bay rum.

Canella and allspice grow on these islands and also the wax palm which is found in Brazil.

Many of the common plants native to the British Isles and to north Europe and Asia are present also in N America. Amongst these are the eyebright which is the best of all plants to give a sparkle to the eyes; and lady's mantle, a decoction of which, applied to the breasts will bring about their firmness. The Black elder with its world wide distribution is a common plant of N America and of north Europe. From the flowers an effective astringent lotion is obtained.

Those plants of northerly climes, north of latitude 45° from north Italy and the Black Sea to the British Isles, Iceland and Scandinavia, include the Angelica and Lady's Mantle; Chickweed and Tormentil; Brooklime and

Sow Thistle, whose milky juice, in a little warm water or milk is an admirable skin cleanser.

Those plants of colder parts used for health and beauty mostly take on a different form from those growing in warmer climes. These are of a woody nature: they do not die back in winter as do those of northern parts as protection from the cold. These plants are mostly used fresh in spring and summer and for the various preparations made from them which will last for a year or more.

The useful plants for cosmetics are not of dense forests and deep valleys but of waste ground and embankments, of hedgerows and fields. Some are annual and some perennial, but with few exceptions all die back in winter, and there are few plants able to ripen their seeds before doing so. For all that they provide a wide range of beauty aids. Of woodland trees, the distillation of lime tree blossom rivals that of the elder as an astringent and after shave; and box leaves promote the growth of new hair better than anything else. A decoction of the lesser celadine is an effective astringent, and fumitory makes an efficient complexion water. The flowers of mullein, boiled in milk for a few minutes, make an excellent complexion milk and those of succory, infused in milk or warm water, give a sparkle to the eyes. There is no part of the world which does not make its contribution to the beauty and allurement of mankind.

A practical guide to the plants and their use

Reference Section I
In the following pages the reader will find, listed in alphabetical order, 172 selected plants for natural beauty. Besides each plant is a list of cosmetic applications (such as "to soothe tired eyes") for which the plant has been found helpful. The reader can look up specific instructions and preparations in Reference sections II and III.

In the same way that herbs have an important part to play in modern medicine, if only because of the ever-increasing cost of synthetic cures, so too are natural preparations, which are just as effective as toxic chemicals minus their unpleasant side effects, returning to the modern beauty parlour and hair salon. The beauty houses the world over are now being compelled by public demand, to use more natural products in their preparations and less of those manufac-

from the chemist or drug store than to make them from plants of the countryside or garden. Those who had to find their own plants knew from experience exactly the right time to collect them, when they would be most effective either as medicine or simply for personal enjoyment. The weather too, played a big part in their collecting, drying and storing which had to be done with care for the plants to retain their best qualities.

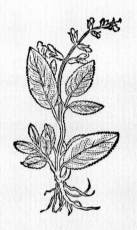 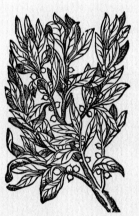 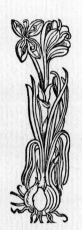 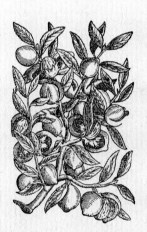 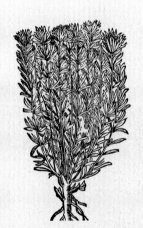

Above, woodcuts of some of the plants used since ancient times for their medicinal properties as well as for their essential oils – salvia, bay laurel, saffron, cloves, rosemary.

tured by the chemicals industry. Both in her eating habits and in her make up, modern woman is going back to nature, the healthy complexion of the country maid is now again in vogue. Whereas the well-to-do have generally sought their beauty preparations and treatments at salons, the less well-off have had to turn to the cosmetics of the countryside: free for the taking, though taking longer to prepare. The affluent of society came to reject nature's beauty products just as they rejected nature's medicine's. It is, after all, less irksome and time consuming to buy one's medicines

Correctly made, home-made natural beauty preparations will prove as effective as those obtained commercially. And today's stores and supermarkets offer such a wide variety of fruits and vegetables that people who have neither the time nor desire to collect their materials may nonetheless make up their own preparations, to be assured of their purity and to save expenses.

Plant number (see Lexicon, page 30)	Plant name	Principal cosmetic uses	Plant number (see Lexicon, page 30)	Plant name	Principal cosmetic uses
1	ACACIA	Perfumes	120	BAY RUM	Shampoos Hair tonics
4	AGRIMONY	To brighten and soothe the eyes	5	BEAR'S FOOT	Astringents To firm the breasts
11	ALKANET	Rouge	157	BENZOIN	Astringents Perfumes
78	ALL HEAL	To heal and soften the skin	23	BIRCH	Complexion waters Perfumes
121	ALLSPICE	Perfumes Toilet soaps	110	BITTERCRESS	Complexion waters A relaxing bath
9	ALMOND	Face creams	136	BLACKTHORN	To whiten the teeth
12	ANGELICA	Toilet waters	131	BLOODROOT	Face creams To brighten and soothe the eyes
24	ANNATTO	Lip sticks			
143	APOTHECARY'S ROSE	Toilet waters	25	BOLDO	Scented powders Perfumes Toilet soaps
98	APPLE	Hair rinse To whiten the teeth	27	BOX, BOXWOOD	Hair tonics
134	APRICOT	To brighten and soothe the eyes	65	BRIDEWORT	Complexion waters To brighten and soothe the eyes
14	ARNICA	Deodorants Hair tonics Care of the feet and legs	171	BROOKLIME	Complexion waters
119	AVOCADO	Face creams	160	BUTTONS	Complexion waters To heal and soften the skin
101	BALM	Toilet waters	99	CAJUPUT	To heal and soften the skin Perfumes
108	BALSAM OF PERU	Perfumes Toilet soaps	30	CANANGA	Hair lacquers and brilliantines Perfumes
130	BALSAM POPLAR	Toilet soaps perfumes	106	CANDLEBERRY	Face creams To heal and soften the skin
105	BANANA	Face masks To soften and smooth the skin			
76	BARLEY	Face packs	3	CANDLE TREE	For a relaxing bath
87	BAY	To heal and soften the skin For a relaxing bath To make Toilet soaps Care of the feet and legs	32	CANELLA	Scented powders Perfumes

Plant number (see Lexicon, page 30)	Plant name	Principal cosmetic uses
34	CARAWAY	Complexion waters Shampoos Toilet soaps
57	CARNATION	Perfumes
49	CARNAUBA WAX	Face creams Hair lacquers and brilliantines
38	CARRAGEEN MOSS	To heal and soften the skin Hand lotion
56	CARROT	Face packs
33	CARTHAMINE	Rouge
41	CASSIA	Hair tonics Perfumes
1	CASSIE	Perfumes
141	CASTOR OIL PLANT	Eyebrow pencil Hair lacquer and brilliantines
70	CATCHWEED	Rouge To clear the skin
111	CATMINT, CATNIP	Hair tonics
35	CEDARWOOD	Scented powders To heal and soften the skin
61	CENTAURY	Astringents
13	CHAMOMILE	Shampoos Hair tonics
103	CHAMPAC	Hair lacquers and brilliantines Perfumes
75	CHERRY PIE	Perfumes
37	CHERVIL, SWEET CHERVIL	Astringents
156	CHICKWEED	To heal and soften the skin
40	CHICORY	To brighten and soothe the eyes

Plant number (see Lexicon, page 30)	Plant name	Principal cosmetic uses
41	CINNAMON	Hair tonics
2	CINNAMON IRIS	Scented powders To heal and soften the skin Toilet waters
54	CITRONELLA	Perfumes Toilet soaps
146	CLARY/ CLEAR EYES	Complexion waters To brighten and soothe the eyes For a relaxing bath
70	CLEAVERS	Rouge To clear the skin
63	CLOVE	Scented powders Toilet soaps
47	COCONUT PALM	Face creams Sun tan oils Hair lacquers and brilliantines Shampoos Hair tonics
124	COMMON PLANTAIN	Face creams To brighten and soothe the eyes
78	COMMON ST. JOHN'S WORT	To heal and soften the skin
50	CORIANDER	Body lotion Toilet waters After shaves
36	CORNFLOWER	Astringents To brighten and soothe the eyes
159	COSTMARY	Face creams Complexion waters Toilet waters
132	COWSLIP	Face creams Complexion waters
98	CRAB APPLE	Hair rinse To whiten the teeth

Plant number (see Lexicon, page 30)	Plant name	Principal cosmetic uses	Plant number (see Lexicon, page 30)	Plant name	Principal cosmetic uses
52	CUCUMBER	Face creams	6	GARLIC	To heal and soften the skin
17	CUCKOO-PINT	Complexion waters	57	GILLY FLOWER	Perfumes
137	CYDONIA	Face creams For a relaxing bath	154	GOLDEN ROD	Astringents Complexion waters
142	DAMASK ROSE	Perfumes	70	GOOSEGRASS	Rouge To clear the skin
161	DANDELION	Skin lotion To clear the skin	16	GREEN GINGER	Hair tonics
11	DYER'S BUGLOSS	Rouge	112	GROUND IVY	Astringents Complexion waters To brighten and soothe the eyes
4	EGRIMONY	To brighten and soothe the eyes			
43	EGYPTIAN MELON	To refresh the skin	20	GUM TRAGACANTH	Mascara To heal and soften the skin
147	ELDER	Astringents To brighten and soothe the eyes After shaves	75	HELIOTROPE	Perfumes
31	ELEMI	Perfumes	89	HENNA	Hair colourants
64	EUPHRASIA/ EYEBRIGHT	To brighten and soothe the eyes	72	HERB BENNET, HOLY HERB	Complexion waters To clear the skin
66	FENNEL	To brighten and soothe the eyes	94	HONEYSUCKLE	Complexion waters To clear the skin
39	FEVERFEW	Complexion waters			
122	FIR	For a relaxing bath After shaves Toilet soaps	77	HOP	Astringents
			3	HORSE CHESTNUT	For a relaxing bath
92	FLAX WEED	Face creams Astringents	46	HORSERADISH	Face creams Complexion waters
81	FLORENTINE IRIS	Scented powders Perfumes	60	HORSETAIL	Complexion waters
			55	HOUND'S TONGUE	To heal and soften the skin Hair tonics
125	FRANGIPANI	Perfumes			
26	FRANKINCENSE	Perfumes	26	INCENSE	Perfumes
69	FUMITORY	Complexion waters	80	INDIGO, INDICUM	To blacken the hair
7	GALANGA	Scented powders	38	IRISH MOSS	To heal and soften the skin Hand lotion

Plant number (see Lexicon, page 30)	Plant name	Principal cosmetic uses	Plant number (see Lexicon, page 30)	Plant name	Principal cosmetic uses
127	JACOB'S LADDER	Hair dressing To blacken the hair	48	LILY OF THE VALLEY	Astringents Complexion waters
82	JASMINE	Perfumes	163	LIME TREE	Complexion waters
31	JAVA ALMOND	Perfumes	24	LIPSTICK TREE	Lip sticks
109	JONQUIL	Perfumes	140	LITTLE DARLING	Body lotion Perfumes
53	KACHOORA, KURKUM	Scented powders	91	MADONNA LILY	Face creams Astringents
42	LABDANUM	Perfumes	84	MAPATO	To whiten the teeth
5	LADY'S MANTLE	Astringents To firm the breasts	28	MARIGOLD	Face creams To brighten and soothe the eyes
127	LADDER-TO-HEAVEN	Hair dressing To blacken the hair	115	MARJORAM	Complexion waters Toilet waters Shampoos For a relaxing bath Hair tonics Care of the feet and legs
88	LAVENDER	Hair tonics Perfumes			
45	LEMON	Hair tonics			
101	LEMON BALM	Toilet waters For a relaxing bath	8	MARSHMALLOW/ MALLARD	Face creams To heal and soften the skin To brighten and soothe the eyes
54	LEMON GRASS	Perfumes Toilet soaps	123	MASTIC	To whiten the teeth Perfumes
62	LEMON GUM TREE	Perfumes	65	MEADOWSWEET	Complexion waters To brighten and soothe the eyes
14	LEOPARD'S BANE	Deodorants Hair tonics Care of the feet and legs	100	MELILOT	Toilet waters To brighten and soothe the eyes
139	LESSER CELANDINE	Astringents	140	MIGNONETTE	Body lotion Perfumes
117	LICHWORT	Complexion waters To heal and soften the skin Hand lotion Hair tonics	1	MIMOSA	Perfumes
158	LILAC	Perfumes	102	MINT	To whiten the teeth For a relaxing bath After Shaves Toilet soaps

Plant number (see Lexicon, page 30)	Plant name	Principal cosmetic uses
104	MORINGA	Sun tan oils Face creams For hair lacquers and brilliantines
46	MOUNTAIN RADISH	Face creams Complexion waters
169	MULLEIN	Body lotion Hair colourants
22	MYRRH	Perfumes Toilet soaps
109	NARCISSUS	Perfumes
44	NEROLI	Toilet waters Perfumes
107	NUTMEG	Scented powders Toilet soaps
113	NUTMEG PLANT	Scented powders To firm the breasts
21	OAT	Face packs
138	OAK	To clear the skin
59	OIL PALM	Perfumes Toilet soaps
114	OLIVE	Face creams Hair tonics
81	ORRIS	Scented powders Perfumes
116	PANDANG	Hair tonics Perfumes
126	PATCHOULI	Scented powders
135	PEACH	Face masks
117	PELLITORY-OF-THE-WALL	Complexion waters To heal and soften the skin Hand lotion Hair tonics

Plant number (see Lexicon, page 30)	Plant name	Principal cosmetic uses
135	PERSIAN APPLE	Face masks
121	PIMENTA	Perfumes
122	PINE	For a relaxing bath After Shaves Toilet soaps
123	PISTACIA	To whiten the teeth Perfumes
105	PLANTAIN FRUIT	Face masks To soften and smooth the skin
153	POTATO	Astringents
161	PRIEST'S CROWN	Skin lotion To clear the skin
133	PRIMROSE	Face creams Astringents
90	PRIVET	To heal and soften the skin Toilet waters
97	PURPLE LOOSESTRIFE/PURPLE WILLOW HERB	Complexion waters To brighten and soothe the eyes Hair colourants
137	QUINCE	Face creams For a relaxing bath
29	RAMPION	Complexion waters
164	RED CLOVER	To heal and soften the skin
166	RED ELM	Face creams Face packs After Shaves
143	RED ROSE	Toilet waters
84	RHATANY, RED RHATANY	To whiten the teeth
113	ROMAN CORIANDER	Scented powders To firm the breasts

Plant number (see Lexicon, page 30)	Plant name	Principal cosmetic uses
144	ROSEMARY	Astringents
		Deodorants
		Toilet waters
		For a relaxing bath
		Hair tonics
		After Shaves
151	ROSE-ROOT	Astringents
		Toilet waters
33	SAFFLOWER	Rouge
51	SAFFRON	Toilet waters
		Hair colourants
		Care of the feet and legs
145	SAGE	Hair colourants
149	SANDALWOOD	Mascara
		Hair lacquers and brilliantines
		Perfumes
148	SANICLE	To heal and soften the skin
150	SASSAFRAS	Perfumes
		Toilet soaps
10	SCARLET PIMPERNEL	Complexion waters
118	SCENTED-LEAF GERANIUM	Face creams
		To make toilet soaps
116	SCREW-PINE	Hair tonics
		Perfumes
68	SEA-KELP	Face packs
152	SESAME	Face creams
		Sun tan oils
136	SLOE	To whiten the teeth
129	SOLOMON'S SEAL	Complexion waters
		Toilet waters
15	SOUTHERNWOOD	To heal and soften the skin
		Hair tonics

Plant number (see Lexicon, page 30)	Plant name	Principal cosmetic uses
155	SOWTHISTLE/ SPROUT THISTLE	Complexion waters
79	STAR ANISE	Hair lacquers and brilliantines
156	STARWEED	To heal and soften the skin
167	STINGING NETTLE	Astringents
		Hair tonics
151	STONECROP	Astringents
		Toilet waters
67	STRAWBERRY	Face packs
		To whiten the teeth
40	SUCCORY	To brighten and soothe the eyes
74	SUNFLOWER	To heal and soften the skin
		Hand lotion
9	SWEET ALMOND	Face creams
87	SWEET BAY	To heal and soften the skin
		For a relaxing bath
		Toilet soaps
		Care of the feet and legs
100	SWEET CLOVER	Toilet waters
		To brighten and soothe the eyes
37	SWEET FERN	Astringents
2	SWEET FLAG	Scented powders
		To heal and soften the skin
		Toilet waters
54	SWEET GRASS	Perfumes
		Toilet soaps
93	SWEET GUM	Perfumes
160	TANSY	Complexion waters
		To heal and soften the skin
162	THYME	Deodorants
		Hair colourants

Plant number (see Lexicon, page 30)	Plant name	Principal cosmetic uses
92	TOADFLAX	Face creams Astringents
95	TOMATO	Face packs
58	TONQUIN/TONKA BEAN	Scented powders Perfumes
131	TORMENTIL	Face creams To brighten and soothe the eyes
128	TUBEROSE	Perfumes
168	VANILLA	Perfumes
170	VERVAIN	To brighten and soothe the eyes Hair tonics
172	VIOLET	Face creams Perfumes
19	WALL RUE, WALL MAIDENHAIR	Hair tonics
83	WALNUT	Astringents Hair colourants
110	WATERCRESS	Complexion waters For a relaxing bath
43	WATER MELON	To refresh the skin
171	WATER PIMPERNEL	Complexion waters
1	WATTLE	Perfumes
106	WAX MYRTLE	Face creams To heal and soften the skin
49	WAX PALM	Face creams Hair lacquers and brilliantines
10	WEATHERGLASS	Complexion waters
120	WEST INDIAN BAY	Shampoos Hair tonics

Plant number (see Lexicon, page 30)	Plant name	Principal cosmetic uses
165	WHEAT	Face creams Face packs
32	WHITE CINNAMON	Scented powders Perfumes
81	WHITE IRIS	Scented powders Perfumes
91	WHITE LILY	Face creams Astringents
17	WILD ARUM	Complexion waters
56	WILD CARROT	Face packs
85	WILD LETTUCE	To heal and soften the skin
96	WILLOW-WORT	Face creams Astringents
71	WINTERGREEN	To make toilet soaps
73	WITCHHAZEL/ WINTERBLOOM	To clear and soften the skin
72	WOOD AVENS	Complexion waters To clear the skin
94	WOOD BINE	Complexion waters To clear the skin
18	WOODRUFF	Complexion waters Toilet soaps
16	WORMWOOD	Hair tonics
86	YELLOW ARCHANGEL/ YELLOW DEADNETTLE	Complexion waters
96	YELLOW LOOSESTRIFE	Face creams Astringents
30	YLANG-YLANG	Hair lacquers and brilliantines
53	ZEDOARY	Scented powders

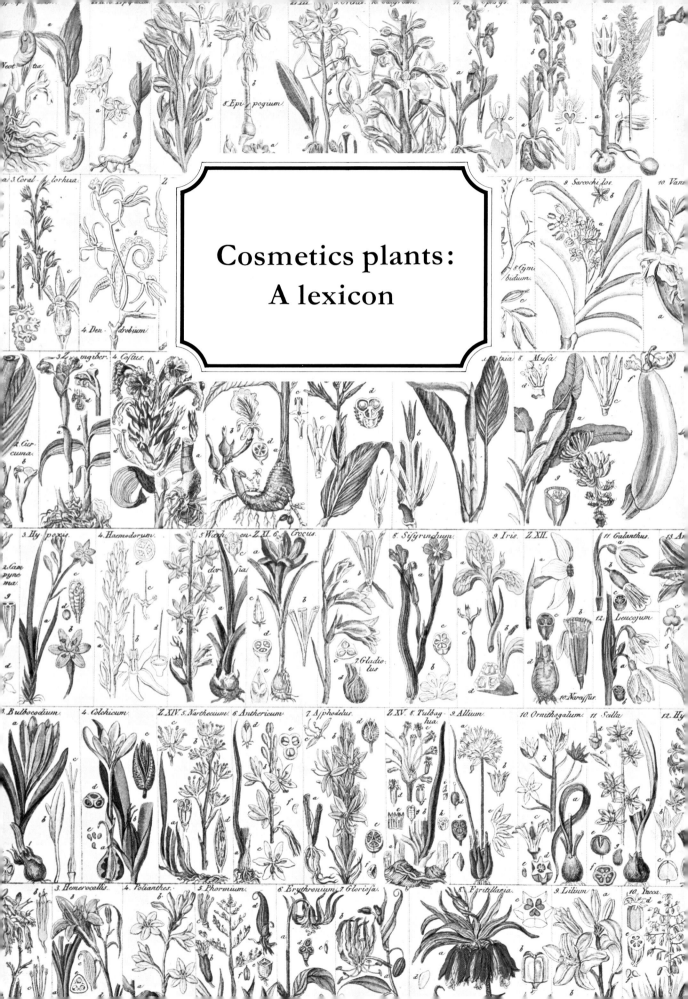

Cosmetics plants:
A lexicon

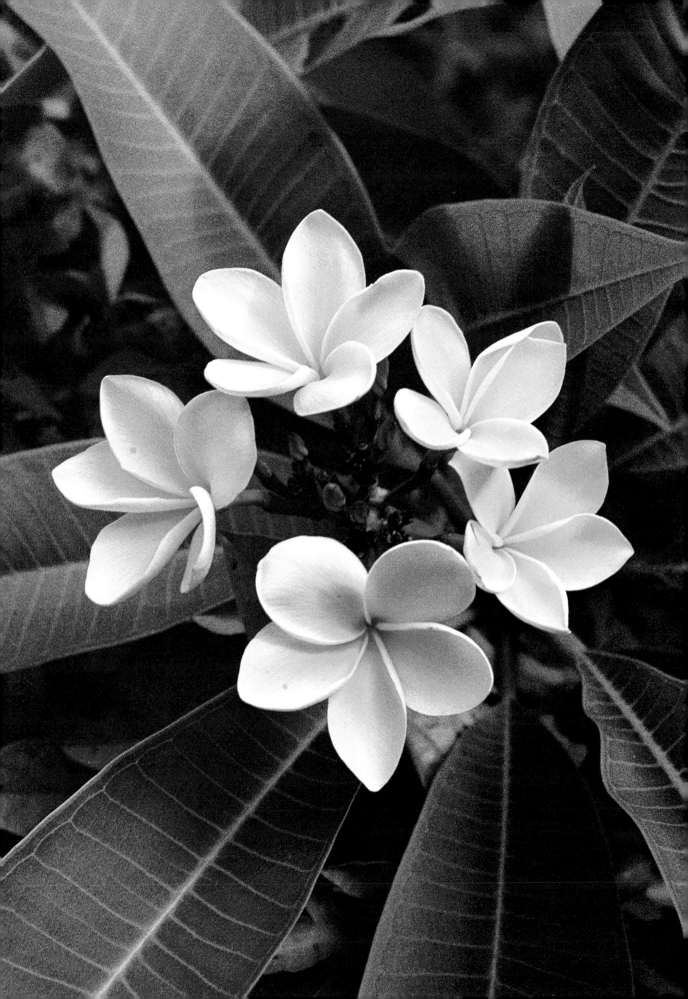

The picture on p. 25 is a composite of plates from Oken's *Allgemeine Naturgeschichte für alle Stände*, published in Stuttgart in 1843. The Iris florentina depicted below is from an early 19th century manuscript in the Bodleian Library in Oxford. Right, *Rosa centifolia* in a painting by Dr. F. Losch from *Les Plantes Médicinales*, published in 1888.

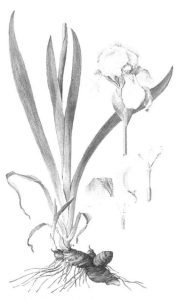

Meticulously drawn and hand painted illustrations from old herbals are often clearer than many modern diagrams.

The flowers of the Frangipani (opposite) have long been associated with the most famous and classical of European perfumes. It takes its name from Mercutio Frangipani, a botanist travelling with Columbus on his 1492 voyage.

This section includes basic descriptions, primarily botanical in nature, of the 172 plants that constitute the basic material of the book.

CONTENTS OF THE PLANT LEXICON

For each plant we provide the Latin name, common English names, the plant family to which it belongs, and indications of its geographical distribution. Classification of plants is by no means as simple as it was in the day of Linnaeus. An attempt has been made to adhere as closely as possible to this classification, but other systems of nomenclature are also used at times. The text on each plant explains its name and gives a detailed account of its appearance and characteristics (growth, blooming, seed-bearing, and so on). Indications of the plant's *active principles* (i.e., active constituents) and cosmetic uses are also given. The reader will find further information in Reference Sections I and II.

Indispensable to any plant description is, of course, an illustration that can guide us in recognizing and identifying the plant in its natural site. Particular care has been given to the selection of photographs, and of hand-painted illustrations from herbal guide-books of the last century, which are both accurate and beautiful.

HOW TO LOCATE A PLANT IN THE LEXICON

Because English common names of the plants are so unstandardized and variable, the 172 plants of the Lexicon have been arranged in alphabetical order according to their standard *Latin names* and each plant has been assigned a number from 1 to 172. This number can be located in the list of English names on the next two pages. The reader can look up the more common English names in this

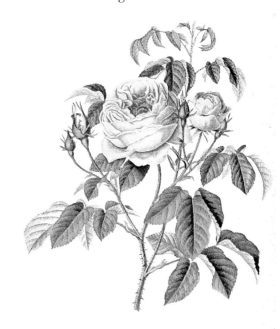

list; if a particular name is not listed, it can be sought in the English Plant Index at the end of the book, where a further range of alternative English names are given, with cross-references to their number in the Lexicon.

Index and Key to the Plant Lexicon

Common English names of the 172 plants are listed here with the number designating each plant's location in the Lexicon.

Each text in the Plant Lexicon includes the following information in its heading:
Latin name, English name, plant family, plant number (in colour box; in other reference sections, circled), and references to the plant's geographical distribution. The distribution is indicated in two lines. The first line gives the plant's original habitat or place of provenance; the second, in italics, indicates areas in which the plant has been introduced by man. The following abbreviations are used:

N   North
S   South
W   West
E   East
C   Central
–   parts of (Example: W–C Asia = western parts of Central Asia)

Af   Africa
Am   America
Aus   Australia
Eur   Europe
Medit   Mediterranean Region

trop   tropical
subtrop subtropical

A

1   ACACIA
4   AGRIMONY
11 ALKANET
78 ALL HEAL
121 ALLSPICE
9   ALMOND
12 ANGELICA
24 ANNATTO
143 APOTHECARY'S ROSE
98 APPLE
134 APRICOT
14 ARNICA
119 AVOCADO

B

101 BALM
108 BALSAM OF PERU
130 BALSAM POPLAR
105 BANANA
76 BARLEY
87 BAY
120 BAY RUM
5   BEAR'S FOOT
104 BENJAMIN
157 BENZOIN
23 BIRCH
110 BITTERCRESS
136 BLACKTHORN
131 BLOODROT
25 BOLDO
27 BOX, BOXWOOD
65 BRIDEWORT
171 BROOKLIME
160 BUTTONS

C

99 CAJUPUT
30 CANANGA
106 CANDLEBERRY
3   CANDLE TREE
32 CANELLA
34 CARAWAY
57 CARNATION
49 CARNAUBA WAX
38 CARRAGEEN MOSS
56 CARROT
33 CARTHAMINE
41 CASSIA
1   CASSIE

141 CASTOR OIL PLANT
70 CATCHWEED
111 CATMINT, CATNIP
35 CEDARWOOD
61 CENTAURY
13 CHAMOMILE
103 CHAMPAC
75 CHERRY PIE
37 CHERVIL/SWEET CHERVIL
156 CHICKWEED
40 CHICORY
41 CINNAMON
2   CINNAMON IRIS
54 CITRONELLA
146 CLARY/CLEAR EYES
70 CLEAVERS
63 CLOVE
47 COCONUT PALM
124 COMMON PLANTAIN
78 COMMON ST. JOHN'S WORT
50 CORIANDER
36 CORNFLOWER
159 COSTMARY
132 COWSLIP
98 CRAB APPLE
17 CUCKOO-PINT
52 CUCUMBER
137 CYDONIA

D

142 DAMASK ROSE
161 DANDELION
11 DYER'S BUGLOSS

E

4   EGRIMONY
43 EGYPTIAN MELON
147 ELDER
31 ELEMI
64 EYEBRIGHT/EUPHRASIA

F

66 FENNEL
39 FEVERFEW
122 FIR
92 FLAX WEED
81 FLORENTINE IRIS
125 FRANGIPANI
26 FRANKINCENSE
69 FUMITORY

ACACIA FARNESIANA

ACACIA
Cassie, Mimosa

Leguminosae

1	Australia, S. Africa, S.E. Asia

ACORUS CALAMUS

SWEET FLAG
Sweet rush

Araceae

2	S.E. Asia *Europe, E. Africa, E.-N. America*

AESCULUS HIPPOCASTANUM

HORSE CHESTNUT

Sapindaceae

3	S.E. Europe, W. Asia *C. Europe, N.-N. America*

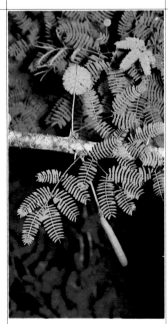

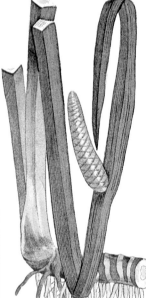

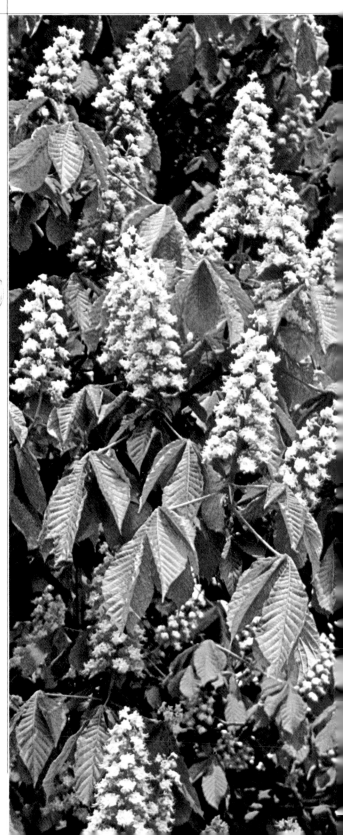

Of more than 400 species, *A. farnesiana* is that which provides most of the essential oil for perfumery. It grows to a height of 7–12 ft (2–4 m) and will spread out its branches to half its height. A fully grown tree when 10–12 years old will yield about 20 lb (9–10 kg) of blossom each season which is during October and November. The tree, like most acacias, is spiny, the emerald green leaves bipinnate and fern-like and assuming a vertical position at nightfall. The deep yellow flowers, made up of numerous long yellow stamens and growing in sprays, have a violet-like perfume. The scent is extracted by enfleurage and, as the flowers open in succession, this enables repeated changes of blossom to be made so that the fat is fully charged over a long period. It takes about 10 lb (4–5 kg) of flowers to yield 2 oz (28 g) of otto, which is included in François Coty's L'Aimant perfume.

The erect sword-like leaves resemble those of the yellow iris to which it is in no way related, being of the Arum family, its botanical name being from the Greek *calamos* (a reed). The waved margins distinguish it from the yellow iris. The tiny flowers appear in a spadix, packed tightly together. They are greenish-brown with the surface covered in a golden mosaic. They emit a most unpleasant smell to draw midges for their pollination. From the roots, a fragrant aromatic oil is obtained by distillation and is used in perfumery and in toilet soaps. The oil is a carminative and from the root a tonic medicine is made. The powdered root is used to impart its scent to hair powders, in the same way as orris, and to talcum powders to use after bathing. With its spicy flavour, the root is used as a substitute for ginger, and as a lotion to ease sore skin caused by exposure to sun or wind. It is supreme in the floral kingdom.

AGRIMONIA EUPATORIA

AGRIMONY
Egrimony

Rosaceae

| 4 | Europe, N. Africa, W. Asia *N. America* |

ALCHEMILLA VULGARIS

LADY'S MANTLE
Bear's foot

Rosaceae

| 5 | Europe, N. Africa, Asia, N. America |

ALLIUM SATIVUM

GARLIC
Common garlic

Liliaceae

| 6 | C. Asia *Warm Temperate Zones* |

One of the most handsome of deciduous trees, it is one of a genus of 13 species indigenous to S.E. Asia and N. America. The Horse Chestnut is native to E. Europe and W. Asia. It is a light-loving tree, rarely found in woodlands, almost always in hedgerows or growing singly in fields and usually in a sandy soil. It will attain a height of 100 ft (30 m) with a girth of up to 16–17 ft (5 m) with smooth light brown bark. The dark green palmate leaves are composed of 5–7 lance-shaped leaflets joined at the same point and held on long footstalks. They turn gold, then brown before they fall in autumn. The flower buds are borne in the axils of the leaves of the previous season, the buds being covered with overlapping scales protected by a sticky resinous substance. The white flowers are borne in a large upright inflorescence in May and are visited by bees. They are followed in autumn by large, shining dark red single fruits enclosed in a prickly green leathery capsule which school-boys remove, fastening the fruits to string to play the game known as conkers. From the fruits, after removing the hard polished outer skin, the juice is extracted and used in bath oils for a foam bath which will tone the flesh and make it soft and supple. Fruits of the Red Buckeye, *A. pavia*, of N. America are used in the same way.

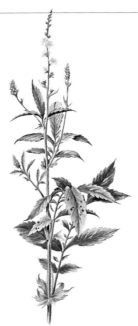

It is usually found in hedgerows and by the side of woodlands. It takes its name from the Greek *argemone* (shining), for the ancients believed that a decoction of the fresh leaves used for bathing the eyes would prevent cataract. This may not be so but it gives a sparkle to the eyes in the same way as the more common Eyebright (*Euphrasia officinalis*). A slender plant, the stems are covered in soft hairs, the leaves being composed of 3–6 pairs of leaflets with toothed edges. It blooms in July and August, the small bright yellow flowers being borne in long spikes or racemes, hence its country name of "church steeples". Where not common in the countryside, it is readily raised in the garden from seed sown in spring in rows 12 in (30 cm) apart. To encourage the plants to form more leaf, do not let them flower. They will die back at the end of summer.

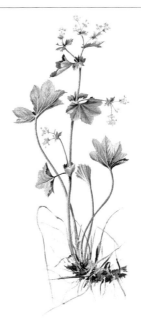

Its association with the Virgin Mary earned it the name of Our Lady's Mantle which Linnaeus was to adopt, the leaf lobes resembling the scalloped edges of a mediaeval mantle. The hairy, many-lobed leaves were also thought to resemble a bear's foot. All parts of the plant are covered in short hairs whilst the leaves may be divided into as many as 10 or 11 lobes, as Culpeper said, "making them seem like a star". The flowers, which bloom all summer, are greenish yellow and cluster together at the end of short stems. They are without petals. The rootstock is long and black and a decoction of it was used since earliest times to stop bleeding caused by skin abrasions. The whole plant has astringent and styptic properties and, dabbed onto the face, will heal a sore skin and prevent wrinkles. Northern women use a decoction to firm the breasts after breast feeding.

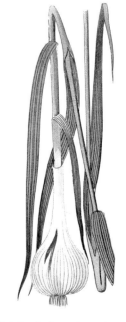

Rich in alkaline salts and sulphur compounds, garlic is a blood purifier and keeps the skin clear of spots and pimples. The juice added to warm lard or olive oil and applied to a spotty skin or where there is soreness, will bring about rapid healing. The bulbs are composed of numerous bulblets enclosed within a white skin which holds them together like a single bulb. The bulblets are known as cloves and are separated when the bulbs are lifted in autumn when ripe. The grass-like leaves are long and narrow, tapering to a point, and from the bulb arises the stem which bears the small white flowers in a capitate head in July and August. To prevent the plants running to seed at the expense of the bulbs, the stems should be bent over when they begin to flower. The bulbs are lifted when the leaves turn yellow and are spread out to dry in a shed or attic, using the cloves when required.

ALPINIA OFFICINARUM

GALANGA
Galingale

Zingiberaceae

7 S.E. Asia

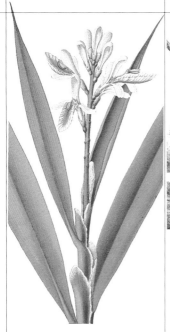

A. officinarum forms a thick tuberous root with alternate leaves about 12 in (30 cm) long, narrowly lanceolate and unfolding from a smooth sheath of brilliant green. The flowers, which appear before the monsoons, are white, veined with red, and are borne in a dense terminal spike. The reddish brown roots have an aromatic taste and smell due to resin and an essential oil. In the East, they are dried and ground to use, with orris and sandalwood, in talcum powders. *A. sessilis* has more sweetly scented roots and is more popular in talcum powders, which Hindu women have long appreciated. The roots are marketed in the east as Kamala. The plant has lanceolate leaves and bears white flowers which have a purple dot on each of the petal edges. *A. aromaticum* has scented roots and bears pale yellow tuberous flowers followed by seeds which are used as a substitute for cardamon.

ALTHAEA OFFICINALIS

MARSHMALLOW

Malvaceae

8 S.E. Europe
S. + W. Europe, W. Asia, N.E.-N. America

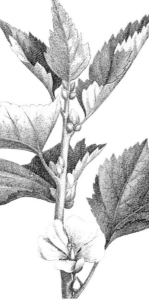

It makes a branched plant with downy stems and 3–5 lobed leaves 2–3 in (5–7·5 cm) long which are downy on both sides. The plant dies down in winter and comes up again in spring. The large 5-petalled flowers are borne in panicles during July and August and are of a lovely shade of soft pink. They are followed by large round seed receptacles, like cheeses, the seeds arranged in rows having a crisp, nutty taste. The plant takes its name from the Greek *altho* (to cure) on account of its demulcent properties used internally and externally for the roots contain more than half their weight of saccharine viscous mucilage. Gerard wrote that the roots "will take away aches and pains when used in a bath". A decoction of the cleaned roots is soothing for inflamed eyes if used when slightly warm, whilst fomentations placed on a sore face caused by cold wind or too long exposure to the sun, will give instant relief.

AMYGDALUS COMMUNIS VAR. DULCIS

ALMOND
Sweet Almond

Rosaceae

9 W.-C. Asia, Mediterranean
Warm Temperate Zones

Native of Persia and the Near East the fruit, since earliest times, was appreciated for its high nutritional value. "No man who can fill his pockets with almonds need starve on a journey" is an eastern saying. The nuts are roasted in butter and eaten with salt, and ground to bake into cakes. Eastern women have long realised the value of massaging the oil obtained from the nuts, into the skin, to give it elasticity and to prevent wrinkling. Its fame spread into Europe long before the Christian era. It was used by the women of Athens and Rome and in mediaeval times, records show that in one year alone (1372), 500 lb (227 kg) of almonds were purchased by the Queen of France for the extraction of oil to massage into the skin to keep the face soft and young looking. In warm parts, the trees bloom in January before the appearance of the leaves, when the twiggy stems of the sweet almond are as if covered with snow. The flowers of the bitter almond are white, the small lance-shaped leaves being finely toothed. The fruit is borne on short spurs and has the appearance of an unripe apricot. When ripe, the green case splits open to reveal the nut enclosed in its rough shell which is yellow and pitted with holes. The shell is hard and woody, the fruit flat and ovoid, round at

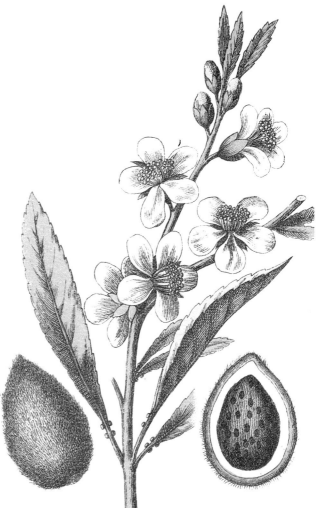

ANAGALLIS ARVENSIS

SCARLET PIMPERNEL
Weatherglass

Primulaceae

10 N. Asia, N. Europe

ANCHUSA OFFICINALIS
Anchusa tinctoria

ALKANET
Dyer's bugloss

Boraginaceae

11 S. Europe, W. Asia

ANGELICA ARCHANGELICA

ANGELICA
Angel's Food

Umbelliferae

12 N. + E. Europe, N. Asia
N.-N. America

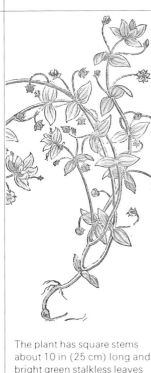

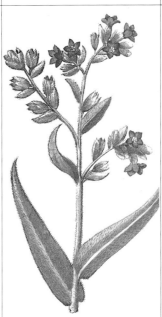

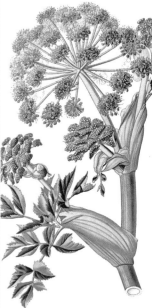

one end, pointed at the other and covered in a brown skin. The nuts contain about 20% protein and no starch. On expression they yeild almost half their weight in oil. The seeds are first ground, then the oil is extracted by pressure, then filtered and bleached by exposure to light. It is pale yellow and odourless and is added to the best toilet soaps owing to its ability to soften the skin. As long ago as the 16th century, the English botanist Gerard wrote: "oil of almonds makes smooth the hands and face of delicate persons, and cleanseth the skin from all spots and pimples". There is a record of hand creams made from almond oil being popular at the time, used in the same way as in modern beauty parlours. Almond cream figures in the bills paid for perfumes for the use of the Emperor Napoleon's wife, Josephine, the creole daughter of a French merchant born in Martinique where fragrant creams and oils are massaged into the skin to prevent it drying in the hot sun. Macasssor oil, once popular to rub into hair to prevent dryness and eventual baldness, was made from almond oil, coloured with alkanet root and scented with a little oil of cassia (cassie oil). Or simply use oil of almonds to massage into the scalp. Almond meal makes an excellent face mask to remove blackheads and pimples. Milk of almonds is also a valuable skin tonic if applied to the face at bed-time.
For the hands, honey and almond oil mixed well together and worked into the hands at bed-time, has no equal for smooth, white hands.

The plant has square stems about 10 in (25 cm) long and bright green stalkless leaves which always turn to the sun. The flowers appear singly, from the leaf axils, throughout summer and are brilliant red with a purple spot at the base of each of the five petals which form the corolla. They, too, always turn towards the sun. The plant was named by Dioscorides from the Greek *anagelao* (to laugh) for an infusion of the whole herb, taken inwardly, acts on the liver and brings about a cheerful countenance, itself one of the first of all beauty requirements. Culpeper advised using its distilled water to improve the complexion, for it clears the skin of freckles and soreness brought about by exposure to the sun or strong winds. The plant has a pleasant bitterness and included in a salad will cleanse the blood of impurities.

The name is derived from the Greek *anchousa*, "paint", for the red dye obtained from the roots. The roots are large and carrot-like and it is from the rind that a red dye is obtained. It is extracted by oil and spirit of wine after drying the roots in the sun or in a warm oven. The dye has been used since earliest times for colouring medicines. *A. officinalis*, often seen as a garden plant, and which may be classed as partly perennial, has angular stems and narrow lanceolate leaves. During June and July it bears bright blue flowers in forked cymes. All parts of the plant are covered in small stiff hairs. *A. tinctoria* is similar but of less vigorous habit. It bears small purple-blue flowers with a calyx which enlarges when in fruit. They are waste ground plants and grow in an open position and sandy soil.

The plant grows on waste ground and by the banks of streams, usually in partial shade and moist soil like the more widely dispersed *A. sylvestris* from which it differs in that its smooth stems are free from purple markings. The plant is only part-perennial for it usually dies in its third year after flowering for the first time but endures by self-sown seedlings. The leaves are divided into numerous segments and measure 2 ft (60 cm) across whilst the umbels of small greenish-white flowers appear in July. The stems are brilliant green after candying and are used in confectionery. They are also used to impart their muscat flavour to jams and preserves whilst the seeds are included by the Monks of La Grande Chartreuse in their distinctive flavoured liqueurs. The fruits are pale yellow when ripe and are oblong, flat on one side and with 3 convex ribs on the other. They have a muscatel flavour and taste.

ANTHEMIS NOBILIS

CHAMOMILE
Maythen

Compositae

13 S.W. Europe, N.W. Africa
Europe, N. America

ARNICA MONTANA

ARNICA
Leopard's bane

Compositae

14 Europe

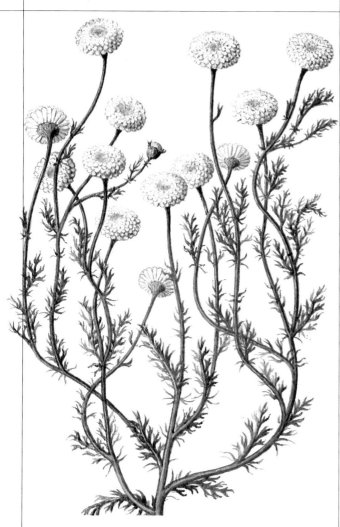

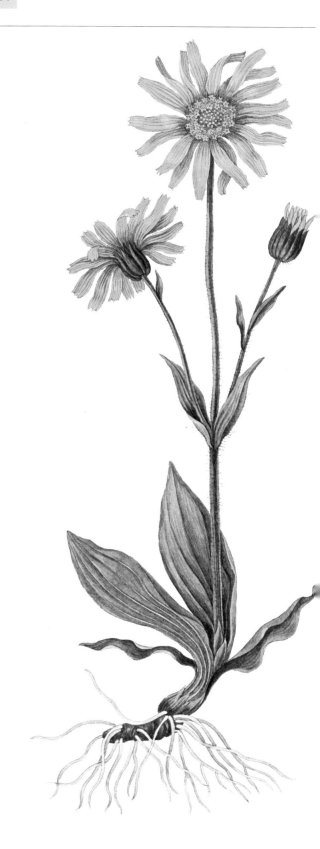

It takes its name from the Greek *kamai* (ground) and *melon* (apple) or ground-apple, from the apple-like fragrance it releases when trodden upon. For it is an almost prostrate plant which forms a dense mat, entirely covering the ground, and inhabits sandy soil and waste ground. *A. Nobilis* has a much-branched stem and leaves almost free from down and divided into thread-like segments, which give the plant a feathery appearance. The flowers, with their white ray petals and yellow centres, are borne solitary on erect stalks late in summer. The medicinal value of the plant is concentrated in the yellow disc of the flowers, an infusion of which, taken at night as a tea, acts as a sedative and encourages sleep. The flowers also have tonic properties. The whole plant is used for making tonic beers and, in muslin bags immersed in a warm bath, relieves tired limbs. Its dried leaves make a pleasant herbal smoke and an infusion of the flowers rubbed into the hair stimulates the growth and gives it a blond sheen.

ARTEMISIA ABROTANUM	ARTEMISIA ABSINTHIUM	ARUM MACULATUM
SOUTHERNWOOD Citronelle	**WORMWOOD** Green Ginger	**CUCKOO-PINT** Wild arum
Labiatae **15** S. Europe	Compositae **16** C. + S. Europe, N. Africa, C. Asia *Temperate Zones*	Araceae **17** C. Europe, Mediterranean *North Temperate Zones*

It is a native of the alpine regions of C. Europe extending into W. Asia where it grows in woodlands and on mountain pastures. It forms a rosette of flat leaves from the centre of which arises a flower stem up to 2 ft (60 cm) tall, at the end of which is borne a large orange daisy-like flower. The root is a dark brown cylindrical rhizome and yields tincture of arnica which contains the bitter yellow principle, arnicin, and a volatile oil. It also contains tannin, which the flowers do not. Known in Europe as a stimulant to circulation, extracts of arnica were even purportedly used by Goethe to strengthen his weakening heart. In addition to its boon to the circulatory system, arnica is also used in compresses and tinctures to help promote the healing of bruises and contusions. As the plant is toxic, it should be used internally with the utmost caution in its treatment of epilepsy. Externally, a few drops applied to the scalp and massaged in can promote the growth of hair, whilst for tender feet, caused by walking over rough ground, a few drops in a foot bath of warm water will give instant relief. Afterwards, the feet should be rubbed down with surgical spirit. Where there is a lot of walking to be done, this treatment should be given at the end of each day when it will keep the feet free of soreness.

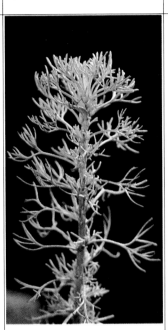

A plant of upright shrubby habit, its lower grey-green leaves are twice pinnately dissected and it bears its small yellow flowers in a panicled cyme, though rarely does it bloom away from S. Europe where it grows on wasteland, in sandy soil and in full sun. It takes its name from its habitat, which distinguishes it from the artemisias of more northerly parts, yet it is as hardy as other species. The plant is also called Lad's Love for it was included in every lover's posies because of its refreshing lemony fragrance in summer; hence the French call it *Citronelle*. The Monk Walfred Strabo, from his monastery on the shores of Lake Constance, considered the plant to have as many virtues as the dissections of its leaves. Its dried leaves in muslin bags placed under a pillow-slip will encourage sleep and an infusion of the leaves in hot water will, if massaged into the scalp, prevent hair from falling out.

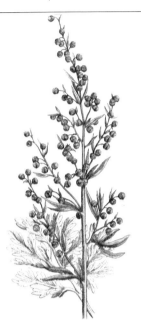

The plant forms woody stems, its leaves divided into numerous narrow segments and, like the stems, covered in silky hairs, giving the plant a handsome grey-green appearance. The dull greenish yellow flowers appear late in summer and are borne in leafy panicles. It is a plant of waste ground, exposed to full sunlight. The plant contains the bitter glucocide absinthin and from it the liqueur absinthe is made; it is also used in the preparation of Vermouth. Before hops were used for brewing, wormwood was used to impart a bitterness to ale. An infusion of the leaves and flower tops, sweetened with honey, makes a tonic drink and can clear the blood of impurities and the skin of blemishes. An infusion, mixed with rosemary, will prevent falling hair if regularly rubbed into the scalp. Sea Wormwood, *A. maritima*, a plant of salt marshes, distributed over Europe and Asia, has similar properties.

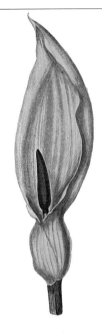

A glabrous plant with a short fleshy rhizomatous root and leaves shaped like an arrow head. They are net-veined with long footstalks and waved margins. The plant produces a sheath-like leaf, the spathe, which encloses a yellowish-purple column, the spadix. As the spathe opens, in April or May, the spadix begins to rise in temperature, often 20° F (10° C) above the surrounding air temperature, and emits an unpleasant urinous smell, to attract a species of midge (*Psychoda*) for its pollination. They are held captive by downwards pointing hairs until pollination has taken place. The hairs then wither and release the insects. The spadix is replaced by a bunch of bright red berries which are highly poisonous. So is the root until some of the starchy matter has been removed by long soaking and boiling. Arum starch was the ingredient of the Cyprus powder used on the face by French women in the early 19th century.

ASPERULA ODORATA

WOODRUFF
Wood-nove

Rubiaceae

18 N. + C. Europe

ASPLENIUM RUTA-MURARIA

WALL RUE
Wall Maidenhair

Filices

19 Europe, Asia
Temperate Zones

ASTRALAGUS GUMMIFERA

GUM TRAGACANTH
Syrian Tragacanth

Leguminosae

20 *Warm and temperate Zones*

It grows in deciduous woodlands, usually in a chalk or limestone soil. An almost glabrous prostrate plant with erect four-angled stems and lanceolate leaves produced in star-like whorls of 6–9 with prickles at the margins. It's name is derived from the French *rovelle* (a wheel) an allusion to the circular whorls of leaves, or from the Anglo-Saxon *rofe*, (a ruff), and "wood" denotes its habitat. It is mostly found in shady places, where the sun cannot penetrate, and is deep green in colour. The tiny white flowers are borne in terminal heads in early summer and like the whole plant have the rich scent of newly mown hay. This is due to the chemical principle coumarin which is present in sweet vernal grass of meadows and gives its peculiar scent to freshly dried hay. Its perfume increases as it dries (just like well-made hay) and persists for several years. It also has the ability to fix other odours and is used in perfumery and in the manufacture of soaps. When dry, the powdered leaves of woodruff are included in snuffs and in sweet bags to place amongst clothes.

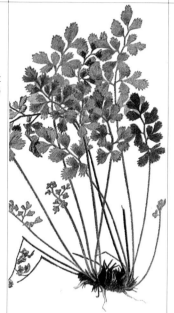

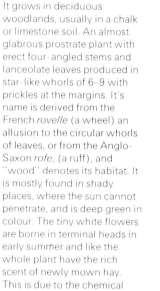

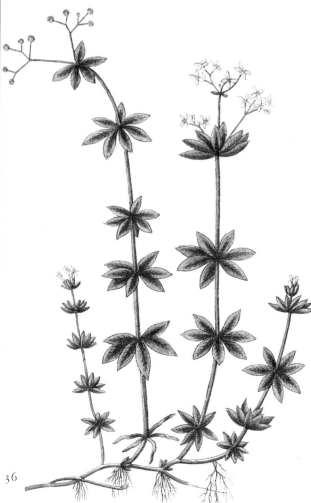

This little fern is distributed throughout many parts of the N. temperate regions of Europe and Asia and is found growing between the stones of dry walls. It grows in tufts, often deep inside a wall, its wedge-shaped pinnules resembling those of the rue both in colour and form. Though growing only where there is ample drainage, it enjoys protection from full exposure to the sun, afforded by the wall. A decoction of the fronds is good for kidney troubles and, boiled with chamomile flowers, makes a lotion that will rid the head of scurf and prevents falling hair. Add a little oil of rosemary for greater efficiency. The Common Maidenhair, *A. trichomanes*, is also a plant of dry walls and has much the same qualities. Its pinnate fronds grow taller and are sweet and mucilaginous. From an infusion, a thick paste is obtained which, when massaged into the scalp removes dandruff and prevents falling hair.

A large genus of more than 1600 species, it is distributed throughout the warm temperate regions of the world except Australia. Mostly bearing purple-blue flowers pollinated by bees, *A. gummifera* is a low growing, much-branched thorny shrub, its woolly stems armed with large spikes and bearing yellow pea-like flowers from the leaf axils. The entire plant is scentless; likewise the gummy exhudation, until it is burnt to fumigate clothes or use as incense in the home. To obtain the gum, vertical slits are made in the bark, the gum exhuding as flat ribbon-like pieces which are colourless and hard. When placed in cold water the gum swells to form a

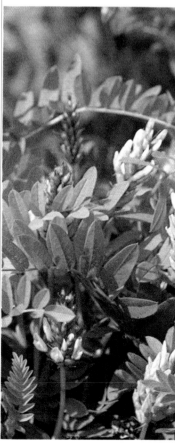

AVENA SATIVA

OAT
Groat, Wild oat

Gramineae

21 *Temperate Zones*

BALSAMODENDRON MYRRHA

MYRRH
Myrrha

Burseraceae

22 Tropical Africa

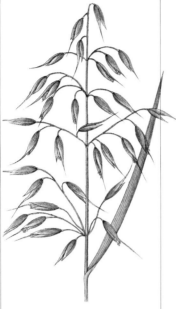

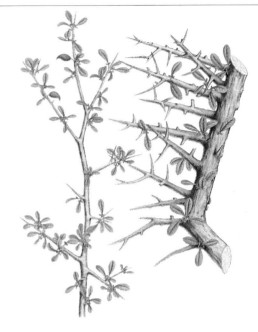

gelatinous mass but no more than 10% dissolves. Its value lies in its mucilage which is used to suspend insoluable materials and for this reason it is used as a base for liquid mascaras and other beauty aids. The mucilage is soothing when applied to a sore skin or when burned by the sun.

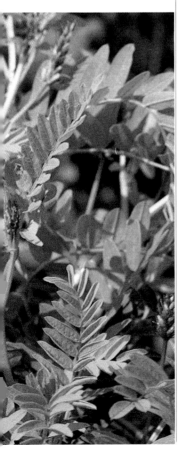

The hardiest of the grains, the 70 species of oat are distributed throughout the temperate world. Ground oats form oatmeal to bake into bread, whilst crushed oats boiled in water, make a nourishing porridge. The seeds are enclosed in a protective cover or paleae which, after harvesting, is removed by winnowing before the seed is used. *A. sativa* is the cultivated form of the wild oat, *A. fatua*, found in arable land and by the wayside and which has broad rough lanceolate leaves and branched flower heads, each spikelet having a tuft of brown hairs which rustle in the wind. *A. sativa* has smooth stems and the pendulous spikelets are two-flowered. *A. strigosa* grows wild on the west coast of Ireland and is without the tuft of brown hairs. Oats are valuable food for horses as well as humans and have many uses in beauty treatments both raw and when cooked. Oatmeal has no equal as a skin improver and there are many recipes for its use.

A small twiggy bush found only in Saudi Arabia, Somalia and Ethiopia, on either side of the southernmost shores of the Red Sea, where it is known as kurbeta. To the ancient world it yielded one of its most prized substances (gold, frankincense and myrrh), for only myrrh provided a strong and lasting perfume. It was used throughout the Near East for embalming and, as told in *Proverbs*, was placed amongst clothes and linen to impart its resinous perfume. Small pieces were placed in muslin bags and suspended on a cord between women's breasts to release its fragrance with the warmth of the body by day and by night. Before animal fixatives were used, myrrh was the only substance able to provide a lasting perfume to pomades and scents and for this reason is still used in modern perfumery. In his *Natural History*, Pliny gives the composition of the famous Greek ointment, susinum, used to rub onto the body after bathing. It included

cinnamon, saffron and myrrh which were also the ingredients of Megaleion, made by the Athens perfumer, Megallus, during the time of Alexander the Great. There are two forms of *Commiphora*. One is a dwarf shrub with dark green serrated leaves; the other *C. kataf*, a small twiggy tree growing 8 ft (2·5 m) tall. In the intense heat, the plants yield a yellow gum which exudes from the bark and glandular hairs on the leaves and is collected on the beards of browsing goats to make into cakes exactly as in ancient times. In this way it is exported to all parts of the world. Distilled with alcohol, it is used to make quality soaps and shampoos and also as a fixative in perfumery.

BETULA ALBA	BIXA ORELLANA	BOLDOA FRAGRANS
BIRCH Sweet Birch	**ANNATTO** Lipstick tree	**BOLDO** Chile boldo
Betulaceae	Bixaceae	Nyctaginaceae
23 Europe, W. Asia *N.-N. America*	**24** Tropical America	**25** Chile

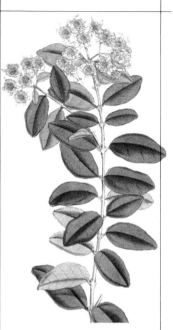

A tall tree, native of tropical America and represented by a single species, is now cultivated throughout tropical America. The seeds are covered in a fleshy orange coat which yields a dye widely used to colour lipsticks; hence it derives its name of lipstick tree. The dye is also used to colour cheese and margarines, whilst the seed is used both as a colouring and a condiment for Indian rice dishes. The handsome arrow-headed alternate cordate leaves are dark green and held on long footstalks so that they continually move. The small pinkish white flowers are borne in panicles at the end of the branches. They have five sepals and five petals and numerous stamens. The fruit, known technically as spinose, is a capsule containing numerous seeds enclosed in fleshy orange-red pulp containing a dye known to commerce as annatto. It blends well with the waxes and oils used to make lipsticks to which it imparts a brilliant reddish orange colour. It is one of the few natural dyes still in commercial use.

A genus of 60 species of deciduous trees, several yield a sugary sap which is employed in the brewing of a tonic beer, fermented with yeast. Birch tar oil is identical with oil of wintergreen and is used for making medicated soaps. A decoction of the leaves makes an astringent skin lotion. *B. alba*, the Silver birch, is conspicuous by its silvery bark which continually peels off in layers. The leaves are grey-green with thin stalks and turn yellow in autumn. They are small and triangular, terminating in a point and unevenly serrated. The flowers are drooping catkins and form in the autumn, the males being dark red and pendulous; the females, yellow and erect. *B. lenta* can reach a height of 80 ft (5 m). The wood and bark is cut in summer and distilled in vats, in the same way as sassafras, to yield the essential oil which has the smell of wintergreen. From the serrated heart-shaped leaves an astringent skin lotion is obtained.

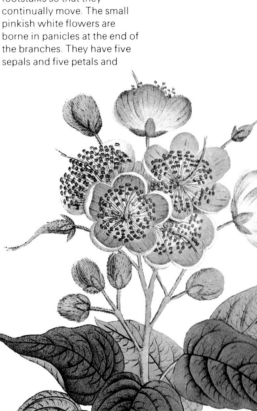

A genus of a single species, it grows in isolation, never in forests. It is a slow growing tree with cylindrical branches covered with smooth brown bark, though the young twigs are rough and hairy. The bark and twigs are pleasantly aromatic and are dried and ground and used in talcum powders. The opposite leaves are broadly oval and about 2 in (5 cm) long. They are thick and dark green, rough on both surfaces, with wart-like projections which on the under-surface are set with stiff hairs. The leaves have cells containing an essential oil which is transparent in the green leaf, though green when the leaf is dried (while the leaf takes on a reddish colour). The leaves have valuable tonic properties and yield a highly scented essential oil used in perfumery and soap making. Its scent is like Sweet gale. The greenish yellow flowers are borne in terminal and axillary cymes during autumn and winter and are followed by fragrant pea-size fruits.

BOSWELLIA SERRATA

FRANKINCENSE
Incense

Burseraceae

26   Africa, S.E. Asia

BUXUS SEMPERVIRENS

BOX
Boxwood

Buxaceae

27   S. Europe, tropical + S. Africa, C. + S.E. Asia

CALENDULA OFFICINALIS

MARIGOLD
Pot marigold

Compositae

28   S. Europe, N. Africa, W. Asia
Temperate Zones

A genus of 24 species of aromatic plants. All parts of the plant are fragrant and furnish the frankincense used to make the holy incense to burn in temples. In the ancient world it was valued with gold and myrrh, the three most precious things then known to man and carried by the three eastern kings to offer to the infant Jesus in recognition of His Divinity. "And when they were come into the house, they saw the young child with Mary his mother, and fell down, and worshipped him: and when they had opened their treasures, they presented unto him gifts; gold and frankincense, and myrrh." It is mentioned on 22 occasions in the Bible, sixteen times in relation to its use in religious worship. Frankincense is the gummy resin discharged from the shrub *B. serrata*, so named because the compound leaves are divided into numerous serrate leaflets arranged into 10 or more opposite pairs. The greenish white flowers tipped with pink open star-like and appear in the axils of the small oval privet-like leaves which are covered in glandular dots and when handled release an invigorating resinous smell. The small leaves and twiggy habit of the shrubs reduce transpiration to a minimum and enable them to grow in the most barren soils, on rocky hillsides and in ravines.

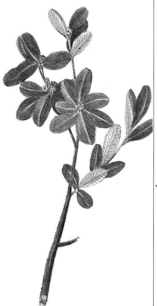

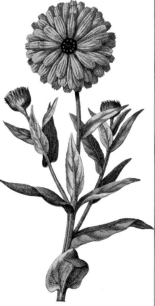

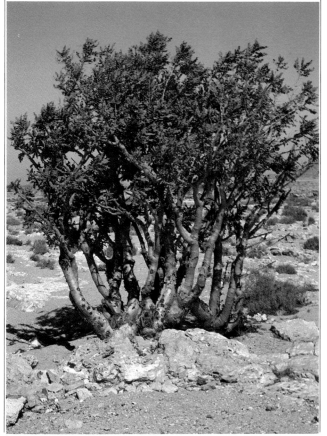

A well-known evergreen, one of a genus of 70 species distributed in the British Isles and S. Europe, tropical and S. Africa and C. and S.E. Asia, its foliage is quite pungently scented, especially when it is wet. They are small leafy trees or shrubs of slow growth with small ovate dark green leaves and bearing small white flowers in terminal heads. Hardy plants, they are present in open woodlands, usually in a limestone soil. Box plantations are a familiar sight of S. England. The yellow wood of its stems and roots has long been in demand by cabinet makers in England and France. At one time the leaves and wood shavings were boiled to dye hair a rich auburn colour, whilst John Wesley, founder of the Methodist Movement, said that a decoction of the leaves rubbed into the scalp was the best of all hair restorers. Modern science has proved him correct, for the leaves contain buxine which stimulates the hair nerves around the hair follicles and promotes growth.

It is found on railway embankments and waste ground, usually growing in sandy soil. Though annual, the plant will often bloom the whole year, being seen in bloom on the first day of each month, the calends, hence its botanical name. The petals and young leaves are anti-scorbutic and are included in salads, though sparingly for they are bitter. The yellow or orange flowers produce a dye for the hair which women used in 16th-century Europe. William Turner, Dean of Wells, wrote in *The New Herbal* (1551): "Some women use to make their heyre yellow with the flowers of this herb, not being content with the natural colour which God hath given them." Today it has greater use, to make a soothing face cream with the essence of the flowers, whilst marigold water brings relief to sore eyes. It is a strong but pleasantly smelling plant with pale green oblong sessile leaves and flowers about 2 in (5 cm) in diameter with yellow or orange ray petals and brown disc florets.

CAMPANULA RAPUNCULUS

RAMPION
Ramps

Campanulaceae

29 Europe, N. Africa, W. Asia
Temperate Zones

CANANGA ODORATE

YLANG-YLANG
Cananga

Annonaceae

30 S.E. Asia, Australia

CANARIUM COMMUNE

ELEMI
Java almond

Burseraceae

31 W. Africa, S.E. Asia, N. Australia

CANELLA ALBA

CANELLA
White wood

Canellaceae

32 C. America

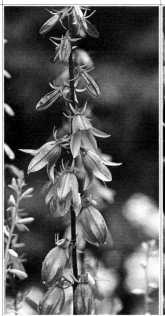

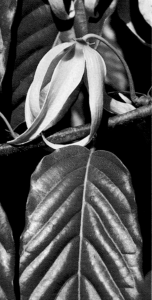

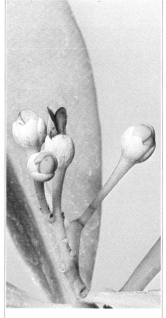

One of the most handsome of wild flowers, it is found in gravelly soil on chalkland and about rocky outcrops, making a stout unbranched plant with broad ovate leaves 2–3 in (5–7 cm) long and bearing white or purple flowers in erect panicles. It is the largest of the bell flowers and blooms in June and July. It takes its name from the Latin *rapa* (turnip) for the roots are large and round and when boiled and served with white sauce have a pleasant sweet nutty taste. They should be earthed up before lifting and using in winter. The young shoots can be blanched in early summer to cook like asparagus and the leaves, included in a salad, clear the blood of impurities and the skin of blemishes. From the leaves and flowers, a toilet water is distilled which, in the words of one writer, "maketh the face very resplendent". If applied at night, it will leave the skin soft and white by morning. It is dabbed onto the face after make-up is removed.

A genus of a single species, it is a native of S.E. Asia and Australia, especially Burma, Malaysia and the Philippines where it is known as Ylang-Ylang or Flower of Flowers. The redolent perfume made from its flowers, which has the scent of jasmine but with spicy undertones, is also known as Ylang-Ylang. Found on exposed hillsides growing amongst rocky outcrops, it makes a small twiggy tree with dark green oval leaves. All through the summer, it bears masses of dull greenish yellow flowers with thin, narrow petals terminating in a point. Although these flowers are highly scented on the tree, a considerable quantity of them is required to make an otto of lasting fragrance. For this reason it is usually mixed with oil of cloves or pimento to give it more substance. In the East, the perfume is as fashionable as it ever was and its clove-scented oil is included in the famous Macassar oil, which imparts its pleasing scent and fixative qualities when used as a western hair dressing.

A genus of more than 100 species of the same family which includes the resinous gums, frankincense and myrrh. The finest elemi, used in perfumery, coming from Manilla. *C. commune* makes a tree about 40 ft (12 m) tall and is deciduous. It is present about wooded hillsides and valleys in the island of Luzon. It is hard wooded and from cuts made in the bark, a white granular resinous gum, known as Brea, exudes. It is soft and sticky, with a sharp lemony scent, like oil of water fennel, the principle constituent being Phellandrine which is also present in angelica roots. *C. commune* has deeply veined oval leaves up to 12 in (30 cm) long and it bears greenish white flowers in panicles during May and June. Before they open, the flower buds are enclosed in bracts which are covered with sticky tomentum. *C. edule*, native of W. Africa, emits from its bark a verbena-scented gum which is used by the native population to place amongst clothes. When dried and powdered it is used for fixing sachet powders.

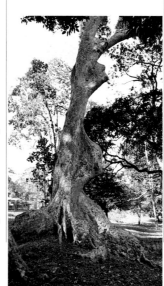

A genus of a single species, its bark is exported as long quills, the name *canella* meaning a reed which the rolled bark is thought to represent. It is a tall upright tree, branching only at the top, and inhabits dense forests, often near the coast. It is readily recognised by its silver-grey bark, collected by beating the tree with a stick to detach the outer layer, which is peeled off and dried in the shade. When dry it is yellowish brown with a warm clove-like aroma. The essential oil contains eugenol, the principle substance of cloves. It figured in the earliest known recipe for lavender water. *C. alba* has alternate shortly-stalked leaves, about 4 in (10 cm) long, blunt at the apex and thick. They are bright green and glossy above, dull green below and covered with pellucid glands which release a resinous scent. The purple flowers are borne in clusters at the ends of the branches and diffuse a powerful clove perfume.

CARTHAMUS TINCTORIUS

SAFFLOWER
Carthamine

Compositae

33 S. Europe, C. + S. Asia, Africa

CARUM CARVI

CARAWAY
Carvi

Umbelliferae

34 Europe, C. + N. + W. Asia *N. America*

CEDRUS LIBANOTICA
Cedrus libani

CEDARWOOD
Cedar of Lebanon

Pinaceae

35 Mediterranean

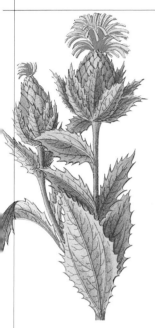

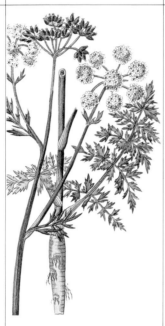

A genus of only four species appreciated since earliest times for their durable wood and fragrance and burnt in the temples of Egypt and Greece as incense. Amongst the largest of all trees, it has a horizontal spread of 100 ft (30 m) or more. Its needle-like leaves are produced in long and short shoots or tufts. They do not bear cones until at least 40 years old and the cones take three years to ripen. The temple of Solomon in Jerusalem, begun by David, was built entirely of the timber of *C. libanotica* and to satisfy the needs of the builders, more than a quarter of a million men plundered the forests of the Lebanon, which never recovered. The wood was also shipped to Egypt in large quantities and used to make mummy cases which have retained their fragrance after 4000 years. The wood was later used to build the temple of Diana at Ephesus. Cedarwood oil extracted from the timber was used in Mediterranean countries to massage into the body to give elasticity and a lasting fragrance. Modern "cedarwood" oil is extracted from the Virginian Juniper of N. America, *Juniperus virginiana*, called the red cedar because of the colour of its wood. The wood burnt on a low fire will sweeten a room and from it an oil is extracted to impart its perfume to toilet soaps and to bath oils.

One of 13 species, it belongs to the thistle family and has been cultivated in Asia, especially India, since earliest times for its flowers which yield pink and red dyes for colouring cloth and silk. The dye obtained from the flowers is mixed with talc to make powdered or solid rouges. An infusion of the flowers is also given for skin complaints, whilst the seeds have culinary uses. The high proportion of linoleic acid in its oil makes it ideal for the low cholesterol diet. A spiny thistle-like plant, it has a stout upright almost white stem, branched near the top and with alternate oval sharply-pointed stem-clasping leaves, prickly at the margins. The flowers have reddish petals from which the dye is obtained by steeping in water. They are followed by shining white, almost four-sided fruits which also yield a red colouring matter. In ancient Egypt, clothes used for mummified bodies were dyed with it.

It is a glabrous plant with hollow stems and a parsnip-like root running deep into the ground. When boiled as a vegetable, the root has an aromatic smell and taste like the parsnip. The 2-pinnate leaves are cut into linear lobes, like parsley. The white flowers are borne in large irregular umbels in mid-summer and are followed by oblong fruits with small ridges. They have a powerful aromatic scent when fully dry which increases with age. Its essential oil consists of carvene and carvol, the latter an oxidised solid resembling camphor becoming pure upon removal of the carvene by fractional distillation and identical to that obtained in the manufacture of inexpensive soaps. Caraway seeds are included in sachets, mixed with lavender and other sweet smelling herbs to place amongst clothes and the seeds are included in bread and cakes, though the taste is not to everyone's liking.

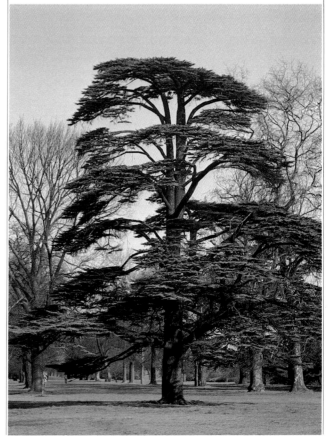

CENTAUREA CYANUS

CORNFLOWER
Blue-bottle

Compositae

36 C. + N. Europe, Asia, N. + S. America

CHAEROPHYLLUM CERIFOLIUM

SWEET FERN
Sweet chervil

Umbelliferae

37 C. Europe, C. Asia *N. America*

CHONDRUS CRISPUS

CARRAGEEN MOSS
Irish moss

Algae

38 N. + W. Europe, E.- N. America

CHRYSANTHEMUM PARTHENIUM

FEVERFEW
Featherfew

Compositae

39 C. + S. Europe, Asia

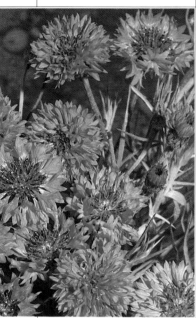

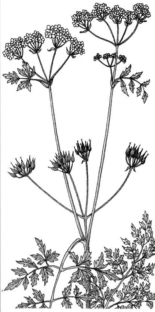

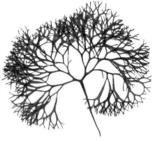

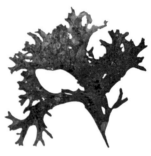

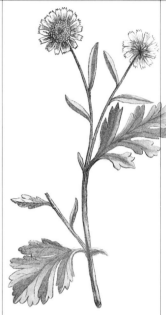

A genus of 600 or more species, *C. cyanus* is present in cornfields and on waste ground, growing in full sunlight. It forms an erect, unbranched stem with alternate lanceolate leaves, the lower ones toothed and bearing bright blue solitary flowers about 1 in (2·5 cm) across during July and August. The ray florets are deeply cut, whilst the whole plant is covered in silky down giving a grey appearance. From the juice of the flowers a blue ink and· paint is made to use in water colouring. From the petals, a distilled water is made which will remove soreness from the eyes and give them a sparkle. It is also an astringent, tightening the skin and removing wrinkles. *C. moschata*, named Sweet Sultan, was said to be "of so exceeding a sweet scent that it surpasseth the finest civet . . ." In the Near East its flowers have the same uses as *C. cyanus.*

Native of mountain pastures and hedgerows, it is a pubescent plant, its hollow stems covered with silky hairs between the nodes, its 3-pinnate leaves pubescent on the underside. When handled, they emit the sweet aromatic smell of aniseed. It blooms in May and June, bearing its white flowers, much visited by bees, in lateral umbels. They are followed by dark brown fruits 1 in (2·5 cm) long. The fern-like leaves taste as if sprinkled with sugar, hence its name Sweet fern. The plant is also known as Chervil, from the Greek *cheirei* and *phyllum* ("that which rejoices the heart"), for the warming qualities of the leaves, used fresh or as a sauce for fish, and also when smelled, give one a feeling of well-being. An infusion of the leaves applied warm to the face will clear it of soreness and blemishes, leaving the skin soft and white. It is more effective if mixed with rose water and is astringent, tightening the skin.

Not a moss but a seaweed, plentiful on both sides of the North Atlantic, especially the west coast of Ireland where it is collected and dried and exported as a demulcent and emollient and included in many herbal toilet preparations. It has much-branched fan-shaped fronds which vary in colour from dark green to purple-brown and which fade with exposure to the air; fronds thrown up by heavy seas are almost white with long exposure. It is this colour when obtained from the herbalist. It is present in deep water and in shallow rock pools. It is washed free of sand then soaked for two hours in cold water before boiling in milk (or fresh water) so that its mucilage dissolves to a thick paste or jelly. It contains neither sugar nor starch but a large amount of glutinous material. Taken hot it is nourishing and is a valuable demulcent. If soaked in glycerine and slightly warmed then allowed to cool, it will set into a stiff cream for soothing the face and hands.

A woody plant, its name being a corruption of "febrifuge" denoting its tonic and fever-dispelling properties. It is a plant of field sides and waste ground, usually growing in sandy soil and in full sun. It is a pubescent, branched plant with alternate yellowish green pinnate leaves, the one or two narrow leaflets divided into lobed segments, giving the plant a feathery appearance, the lower leaves having longer stalks than the upper leaves. They emit an aromatic pungent smell when handled. The flowers are borne all summer in terminal clusters. They have white ray florets and yellow disc-florets which are flat, not conical as in chamomile. The double form is known as Batchelor's Buttons. An infusion of the herb in boiling water and allowed to cool is taken internally for nervous complaints and externally to apply to the face to remove freckles and soreness. It was used in a 17th-century beauty preparation made by Gervase Markham.

CICHORIUM INTYBUS

SUCCORY
Chicory

Compositae

40 Europe, N.W. Africa, W. Asia
Temperate Zones

CINNAMOMUM CASSIA

CASSIA
Safrol, Cassie

Lauraceae

41 S. Asia
S. America

It is present on waste ground, growing around fields, on downland by the road side, usually in limestone soil which is light and gravelly. The plant has a long thick tap root used as a vegetable or a coffee additive. An infusion of the whole herb when in bloom and applied to the face at night will clear the skin of blemishes and of soreness caused by too long exposure to sunlight, leaving it soft and white.

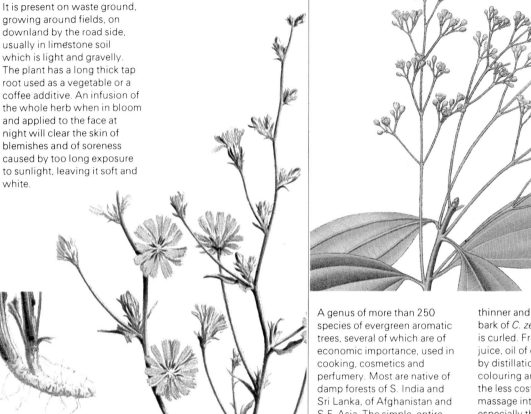

From the blue flowers a water is distilled which when warm is used to bathe the eyes, removing soreness and tiredness and leaving them with a sparkle. The plant is readily distinguished by its branched stems which spread out from the main stem for a considerable distance. The lower leaves are large and hairy and divided into several lobes like the dandelion. The upper leaves are smaller and are stem-clasping at the base. The flowers appear late in summer in twos and threes from the axils of the stem leaves and are about $1\frac{1}{2}$ in (3·5 cm) in diameter. They are a lovely sky-blue colour, each floret being five-toothed.

A genus of more than 250 species of evergreen aromatic trees, several of which are of economic importance, used in cooking, cosmetics and perfumery. Most are native of damp forests of S. India and Sri Lanka, of Afghanistan and S.E. Asia. The simple, entire leaves contain oil glands. *C. cassia*, which grows about 20 ft (6 m) tall with alternate leaves and bears its greenish yellow flowers in axillary inflorescences, is the Cassia of the Scriptures. Today it yields cassie oil for barber shops. It was one of the holy anointing oils mentioned in *Exodus* as being used by Moses on sacred occasions. The bark, young twigs and leaves are removed and tied into bundles for transporting to the distillation centre for boiling. Cinnamon cassia is considered of somewhat lesser quality and of less pronounced taste than proper *cinnamon zeylanicum*. It is usually sold in European and American markets as a powder, but in its flattened prepulverized form it is redder, thinner and smoother than the bark of *C. zeylanicum*, which is curled. From the aromatic juice, oil of cassia is obtained by distillation. It is of amber colouring and is mixed with the less costly olive oil to massage into the body, especially the feet. It is also massaged into the scalp to keep the hair dark and prevent baldness on men. Powdered cassie bark was used in the toilet or talcum powders made for Queen Isabel of Spain, with orris, cloves and a few grains of musk. It was also placed in muslin bags to put amongst clothes and linen. The perfume is long lasting. *C. glanduliferum*, native of N. India and W. China, has similar virtues and is also used to flavour wine. It grows 40 ft (12 m) tall with broad, leathery leaves, pale green above, white beneath and covered with pellucid dots which are oil glands. *C. camphora* of S. India and Japan yields the white crystalline substance, camphor.

CISTUS LADANIFERUS

LABDANUM
Cretan rose

Cistaceae

42 S. Europe

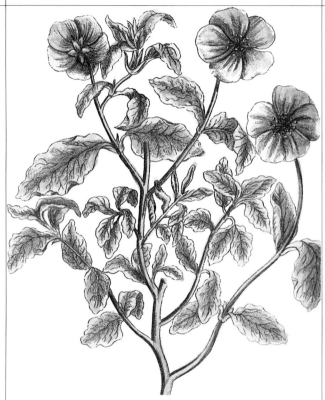

CITRULLUS VULGARIS

WATER MELON
Egyptian melon

Cucurbitaceae

43 N.E. Africa, Tropical Asia, Mediterranean
Warm Temperate Zones

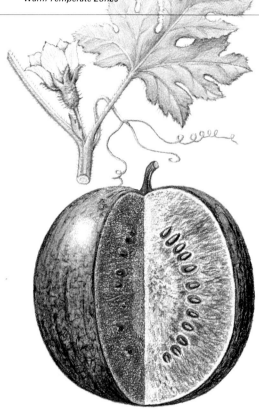

A genus of 20 species of gum-yielding shrubs, it is native of the Mediterranean region, especially the islands of Cyprus, Crete and Rhodes, though the Gum cistus, *C. ladaniferus*, is native also of Spain, Portugal and the Near East. It forms a twiggy bush with narrow dark green leaves about 1 in (2·5 cm) long which release a balsam-like fragrance in the warm sunshine. The single pinkish purple flowers are shaded yellow at the base and open to 4 in (10 cm) across. They bloom in June and July and, though fleeting, appear in continuous succession for at least 8 weeks. The plant grows amongst rocky outcrops in full sun. It has greyish bark, covered in short white glandular hairs which also cover the leaves. Most of the labdanum that is used today comes from Crete and is reddish black with a balsamic scent, similar to ambergris. The exudation, secreted from the glandular hairs on the stems and leaves, sticks to the coats of browsing sheep and goats. From their fleece and from the beards of goats it is collected by shepherds today exactly as described by Dioscorides, living at the time of Christ. The golden yellow resin is made into cakes, like myrrh, and has similar uses. It is transported to all parts of the world to be used as a fixative for perfumes and scents. *C. cyprius* is native of Cyprus where it abounds on mountainous slopes and grows to a height of 6–7 ft (2 m). It has dull grey-green leaves 1 in (2·5 cm) long and blooms in May and June, its large pure white flowers having a crimson spot at the base of each petal. From this species the purest labdanum is collected.

A genus of two species, native of Africa, the Mediterranean and S. Asia, it is a staple food of the Egyptian people and those of the near East and S. Asia since earliest times. The Nile Delta provided the people of Egypt with large crops and it also grew in abundance in the valleys of the Jordan, Tigris, Euphrates and the Ganges, in the alluvial deposits left by the flooding waters. The fruit has a smooth skin (rind) and grows to a large size, being oval in shape, up to 20 in (50 cm) long and about 14 in (35 cm) wide. When ripe, the flesh is red and juicy with black seeds, which are removed before the fruit is used and when dried are nutty and nutritious. The fruits may weigh up to 30 lb when mature and are rich in vitamins A and C. The plants climb by means of tendrils and, in warm climates and not lacking moisture at the roots, make rapid growth. They crop through summer and autumn. The juice, mixed with a little honey and a teaspoonful of lemon juice, is cooling and reduces the body temperature and so is given in times of fever. It also refreshes in hot weather and its culture now extends to most parts of S. Europe and Asia. The queens of ancient Egypt would refresh themselves by cutting a ripe fruit into slices and, lying down on a bed, would spread them over the face and neck. After an hour they would arise refreshed, with the skin tight and re-moisturised. A refrigerated melon is even more efficient especially if the juice of half a lemon is squeezed over it. The eyes are protected by placing an iced damp cloth over them. It takes at least 30 minutes for the treatment to be effective.

CITRUS BIGARRADIA

NEROLI
Bigarrade

Rutaceae

44   China, Japan

CITRUS LIMON

LEMON
Bitter lemon

Rutaceae

45   S.E. Asia, China
      Warm Temperate Zones

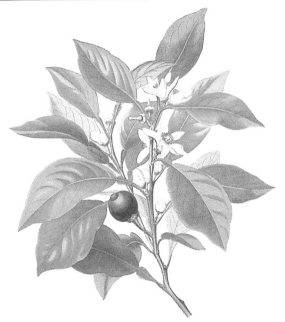

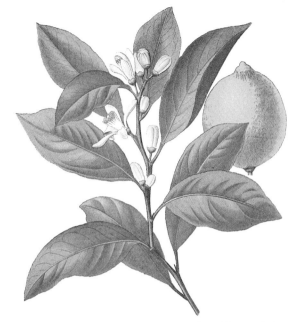

A genus of 12 species of small trees or shrubs, which are often spiny. The blossom most used in perfumery is that of *C. bigarradia*, the Bitter orange, which makes a small bushy plant with alternate elliptic leaves ending in a point and joined to the stem with a winged or flattened footstalk. The large, fragrant, creamy white flowers appear in never-ending succession at the ends of the shoots and at the same time as the fruits, which mature all year round. All parts of the tree yield a fragrant essential oil; that from the upper surface of the petals is known as neroli; that from the leaves, petit-grain; that from the rind of the fruit, bigarrade. Each is used in perfumery, neroli being the main ingredient of eau de Cologne. The name is derived from Flavio Orsini, Prince of Nerola in the 16th century, whose second wife found the perfume much to her liking. Orange trees will begin to bear blossom and fruit when six years old and will attain their maximum productivity at 20 years but will remain so for another 80 or more years. Also included in eau de Cologne, and in many of the most fashionable perfumes, is the essential oil of the rind of the Bergamot orange. It is a variety of *C. aurantium*, the Seville orange, which was introduced into Spain during the Moorish invasion. From the skin (rind) of the small sour unripe fruits, which are pear shaped, oil of Portugal is obtained. Mixed with rectified spirit, essence of bergamot, a popular handkerchief perfume, is obtained. Cedrat is another handkerchief perfume extracted from *C. medica*, the Citron, and usually mixed with essence of bergamot. The Citron has elliptic leaves and large white flowers, purple on the outside. They are followed by pale greenish yellow fruits about 6 in (15 cm) long. An essential oil is extracted from the dried skin and pulp. The first orange to be introduced into Italy is said to have been planted in Rome in 1200 by St. Dominic.

It is native to S. China and S.E. Asia, but was cultivated early in history in S. Europe, N. Africa and the Near East to supply the demands of the rest of Europe, for use in refreshing drinks to quench the thirst and to flavour foods. It is also the best of antiscorbutics, being rich in vitamin C (ascorbic acid) which heals the skin and small blood vessels and is necessary for healthy teeth and gums. The lemon has many uses in promoting beauty. Massaged into the scalp, it prevents loss of hair leading to baldness. For blond hair, a lemon juice rinse in warm water after shampooing, will give lustre to the hair and maintain its colour, for it acts as a mild bleach. Lemon juice will remove or tone down freckles and is even more effective if used with a few grains of powdered borax. A little juice in hot water, taken upon rising each day, will tone the system and give the eyes a sparkle. The common remedy for a sore throat, hot water, honey, and lemon juice, has been a staple of mothers for generations. The tree is found growing on rocky ground in full sun. It has small twiggy branches with spines and grey bark. The glossy leaves are ovate, whilst the flowers, borne in the leaf axils throughout the year, are pinkish white. They are followed all the year round (the plant being in fruit and flower at the same time) by oval fruits about 3 in (7·5 cm) long with a nipple-shaped end. The fruits are green, ripening to bright yellow, and are rich in citric acid which gives them their sharp, bitter taste. The skin, which contains the sunshine vitamin, D, is boiled with sugar and dried to use grated in confectionery. It is also grated into a variety of foods, such as sweet biscuits, cake and Swiss müseli, for its colour, flavour and nutritive value, but is, unfortunately, often injected with a variety of artificial chemicals.

COCHLEARIA ARMORACIA	COCOS NUCIFERA	CONVALLARIA MAJALIS	COPERNICIA CERIFERA
HORSERADISH Mountain radish	**COCONUT PALM** Coco palm	**LILY OF THE VALLEY** Wood lily	**CARNAUBA WAX** Wax palm
Cruciferae	Palmae	Liliaceae	Palmae
46 Europe, Asia *Temperate Zones*	**47** Tropical + subtropical Zones	**48** Europe, Asia *N. America*	**49** Tropical America

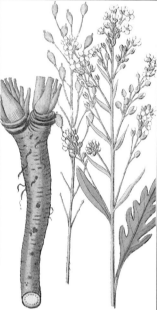

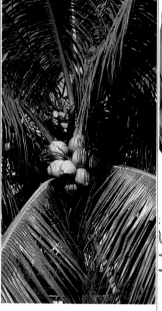

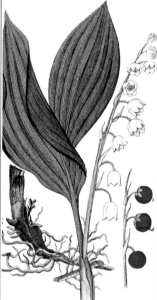

The plant has been appreciated for its medicinal and culinary qualities since earliest times. Gerard (1597) said that "the grated root, with a little vinegar, is used by the Germans for sauce to eat with fish and suchlike meats". The juice extracted from the root can relieve sore skin. The sliced roots boiled in milk and applied as a skin lotion, will clear a spotty face of blackheads and pimples and is especially effective for a greasy skin. Its name was originally "coarse" radish, to distinguish it from the radish with small edible roots. The plant forms a stout cylindrical rootstock, which in old plants is as thick as a man's arm and which penetrates deep into the ground, making it difficult to eradicate. When the root is broken it releases a hot, pungent smell. The large shining dark green leaves are held on 12 in (30 cm) foot-stalks and the small white flowers are borne in dense spikes throughout summer.

It is usually found close to the sea, growing in sandy soil, and has an unbranched slightly curving trunk with the scars of fallen leaves all the way up. At the apex is a head of large pinnate leaves, each about 6 ft (2 m) long. The flowers are white and borne in a dense inflorescence. They are followed by a fruit (the coconut), often 16 in (40 cm) or more in circumference, with a hard shell enclosed in a fibrous pericap. At the base are three circular holes, smooth and thinner than the rest of the shell, which are more easily pierced to obtain the thirst-quenching milk inside. The shell is lined to a thickness of almost 1 in (2·5 cm) with white edible flesh which is highly nutritious. Grated, it is used fresh or dry in confectionery. From the shell (copra), coconut oil is extracted and used in cooking and in the best shampoos. If the oil is massaged into the scalp daily, it will cause thin hair to thicken and take on a pleasing lustre.

It is a glabrous perennial with dark green root leaves, produced in pairs, and a sheathing petiole. The white bell-shaped flowers are borne 6–12 in a one-sided raceme and are heavily scented, lightened by lemony undertones. The flowers are followed by globose red berries. In bloom in May and June, the plant enjoys the cool leafy soil of deciduous woodlands and hedgerows, but is usually confined to calcareous soils. It takes its name from the Latin *convallis* (a valley), for it is found in shady, low-lying land. Today, the distilled water is used on the face after washing to whiten the complexion and tighten the skin, for it is astringent. The essential oil is used in perfumery but is one of the most difficult of perfumes to extract and to imitate. It is included in Jeanne Lanvin's Arpège perfume, introduced in 1925, which still enjoys world popularity.

A genus of 30 species, most important being the Wax palm of Brazil which attains a height of 100 ft (30 m), its unbranched stem ends in a crown of large leaves, its stem ringed with the marks left by the dead leaves. The large palmate leaves give their name to the order and are coated with wax which falls with shaking. Wax is also present on the scales which enclose the leaf buds and is secreted in such abundance at the height of summer that it falls to the ground to be collected. Or the leaf buds are cut off and placed in vats of boiling water when the wax collects on the surface. It is then re-melted and made into cakes. Each tree yields about 4 lb (2 kg) of

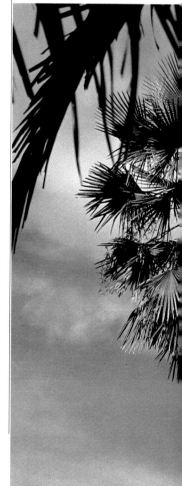

CORIANDRUM SATIVUM

CORIANDER
Coriandre

Umbelliferae

50 S. Europe, Asia, N. Africa
Temperate Zones

CROCUS SATIVUS

SAFFRON
Saferon

Iridaceae

51 S. Europe, W. Asia

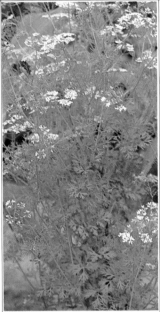

wax during the season which is made into scented candles and gramophone records. Used with olive or almond oil and beeswax it makes an excellent foundation cream and is also present in cake mascaras and solid brilliantines for the hair. The flowers are borne in a large spike enclosed in a large spath which is torn open as the flowers expand. The sessile flowers are arranged in a compact spiral, the pollen from the male flowers escaping in large billowing clouds, pollination being by wind.

It takes its name from the Greek *koros* (a bug) for the unripe fruit (seeds) has the unpleasant smell of the bugs which pollinate the flowers. When the seed is ripe, the unpleasant smell is replaced by a delicious orange scent. It was used to make Carmelite water and a special honey water which George Wilson, an apothecary, made for King James II of England. It is a pleasing after-shave lotion and takes any inflammation from the skin. Its essential oil is pale yellow with a powerful orange scent and is a good fixative in perfumery. The plant is found on waste ground and has solid branching stems which are ridged. The dark green leaves are twice-pinnate with the lower leaves divided into deeply cut segments. The flowers, which appear in mid-summer, are pink or white, the outer petals being longer than the inner. They grow in symmetrical umbels and are followed by round yellow fruits like peppercorns, which fall as soon as ripe.

It is one of the oldest plants still in commercial use, having been used to colour and flavour food since pre-Christian times. It is the Karkom of the Song of Solomon. Like other crocus species, the plant forms a large flat corm from which arise 10 or 12 narrow grey-green leaves, a month before the flower appears. Both leaves and flowers are protected by sheathing leaves at the base. The flowers are collected in September and the yellow stigmas removed, dried and compressed into cakes. Between 4000 and 5000 flowers are required to yield 1 oz (28 g) of the product, from which a perfumed ointment is made to rub into the body after bathing, and the grains infused in hot water, to make a dye which will colour the hair a rich gold. From saffron grains, a fragrant toilet water is to be obtained. Saffron was also used to dye clothes. The Arab people introduced the plant into Spain 1000 years ago, where it has since been cultivated. When once the flowers open, they will never close, and so a dry sunny climate is necessary for the correct ripening of the stigma. Though present in Italy and Greece, it is native to the Near East where, in September, the exposed and barren hillsides are brilliant with its white, pink or blue flowers.

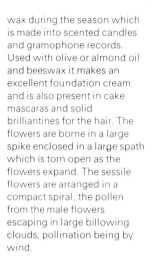

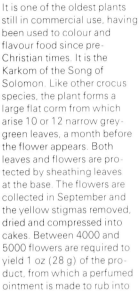

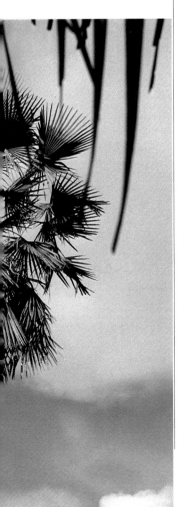

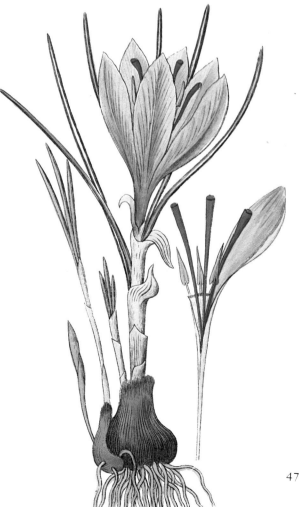

CUCUMIS SATIVUS

CUCUMBER
Cowcumber

Cucurbitaceae

52 Africa, S. + C. Asia
Temperate Zones

CURCUMA ZEDOARIA

ZEDOARY
KURKUM, Kachoora

Zingiberaceae

53 S. Asia
Torrid Zones

CYMBOPOGON CITRATUS

CITRONELLA
Lemon grass

Gramineae

54 N. + S. Africa, S.E. Asia,
India

A genus of 25 species, for centuries plants of *C. sativus*, the cucumber, have provided the people with thirst quenching fruit and the women with aids to their beauty. Elsewhere

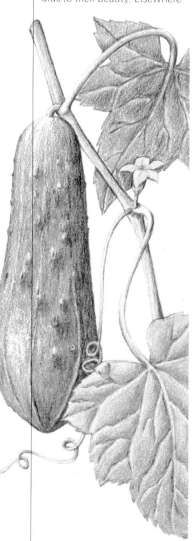

they are cultivated and the fruits used as a vegetable and included in salads. The fruits are also widely used by beauticians in face creams. The fruit, peeled and put through a blender with a carton of yoghurt, makes a cooling and soothing cream and the juice should be included in all astringent lotions combined with witch hazel or rose water. For chapped skin or sunburn, the juice of half a cucumber mixed in a cupful of milk or with a little glycerine and applied to the face with a cotton wool pad will give instant relief and take away the soreness. The high content of Vitamin C – the cucumber's sole claim to being nutritional – is almost entirely within the peel. Skinless, this vegetable can boast neither vitamin, mineral nor protein. *C. sativus* is a hedgerow plant in the wild, climbing by tendrils, but in all warm parts it is grown as a field crop, the plants being allowed to trail over the ground. The fleshy stems are covered in short hairs, the palmately-lobed leaves being long stemmed and also hairy. From each stem node a leaf is formed and a single yellow flower. A tendril grows on the upper side of the leaf base where an extension shoot may be formed. The fruits grow to 16 in (40 cm) long and up to 4 in (10 cm) in diameter, being straight and pointed at one end. They have a hard, thin dark green skin or rind covered with blunt spines. The flesh is pale green and is juicy and cooling when eaten. The soft white seeds, pointed at both ends, are embedded in the flesh and are eaten with it. Before using in beauty preparations, peel off the skin and to obtain the maximum amount of juice from the flesh, slice and simmer for $\frac{1}{2}$ hour or put through a blender. The juice is used in the preparation of high quality toilet soaps which keep the skin soft and smooth.

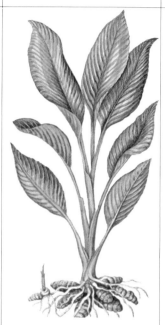

C. zedoaria roots are dried and powdered and, with other aromatics, make a talcum powder used by Hindu women and known as Abir. A similar aromatic powder is obtained from *C. aromaticus*. The genus takes its name from the Persian, *karkum* (Saffron), the reference being to the deep yellow colouring of the roots. The flower stem consists of a sheath of broad lanceolate leaves 2 ft (60 cm) long which are covered with down on the underside. From the sheath arises the short flower spike, some time after, which is of finger thickness. Finally, in June and July appears the yellow and pink tubular flowers which emit the same aromatic fragrance as the roots. Upon distillation, the roots yield 1·3% of essential oil which is used in perfumery. *C. zerumbet* is also famed for its fragrant roots which, as with other species of the genus, consist of palmate tubers and several ovate bulbs.

A genus of perennial grasses distributed throughout N. and S. Africa the Near East, India and Sri Lanka, and S.E. Asia, found on dry, stony ground and wasteland. They form densely tufted plants with the inflorescences crowded at the end of naked stems, with the spikes borne in pairs.
C. citratus, Lemon grass, is present in S. India and Sri Lanka and from it is extracted Lemon-grass otto, which resembles lemon verbena perfume and is extremely potent. *C. nardus*, so named because its hairy root and its perfume resemble those of spikenard, is present in N. Africa, especially Egypt. Here, when riding his elephant during his conquest of Egypt in 332 BC, Alexander the Great became exhilarated by what he thought to be the

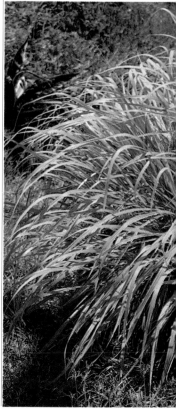

CYNOGLOSSUM OFFICINALE

HOUND'S TONGUE
Dog's tongue

Boraginaceae

55 Europe, W. Africa, Asia
Temperate Zones

DAUCUS SYLVESTRIS

CARROT
Woodland carrot

Umbelliferae

56 Europe, S.W. + N. Asia, N. Africa
Temperate Zones

scent of spikenard, but would more likely have been this species of lemon grass. It makes an inexpensive distillation known as Citronella and is used in perfumery and for scenting "honey" soaps. To the distillers of Khandesh it is called Motiya, when the inflorescence is young and white in colour, and Sonfiya after ripening to crimson-red, the essential oil from the young grass having a more delicate perfume. The grass is mostly cut and harvested in September, after the rains. *C. martini* is found in most parts of India and is known as Indian geranium, for its essential oil has a high Geraniol content similar to that of the rose-scented pelargonium.

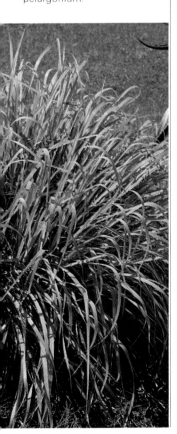

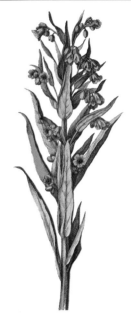

Native of N. and C. Europe and W. Asia, it takes its name from two Greek words *glossa* and *cunos* (dog's tongue) from the shape and furry texture of the leaves. It grows on waste ground, usually of a rocky nature, and has branched hairy stems clothed in downy tongue-like leaves of greyish appearance. The lurid purple-red flowers are borne in June and July in terminal cymes and are followed by large, flat nutlets covered with barbed prickles, like burs, which stick to the clothes and to the coats of animals upon contact. The plant has an unpleasant smell of wet fur. The species *C. germanicum*, native of N. Europe, has leaves which are smooth, not downy and bright green above, so that it is known as the Green leaf Hound's tongue. Both plants have similar properties. The juice from the leaves and stems boiled in olive oil and rubbed into the scalp prevents hair from falling.

A plant of the British Isles, Europe and N. Asia with erect branched stems and finely divided leaves with a sheathing base, its white flowers are borne in an irregular umbel. It blooms June–August and is followed by flattish fruits (seeds) with bristles arranged in five rows. When in bloom, the plant is readily distinguished from other umbelliferae by a small central purple flower. A decoction of the seeds is a carminative and relieves flatulence, whilst the orange coloured roots, pale yellow in the wild form, are the richest of all vegetables (especially the cultivated forms) in vitamin A which strengthens the eyes and improves the vision. It increases the haemoglobin and blood cell level, and, grated into salads provides the intestines with valuable fibre. Vitamin A from carrots is readily assimilated by putting several roots in the blender and adding a little lemon juice to make it more palatable. In addition to its high vitamin A content, the carrot has strong antiseptic qualities, used both internally and externally. The roots, after cleaning, scraping, boiling and mashing into a pulp will sweeten and heal skin blemishes. With a teaspoonful of either almond or olive oil added, the warm pulp makes a toning face mask. It will tighten the skin and remove wrinkles ("crow's feet") from either side of the eyes. It is left on for 30 minutes, then rinsed off. The plant is believed to take its name from *caro* (flesh), which describes the fleshy root. It is present by roadsides and by the side of fields and woodlands, also close to the sea shore. Greek and Latin writers told of the many virtues of the plant, not least an infusion of the green plant as a cure for gout and

rheumatism. More recently, doctors have discovered that carrots have anti-carcinogenic properties.

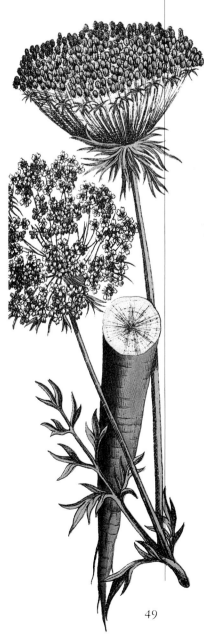

49

DIANTHUS CARYOPHYLLUS

CARNATION
Gillyflower

Caryophyllaceae
57 N. + S. Europe

DIPTERYX ODORATA
Taralea odorata

TONQUIN
Tonka bean

Leguminosae
58 S. America

ELAEIS GUINEENSIS

OIL PALM
African palm

Palmae
59 W. + Equatorial Africa

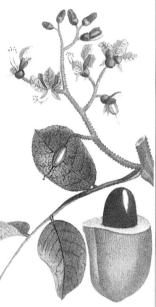

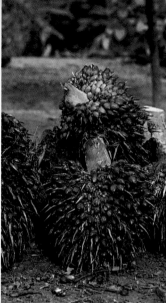

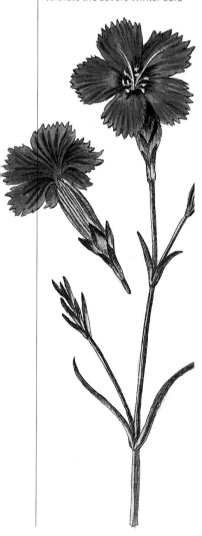

A genus of about 80 species, native of the British Isles, N. and S. Europe, extending as far east as the Caucasus and Balkans, being hardy annual, biennial or perennial plants, with upright linear glaucous or silvery foliage. They bear their flowers either singly or in terminal clusters. They are plants of higher altitudes, of rocky mountainous slopes, especially of a calcareous nature, and require a position open to the direct rays of the sun. The plants are able to tolerate the severe winter cold of Britain and N. Europe. The Athenians, since in Greece and along the southern coast of Europe, *D. caryophyllus* grows in profusion, afforded the plant the highest honour, naming it Dianthos, Flower of Jove. For it was used to impart its delicious clove perfume to wine (hence the poet Chaucer's name for it of "sops-in-wine") and to make garlands and coronets, hence its earlier name "coronation", from which the modern "carnation" is derived. It takes its name "gillyflower" from July-flower, this being the month in which it blooms, and its botanical name from *Caryophyllus aromaticus* (now *Eugenia aromatica*), the clove tree whose dried flowers it resembles in its perfume. Its fragrant petals remain at all times an excellent addition to any pot pourri. In at least one 17th-century pharmacopoeia, clove gillyflowers were mentioned as an antidote to seasickness. From its flesh-pink flowers, which measure about 1·5 in (3 cm) across, the plant gave its name "pink" to the English language. From it and *D. plumarius*, the Fringed pink, the well-known florist's carnation, has been developed and is now grown on a large scale for its clove-scented perfume used in toilet soaps and to make perfumes of a heavy nature. The principle substance of the clove is the alcohol, eugenol or methyl eugenol, the same substance which gives the carnation and pink their unique perfume. The spicy perfumes are built around eugenol, with its warm, heady fragrance, and a blend of musk and carnation.

A genus of eight species, the large trees are remarkable in that they bear single-seeded pods. The flowers, like those of laburnum, are yellow and borne in dense racemes. They are followed by a single-seeded oval drupe or pod of a thick fleshy substance enclosing a black bean which, when dry, shines as if polished. As the bean dries, it emits the powerful scent of newly mown hay, as with sweet vernal grass. The same principle, coumarin, is present in both. It is pure white and is used as a fixative in perfumery and in toilet soaps. In Europe, a fatty substance known as Tonquin butter is sold and the essence obtained in the same way. Since Sir William Perkin made synthetic coumarin in 1868, the tonquin bean has depreciated in value. At one time the ground beans were included in snuffs, to which they imparted a pleasant fragrance, and in sachet powders for, like orris root, its scent increases with age.

A genus of only two species, both being members of the great tree family of mono-cotyledons, which provide fruit, oil and timber for commercial use. The tree forms a thick unbranched stem, the fan-shaped leaves held to the trunk by a strong petiole with a broad sheathing base. The blade remains attached until the petiole eventually decays and falls, leaving conspicuous marks on the trunk. The fruit of the African oil palm is like a small coconut, both the pulp and kernel of which yield, upon compression, a yellowish green oil which has been used in the manufacture of soaps, perfumes and cosmetics for centuries. It has the violet scent of orris which it imparts to its products and for this reason is usually not mixed with other fragrances. It is estimated that more than 50 million pounds of Palm oil are used annually, mostly, it should be added, to use in plating tins used in the canning of food.

EQUISETUM ARVENSE	ERYTHRAEA CENTAURIUM	EUCALYPTUS MACULATA	EUGENIA AROMATICA
	Centaurium erythraea		
HORSETAIL	CENTAURY	LEMON GUM TREE	CLOVE
Bottle-brush	Chironia		
Equisetaceae	Gentianaceae	Myrtaceae	Myrtaceae
60 Europe, N. Africa, N. Asia, N. America	**61** British Isles *Europe, N. Africa*	**62** Australia, New Zealand	**63** S.E. Asia, Madagascar *Tropical Zones*

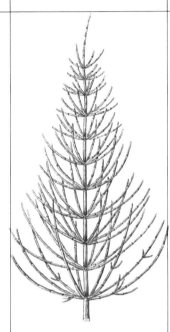

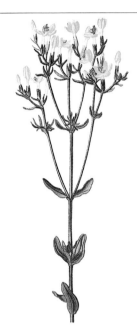

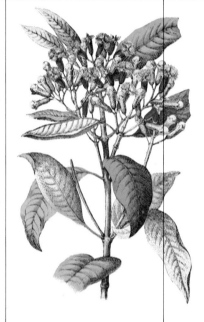

A genus of about 150 species known as the Blue Gums because of their greenish blue foliage and the balsamic resin which exudes from the trunk. The trees are found in marshy land and their ability to absorb large amounts of moisture, making rapid growth, and their valuable antiseptic qualities have made them useful trees to plant in malarial swamps. The trees form a long straight trunk at the top of which an open head forms. The branches are covered with leathery leaves, opposite when young, alternate when the trees become older, and flowers are produced singly or in clusters in the leaf axils. Oil of *E. maculata var. citriodora* is used in perfumery, the fresh leaves yielding about $1\frac{1}{2}$% oil; the dried leaves twice that amount, and consisting almost entirely of citronellon with a small amount of geraniol present, as in *Andropogon nardus*, so that the lemon perfume has pleasant undertones of rose. The tree is found along the coastal districts of Queensland, being especially abundant in the Port Curtis area where distillation of the leaves takes place on a large scale. Oil of eucalyptus was first made official in the British Pharmacopoeia in 1885 for the treatment of lung diseases.

The horsetails are plants of a single genus and amongst the oldest to inhabit the earth. Those found today in corn fields and on wet ground in many parts of the world, are dwarf forms of the giant fossilised plants of the carboniferous era. They are without flowers and require no pollinating insects for their reproduction, relying on spores for their development, like ferns, and underground stolons. They take their name from the Latin *equus* (horse) and *seta* (hair or bristle), since the jointed stems resemble a horse's tail. The plants require plenty of water about their roots and often grow in semi-shade. From the creeping rhizome, two distinct types of stem arise, fertile and barren. The stems are hollow, except at the joints which terminate in sheaths representing leaves. The female stems bear a cone-shaped catkin containing the spores; after releasing them, they die back before the barren stems appear.

A glabrous annual, taking its name from the centaur Chiron, famed in Greek mythology for his skill in medicine. The name Erythraea is from the Greek *erythros* (red), from the colour of its flowers. It is a plant of downlands and chalk cliffs and blooms in mid-summer when it should be gathered. The flowers open only in fine weather and rarely after noon. The plant forms a rosette of pointed pale green leaves from which arises the stem topped by corymbs of rosy-red star-like flowers. The lance-shaped stem leaves grow in opposite pairs. Culpeper said that the flowers are followed by "seeds in little husks, like unto wheat corn", but the plant should be used whilst still in bloom. It is a tonic and blood clarifier and, applied to the face, it takes away blemishes and leaves the skin soft and smooth. The juice of the plant applied to blemishes removes the soreness and heals the skin. The whole plant, like most of the order, is extremely bitter, hence it was known as "gall-of-the-earth".

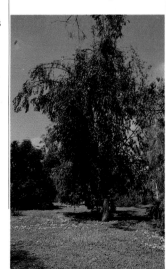

A small genus of evergreen trees or shrubs, *E. aromatica* has smooth grey bark and lance-shaped opposite leaves about 6 in (15 cm) long and covered with oil glands which release a clove-like scent when pressed. The crimson-purple flowers are borne in cymes at the end of the branchlets but are gathered as unopened buds which, when dry, are the cloves of commerce. The season lasts from August to December. At first the buds are yellow, turning pink, then red. Harvesting begins when the trees are six years old and continues for 100 years. The trees grow best in the yellow clay subsoil of the islands of the Indian Ocean and, since earliest times, have been exported to all parts of the world for their culinary and perfumery uses. The world's annual consumption is about 10 million pounds. The cloves are dried, which turns them crimson or black. Zanzibar "red-heads" are superior to other cloves and yield the finest essential oil which is a valuable germicide.

EUPHRASIA OFFICINALIS	FILIPENDULA ULMARIA Spairaea ulmaria	FOENICULUM VULGARE	FRAGARIA VESCA
EYEBRIGHT Euphrasia	**MEADOWSWEET** Bridewort	**FENNEL** Sweet fennel	**STRAWBERRY** Strawberry
Scrophulariaceae **64** Europe	Rosaceae **65** Europe, Asia *N. America*	Umbelliferae **66** S. Europe, N. Africa, W. Asia *Temperate Zones*	Rosaceae **67** Europe, Asia, N.W.- N. America

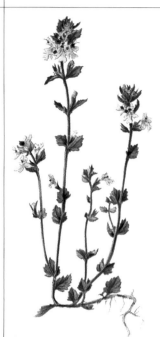

Out of 20 widely distributed species *E. officinalis* is the sole representative in the British Isles. It is a dainty little plant with small, deeply cut leaves which, all summer, bear tiny white or pale lilac flowers with purple veins on the upper and lower lips. The centre lobe of the lower lip is yellow. It is present in alpine pastures, usually in poor soil and often near the sea. It is a variable species sometimes growing only 2 in (5 cm) tall whilst it may reach 8 in (20 cm) in height. The plant is semi-parasitic on grass, with which it is always found growing and on whose roots it relies for part of its food, tiny nodules on the roots extracting nourishment from the grass roots by absorption cells. The plant can clear up any soreness and prevent running eyes. It also accentuates the brightness of the eyes and herbal beauty stores enjoy a greater demand for eyebright lotion than for any other beauty preparation.

A genus of ten species, native of north temperate regions and present in damp meadows and by the side of rivers and ponds, it is also found in open woodlands. Its leaves release the scent of wintergreen, containing methyl salicylate as in wintergreen and willow, which is given for rheumatic complaints in the form of aspirin. It is a plant with furrowed stems, often crimson and with crinkled pinnate leaves, dark green above; grey on the underside and divided into several leaflets. The terminal leaflet is lobed with serrate edges. The creamy white flowers are borne in crowded cymes, June–September, and have a sweet scent but, like the hawthorn, with unpleasant undertones, due to the presence of Trimethylamine. The distilled water of the leaves will take away soreness from the eyes and will comfort them when tired whilst the distilled water from the flowers is an astringent and soothing face lotion. The flowers were used as bridal head decorations, hence its name of bridewort whilst its botanic name is from the Latin, *ulmus* (elm) due to the shape of its leaflets.

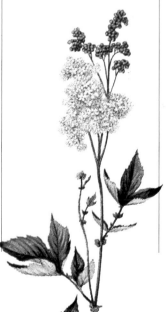

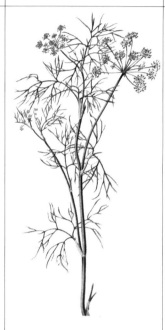

The plant received its name from the Latin *foeniculum* (hay) for it is thought to have the scent of newly mown hay. However, anethol forms the chief constituent of its essential oil which is used to perfume soaps and shampoos. Like dill, fennel water, obtained from the seeds, is a carminative and for 2000 years it has been used slightly warm, to bathe the eyes, removing any inflammation and tiredness and giving them brightness. It is a plant of waste ground, growing best in sandy soil over chalk subsoil and usually close to the sea. It is a stout, erect plant, its 3–4 pinnate leaves divided into numerous narrow segments whilst, from a distance, the plant has a blue-green appearance. The yellow flowers are borne in large terminal umbels during July and August and are followed by narrow ovoid fruits with blunt ends and with eight longitudinal ribs. They are pale green but to obtain their maximum fragrance must be harvested fully ripe and then dried.

F. vesca is native of deciduous woodlands. It is a plant enjoying semi-shade and is a hairy perennial, increasing by runners or string-like growths rooting at the leaf nodes. The trefoil leaves have pointed leaflets and serrate edges, whilst the white flowers with five overlapping petals are borne in clusters on upright stems. The small many-seeded fruits are red or white. Garden strawberries are descended from large fruiting American species, crossed with *F. elatior* of C. Europe, where it is known as the Hautbois. *F. viridis* is also European and has greenish white fruit. It is a plant of alpine meadows, preferring a limestone soil whereas other species enjoy the slightly acid soils of woodlands containing leafmould. Late in the 17th century, a runnerless variant of *F. vesca* appeared near Mt. Cenis in C. Europe which makes a bushy plant and is increased by seed or division and not by runners. It bears small red fruits (berries). Strawberries reduced to pulp and rubbed onto the face and left for an hour will leave the skin smooth and tight.

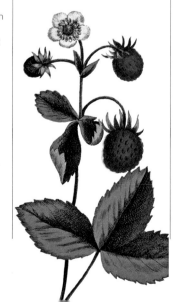

FUCUS VESICULOSIS

SEA KELP
Bladderwrack

Fucaceae

68 N. + W. Europe, E. + W.- N. American

FUMARIA OFFICINALIS

FUMITORY
Earth Smoke

Fumariaceae

69 Europe, N. Africa, W. Asia *Temperate Zones*

GALIUM APARINA

CLEAVERS
Catchweed

Rubiaceae

70 Europe, Asia, N. America *Warm Temperate Zones*

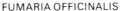

Several species of Fucus, including *F. serratus* and *F. nodosus*, can be used for the extraction of iodine and, after burning, as kelp to use in beauty treatments. The same is true of the seaweed

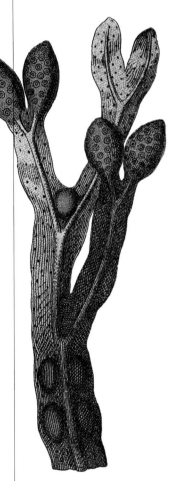

Laminaria digitata, known as "deep sea", "tangle" or "drift-wood" Kelp which is collected on the shore after being washed up by gales and high tides. It contains ten times the iodine content of *F. vesiculosis*, the Bladderwrack, so called because its fruiting bodies are contained in small bladder-like receptacles filled with a transparent mucous. These seaweeds are plentiful only in northern waters, found on both the Pacific and Atlantic coasts of N. America and on the coasts of Britain and N. Europe. Bladderwrack is brownish green and attaches itself to rocks by discs which form at the base of the stalk. The fronds are fan-shaped and flat with a strong mid-rib along which are arranged the "bladders" at regular intervals. It is at its best for drying as kelp and for the extraction of iodine during July, when it dries quickly in the sun and can then be reduced to a fine powder. For some reason, it cannot be dried artificially. The seaweed contains a large percentage of potash and used fresh (chopped up) makes a valuable soil fertiliser. When burnt, it is known as sea kelp and contains mucilage, cellulose, mannite, soda and iodine which make up almost 20% of the ash content. Although a great source of potassium and iodine and an adequate supplier of vitamins A and D, kelp has little protein content, and is not easily digested by humans. Twenty tons of fucus yields about one ton of kelp which yields a litre of iodine. Sea kelp is used in treating obesity by stimulating the thyroid gland in the same way that sea foods also behave. With warm almond or coconut oil, it is massaged into the skin for a revitalising 10 minutes facial and, with yogurt and a beaten egg, imparts a healthy gloss to the hair. Sea kelp (a reddish powder) is obtainable from most health shops and chemists for use in beauty treatment. The manufacture of iodine from kelp was discovered by Prof. Courtois in 1812 and it is still obtained in Scotland, whilst the use of kelp in the manufacture of soap has been superseded by common salt.

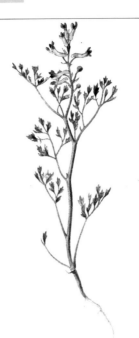

It is a common weed of hedge-rows and ditches, of arable and waste land. Its name is derived from its blue-green colour, seeming at a distance like smoke arising from the ground. For this reason it was a plant surrounded by superstition. A small slender herb climbing by its twisting leaf stalks, its leaves 2–3-pinnate with a bitter taste, its pale pink flowers, tipped with purple, appearing in erect rows all summer. It is self-fertile, setting seed without the aid of insects. Since earliest times, the plant has been known for its purifying powers, cleansing the blood and skin of impuritites when taken internally and used as a lotion on the face. It is perhaps the best of all plants for removing freckles caused by long exposure to the sun, for the plant contains the alkaloid Fumarin. It will leave the complexion white and smooth if used over several weeks. The whole plant may be dried for winter use.

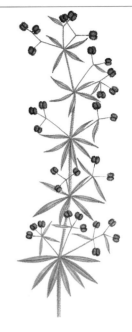

A common weed of hedge-rows and field sides with slender quadrangular stems and leaves arranged in whorls. The whole plant is covered in tiny hooked bristles by which it attaches itself to browsing animals and to people who walk amongst it, hence its name Catchweed. The narrow lance-shaped leaves, which are arranged all the way up the stems, attach themselves (cling) to other plants by their hooks for support and pull themselves up to the sunlight. The small greenish white star-like flowers arise from the axils of the leaves. The seeds, when dried and ground, make an excellent substitute for coffee, a plant of the same order. The plant is distributed throughout temperate Europe and Asia and also North America. The roots yeild a red dye which can be used to give colour to the cheeks. An excellent blood purifyer, it will clear the skin of spots at the end of winter.

GAULTHERIA PROCUMBENS

WINTERGREEN
Checkerberry

Ericaceae

71 E.-N. America

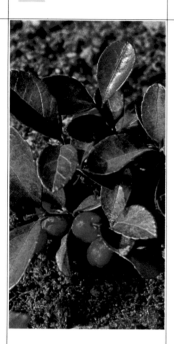

It is a low growing shrubby peat-loving plant usually found in the acid soil of rhododendron woodlands and on heathlands and barren slopes. Several species are Himalayan plants.
G. procumbens is the Creeping wintergreen, especially abundant in the pine woods of North Carolina and New Jersey with small heath-like dark green leaves (bright green when young) which are finely toothed. When handled they emit a penetrating minty aroma, oil of wintergreen, obtained by distillation of the leaves, being included in embrocations to treat sprains and rheumatic pains. The drooping, waxy white flowers are borne on red stalks and are followed by large edible crimson berries which persist all winter. Upon distillation, the leaves yield the otto methyl salicylate which when treated with a warm solution of caustic alkali, yields salicylic acid and methyl alcohol used for perfuming soaps.

GEUM URBANUM

WOOD AVENS
Holy herb

Rosaceae

72 Europe, C. Asia

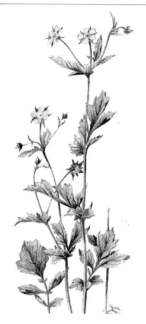

It is distributed throughout the British Isles, Europe and C. Asia, though less common in northern latitudes. It is present in open woodlands and about hedgerows, making a thin upright plant with wiry reddish-brown stems and irregular pinnate (trefoiled) leaves, the terminal leaflet being broad and wedge-shaped, the two others being small and narrow. They are dark green and hairy with toothed margins. In bloom throughout the summer and autumn, the tiny flowers are golden yellow and self-fertile in the absence of insects. The roots are brown and about 2 in (5 cm) long with a clove-like smell and are used, instead of cloves, to flavour apple tarts. They were also used to flavour ale and wine. When dry the roots were placed amongst clothes and vestments to impart their fragrance and to keep away moths. The roots are astringent and have a high tannin content.

HAMAMELIS VIRGINIANA

WITCH HAZEL
Winterbloom

Hamamelidaceae

73 E.-N. America

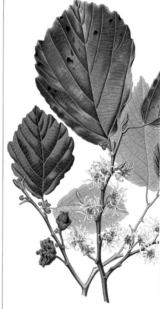

A small family of shrubby plants, *H. virginiana* usually grows in open woodlands. A decoction of its bark and twigs taken as a tea, is still used by tribesmen to check internal and external haemorrhages. The distilled extract of the leaves and twigs is soothing when applied to a chapped or sunburnt skin. It can remove pimples and blackheads. *H. virginiana* is a small twisted tree with smooth silver-grey bark and oval leaves about 4 in (10 cm) long and 3 in (7·5 cm) broad like those of hazel and held on short petioles. After the leaves fall in October, the yellow flowers with their long strap-like petals appear in clusters in the leaf joints and persist through winter. They are followed by black two-chambered nut-like edible fruits containing white seeds. When ripe, the seeds are ejected with a snapping sound, hence its country name.

HELIANTHUS ANUUS

SUNFLOWER

Compositae

74 Mexico, Peru
Temperate Zones

Native of Mexico and Peru, it was introduced into Europe by the Spaniards in the 16th century and has now become one of the most important of economic crops. Its oil has a sweet taste and is used in margarines and cosmetics and has many culinary uses. It is also used in the manufacture of toilet soaps. Every part of the plant has its economic uses. From the flowers a yellow hair dye is obtained and the stems are used in paper making. Bees obtain large quantities of nectar from the flowers and unopened flower buds make a nourishing vegetable. The plant was worshipped by the Aztecs, and on the walls of their temples to the Sun God were sunflowers wrought in pure gold. The plant takes its name from the Greek *helios* (the sun) which the flower represents, its circular head being up to 8 in (20 cm) or

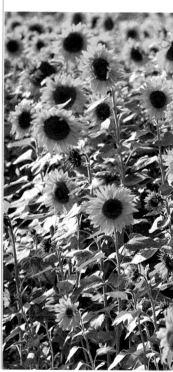

HELIOTROPIUM PERUVIANUM	HORDEUM VULGARE Hordeum distichon	HUMULUS LUPULUS
HELIOTROPE Cherry pie	BARLEY Beerley	HOP Hoppan
Boraginaceae **75** S. America *Warm Temperate Zones*	Gramineae **76** C. Asia *Temperate Zones*	Cannabinaceae **77** Europe, Asia, N. America *Temperate Zones*

more in diameter and composed of numerous small black or brown tubular flowers arranged in a central disc and surrounded by an outer row of broad corolla petals. These are of brilliant golden-yellow, like the rays of the sun. The plant has a thick hairy stem and broad, coarsely toothed leaves up to 10 in (25 cm) long. One of the fastest growing of all plants in the wild, it is found on waste ground and always in full sun. When ripe, the seeds are black and produce a scentless oil which is palest yellow. Massaged into the skin with witch hazel and with the addition of a little honey, it leaves the skin soft and smooth.

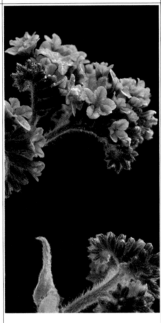

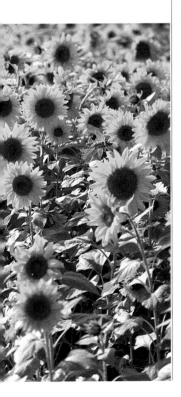

A genus of more than 100 species of warmer parts of both old and new worlds, *H. peruvianum* is a native of Chile and Peru where it is often grown as a hedge reaching 5 ft (1·5 cm) tall and diffusing its unusual perfume over a wide area. The scent is like almond paste, or cherries when baked in a pie, hence its popular name. After treatment with permanganate of potash, it yields heliotropin, a white crystalling powder used to impart the heliotrope perfume to soaps and talcum powders. *H. peruvianum* is a branching plant of shrubby habit with hairy lance-shaped leaves which have a grey appearance and feathery flowers of purple or white borne in terminal cymes. They are followed by fruits containing four nutlets. Though a pleasing handkerchief perfume is obtained from the fresh flowers, it has not been extracted commercially since Messrs Schimmel & Co. of New York discovered the synthetic heliotropin, following the distillation of oil of sassafras which contains 90% safrol.

A genus of 20 species, Barley was cultivated in ancient Egypt to make bread which was of inferior quality to that made from wheat. Egyptian women used barley meal for a face pack, to keep the skin smooth and soft for which purpose it is popular today with women of the western world. The green ears boiled in milk and applied to the skin will remove soreness caused by sun or wind. From the grain, malt is extracted for brewing beer. Extract of malt fortifies in time of illness and malt vinegar, obtained by oxidation of fermented malt wort, has many uses in women's continual search for beauty at all ages. As an astringent there is nothing better. Equal parts with warm water and applied to the face will make the skin firm and reduce large pores. As a rinse, it makes the hair soft and brings out the colour. *H. distichon*, a plant of wastelands, forms an unbranched stem with each spikelet terminating in still awns 1 in (2·5 cm) or more long. *H. vulgare* has its spikelets arranged in six rows.

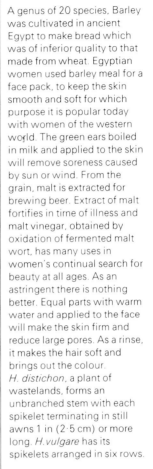

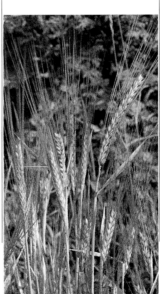

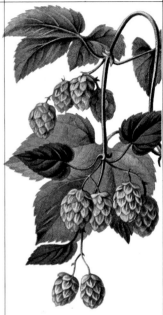

A genus of four species of climbing plants arising each year from a stout rootstock and twining to a considerable height. They are plants with lobed, heart-shaped dark green leaves held on long footstalks. *H. lupulus* is dioecious, the male flowers borne in panicles up to 6 in (15 cm) long appearing on separate plants to the females which are replaced by cone-like catkins, consisting of yellow overlapping bracts covered with glandular hairs, as if sprinkled with a yellow powder, containing 10% lupulin with its valuable tonic properties. The plant takes its name from the Anglo-Saxon *hoppan* (to climb). Hops impart a bitterness to beer and clarify it. Hop bitters and hop tea act as tonic drinks and clear the blood of impurities. From the newly opened flowers, an otto is distilled which is an astringent skin lotion and gives a pleasing fragrance used as a handkerchief perfume.

HYPERICUM PERFORATUM

COMMON ST. JOHN'S WORT
Allheal

Guttiferae

78 Europe, N.W. Africa, N. Asia
Temperate Zones

ILLICIUM PARVIFLORUM

STAR ANISE
Star aniseed

Magnoliaceae

79 S.E. Asia
Warm Temperate Zones

INDIGOFERA TINCTORIA

INDIGO
Indicum

Leguminosae

80 *Warm Temperate Zones*

IRIS FLORENTINA

ORRIS
White iris

Iridaceae

81 S. Europe, N. Africa, India

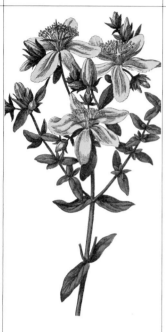

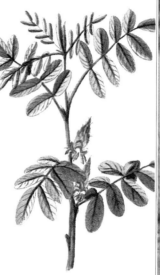

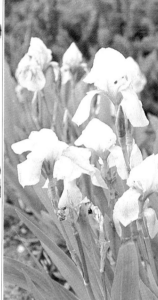

One of a genus of about 300 widely distributed species which has more medical properties than any other plant. The plant takes its name from St. John the Baptist for it usually begins to bloom on his feast day, June 24th. It is an erect plant with a 2-edged stem and small elliptic leaves dotted with pellucid glands and containing caproic acid which gives off the unpleasant smell of wet goat's fur when handled. The French call the plant mille-pertuis, a thousand perforations. The tiny black dots also appear on the sepals and petals of the flowers which are bright yellow and borne in terminal corymbs. The conspicuous stamens are arranged in five bundles. The plant has much the same uses as the common privet and is found in similar places, mostly deciduous woodlands and about hedgerows or shady banks, growing in calcareous soils.

A genus of six species, its botanical name means "allurement", from the fragrance of the trees, whilst its common name is because the flattish fruits are star-like, with eight or more rayed carpels, resembling a star fish and containing scented seeds. Their essential oil consists of eugenol, present in oil of cloves and shikimol, identical with safrol which accounts for its pleasing scent. The oil is used in eastern perfumery and in hair oils; also in toilet soaps, whilst the seeds are used in confectionery. *I. parviflorum*, a low growing shrub, is distinguished from *I. floridanum*, the taller growing Florida aniseed, by its smaller flowers. Both have tapering lance-shaped leaves with long footstalks and when rubbed in the hands leave behind a powerful aniseed scent. The purple-red flowers diffuse a spicy odour, those of *I. floridanum* being followed by fruits with 13 carpels. Similar to *I. parviflorum* in most respects is *I. griffithii* native of the humid forests of E. Bengal but from which it is distinguished by its beaked carpels which number 15.

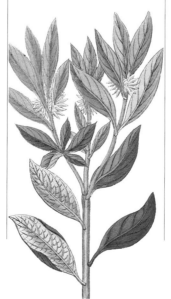

One of a genus of more than 700 species of shrubby plants native of the warmer parts of the old world, with *I. tinctoria* prominent in India and Burma and supplying the purple-black dye, indigo. The pinnate leaves are divided into 6–8 pairs of opposite oval leaflets. The pinkish purple flowers borne in racemes from the leaf axils are followed by thin slightly curved pods containing 8–12 seeds. It is the leaves that yield the dye, the plants being cut almost at soil level just before flowering. They are soaked in vats filled with water for several weeks, the solution turning deep yellow. This is frequently stirred and upon exposure to the air, oxidises to form an insoluble precipitate of indigo, used to intensify the black hair of Indian women who soak the dried (or fresh) leaves in water and usually apply it mixed with henna as a paste. The plants require a dry sandy soil and an open sunny situation.

A genus named in honour of the rainbow goddess Iris, from the variety of colours of its flowers. *I. florentina* figures in the arms of the City of Florence – a white iris on a red shield – though the flower is streaked with purple and has a yellow beard on the fall petals. Since earliest times it has been appreciated by the Italian people to make into powders to apply to the body and face, for contained in the root is the ketone Irone, which gives the flower its violet-like odour and is present in the violet flower. Dried orris root is also included in sachet powders and in tooth powders. Oil of orris, extracted by the distillation of orris root with steam, which is pale yellow, has the exact odour of the violet flower and is included in the most expensive perfumes. The plant takes three years for the roots to form a reasonable size, when the plant will grow about 4 ft (1 m) tall.

JASMINUM OFFICINALE

JASMINE
White jasmine

Oleaceae

82 S. Europe, C. Asia

JUGLANS REGIA

WALNUT
Jove's nut

Juglandaceae

83 S.E. Europe, S.W. Asia
Temperate Zones

KRAMERIA TRIANDRA

RHATANY
Mapato

Krameri

84 S. America

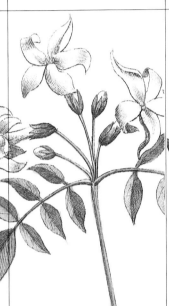

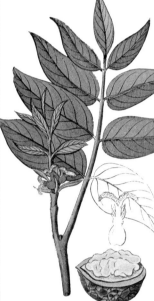

Only one genus comprises this plant order of which there are 25 species of shrubs or perennial herbs named in honour of the Hungarian botanist, Joseph Kramer. All are native of Brazil, Chile and Peru, *K. triandra* being used by the Peruvian Indians as a reliable cure for dysentery and diarrhoea, also as a dentifrice and for strengthening the gums. *R. triandra* is a low growing shrub present on dry mountainous slopes exposed to the direct rays of the sun and at 4-8000 ft (1-2000 m) above sea level. The leaves are pubescent, the large flowers being crimson, borne in axillary racemes and followed by a globose one-seeded fruit covered in spines. It is the roots that have commercial value. When dug up, they are long and cylindrical (known as "longs") or short and stumpy (known as "shorts") and are reddish-brown with thin bark. They are rich in tannic acid and when chewed (to strengthen the gums) colour the saliva red. To make a dentifrice, the hard woody roots are dried in a low oven taking several days to do so. They are then powdered, the powder being reddish-brown and is mixed with gum myrrh and powdered chalk or powdered orris. It removes tartar from teeth and tightens the gums. The root is included in the British Pharmacopaeia and is obtained from drug stores.

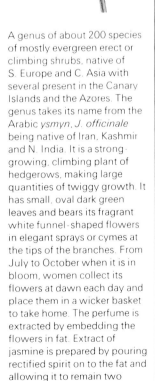

A genus of about 200 species of mostly evergreen erect or climbing shrubs, native of S. Europe and C. Asia with several present in the Canary Islands and the Azores. The genus takes its name from the Arabic *ysmyn*, *J. officinale* being native of Iran, Kashmir and N. India. It is a strong-growing, climbing plant of hedgerows, making large quantities of twiggy growth. It has small, oval dark green leaves and bears its fragrant white funnel-shaped flowers in elegant sprays or cymes at the tips of the branches. From July to October when it is in bloom, women collect its flowers at dawn each day and place them in a wicker basket to take home. The perfume is extracted by embedding the flowers in fat. Extract of jasmine is prepared by pouring rectified spirit on to the fat and allowing it to remain two weeks in the heat of the sun.

One of the most handsome of deciduous trees, its name means Jove's nut or nut of the gods. Some forest trees are 400–500 years old, their large trunks being covered with silver-grey bark, their grey-green pinnate leaves held on long footstalks, being tinted crimson and releasing a sweet resinous scent when handled. The male flowers are borne in drooping catkins; the females in erect terminal spikes. They open early in spring and may be injured by frost. The fruit or drupe is covered in a thick green husk, like a plum, which stains the fingers black when removed to reveal a wrinkled 2-valve shell which encloses a lobed nut (kernel) of purest white covered in a thin brown tunic. The nut, used in confectionery and for dessert, has a delicious milky taste. The husks and nuts yield a dark hair dye.

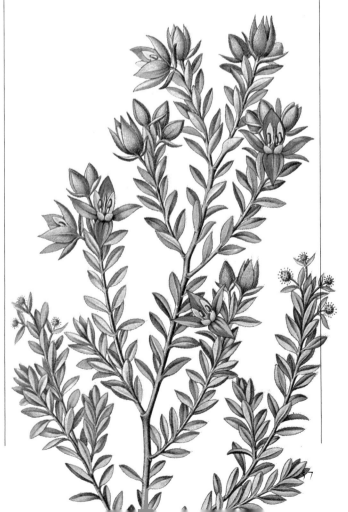

LACTUCA VIROSA

WILD LETTUCE
Acrid lettuce

Compositae

85 N. + C. Europe, Asia
Temperate Zones

LAMIUM GALEOBDOLON
Galeobdolon luteum

YELLOW ARCHANGEL
Yellow Deadnettle

Labiatae

86 Europe, W. Asia

LAURUS NOBILIS

BAY
Sweet bay

Lauraceae

87 S. Europe, N.W. Africa,
S.W. Asia

LAVANDULA SPICA

LAVENDER
Spike

Labiatae

88 S. Europe, N.W. Africa

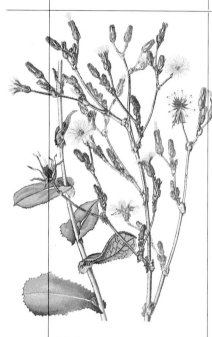

It is found on dry banks and waste ground, often in shade. It takes its name from the Latin *lactus* (milk), for the stems and leaves contain a thick milky juice which is released when the stems are cut. The juice has a bitter taste and narcotic odour, resembling opium and when dry it hardens and turns reddish brown. Collectors cut the plant near the top and collect the juice in bowls. The juice, diluted and applied to the skin, removes blemishes and soreness caused by sunburn or wind, leaving the face soft and smooth. The plant has a thick carrot-like root and a strong erect stem which is smooth and pale green, with prickles on the lower part. The basal leaves are large, often up to 16 in (40 cm) long; the clasping stem leaves being small. The flowers are yellow and are followed by black oval fruits.

It is a plant of woodlands and hedgerows and is distributed throughout S. England, Europe and W. Asia, being closely allied to White deadnettle and so named because, though somewhat similar to the stinging nettle in appearance (though of a different family), the hairs have no sting. Yellow archangel is a slender hairy plant with stalked ovate leaves and coarsely serrate edges, "as if cut or hacked about", wrote Gerard and he added that the distilled water "makes a good colour in the face", meaning that it improves the complexion. The leaves macerated in lard or in olive oil and applied to the face will clear it of blemishes. The flowers are bright yellow with red spots on the lower lip of the 2-lipped corolla and guide the bees searching for the honey contained at the base of the long hairy tube. The flowers are borne during May and June, in axillary whorls. The crushed leaves bound to open sores will cause rapid healing.

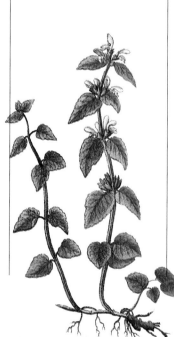

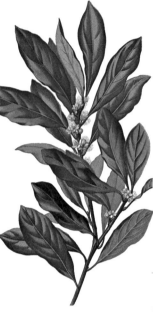

Native of S. Europe and the Levant, where it reaches a height of 50 ft (15 m) but less than half where growing in cooler parts, it never loses its dense, shrubby character. The stems and branches are covered with smooth olive green bark whilst the lance-shaped leaves, about 3 in (7·5 cm) long are dark green and glossy with waved margins. They are covered with small immersed glands which, when pressed or shaken by the wind, release a sweet resinous scent. Its delicious fragrance and the fact that it was available throughout the year, made the sweet bay the most popular plant for garlanding Roman heroes, their poets and generals, hence its name *L. nobilis*. The yellow flowers are produced in small clusters early in summer and are followed by small black oval berries. From these and from the leaves, the greenish oil of bay is obtained by distillation. The oil is used in the preparation of bath oils, toilet soaps and as a skin unguent.

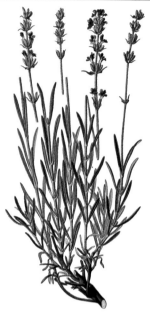

A shrubby plant growing as wide as it grows tall, with narrow lance-shaped leaves, downy on both sides, which gives the plant a silvery-grey appearance. The purple-blue flowers are borne in mid-summer, in whorls of 6–10 on an erect stem or spike about 10 in (25 cm) long. The flowers, when dry, retain their refreshing sweet perfume for many months and since mediaeval times have had many uses. It is a native of S. Europe and Mediterranean islands where it grows in gravelly soil usually of a chalky nature. The commercial distillation of lavender began in the early 17th century. The entire scent of the flowers, the essential oil, being concentrated in the tiny green bracts which enclose the flowers; it is also present in the stems but in smaller amounts and of inferior quality. Lavender water is a refreshing handkerchief perfume and a little in a bowl of warm water is a valuable skin astringent.

LAWSONIA INERMIS

HENNA
Al-herna

Lythraceae

89   N. Africa, Near East

LIGUSTRUM VULGARE

PRIVET
Common privet

Oleaceae

90   Europe, Asia

LILIUM CANDIDUM

MADONNA LILY
Our Lady's lily

Liliaceae

91   S. Europe

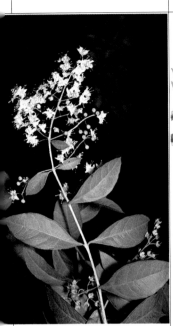

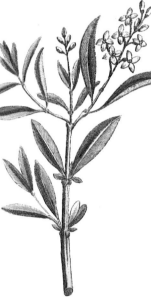

One of the oldest plants known to man still in cultivation, the bulbs have been used for food since earliest times. Because of its whiteness, the early Christian church dedicated it to Our Lady as a symbol of purity. Long before that time, the flower was employed by the ancient Egyptians who were experts in the art of obtaining perfumes by floral extraction, as depicted on the walls of the temple at Edfu on the Nile. The fragrance can be captured in lard or in almond or olive oil by the simple method of enfleurage which retains the full fragrance of the flower. The distilled water of the flowers is a useful astringent, closing the pores and tightening the skin to remove wrinkles. An ointment made from the juice of the bulbs and lard will remove inflammation from blemishes and heal the skin. In its native Palestine, the plant grows about rocky ground and is a lime lover. It also enjoys shade at its roots. The flowers appear in June at the end of erect stems of pencil thickness and clothed with dark green lance-shaped leaves. Each stem carries as many as 12–20 flowers of trumpet shape and of purest white. It is the sweetest scented of all lilies.

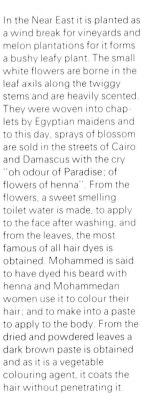

In the Near East it is planted as a wind break for vineyards and melon plantations for it forms a bushy leafy plant. The small white flowers are borne in the leaf axils along the twiggy stems and are heavily scented. They were woven into chaplets by Egyptian maidens and to this day, sprays of blossom are sold in the streets of Cairo and Damascus with the cry "oh odour of Paradise; of flowers of henna". From the flowers, a sweet smelling toilet water is made, to apply to the face after washing, and from the leaves, the most famous of all hair dyes is obtained. Mohammed is said to have dyed his beard with henna and Mohammedan women use it to colour their hair; and to make into a paste to apply to the body. From the dried and powdered leaves a dark brown paste is obtained and as it is a vegetable colouring agent, it coats the hair without penetrating it.

One of 50 species closely related to the olive. *L. vulgare* is found in deciduous woodlands and hedgerows, often in semi-shade and growing in a limestone soil. It makes a straggling bush with small glossy, dark green lance-shaped leaves and its small white tubular flowers are borne in panicles in June and July. Honey is secreted at the base of the tube and is protected from short-tongued insects attracted to the smell by two stamens which fill the mouth of the tube. The flowers are visited by honey bees whose long tongues can reach the honey but whose honey takes on a fishy taste after visiting privet, due to the presence of trimethylamine. Yet this is entirely absent from toilet waters made from the flowers. Where the skin has become chapped by cold winds or exposure to the sun, an infusion of the flowers in olive oil will quickly take away the inflammation.

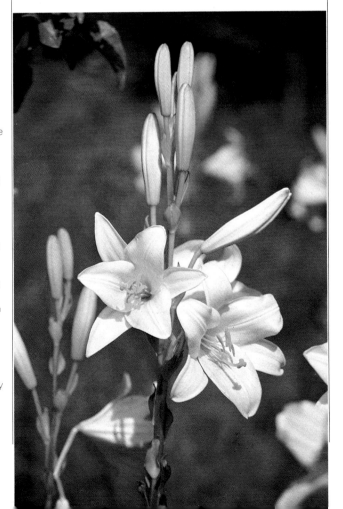

LINARIA VULGARIS	LIQUIDAMBER ORIENTALIS	LONICERA CAPRIFOLIUM
TOADFLAX Gallwort	**SWEET GUM** Storax	**HONEYSUCKLE** Woodbine
Scrophulariaceae **92** Europe	Hamamelidaceae **93** N.E. America, Near East, W. Asia	Caprifoliaceae **94** Europe, Asia, N. + S. America

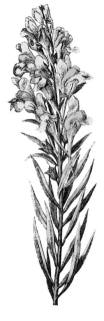

A genus of more than 150 species of annual or perennial plants taking their name from the Latin *linum* (flax) on account of the similarity of the plants before flowering.
L. vulgaris is a plant of hedgerows and the sides of fields, also of waste ground, and is known as yellow toadflax. From the bud formed at the top of the root arises the flower stem, at the end of which is borne a spike of snapdragon-like flowers with an orange lower lip and which are much visited by bees in search of honey secreted at the base of the ovary and which collects in the spur. The glabrous linear leaves are borne alternately all the way up the stem and are slightly glaucous. The leaves have a bitter taste, hence its country name, gallwort. The plant blooms June-October and it is the tops, when the flowers are newly open, that are most effective.

A genus of six species of balsam-bearing deciduous trees with five-lobed maple-like leaves which take on brilliant colourings in autumn. *L. orientalis* is a slow growing shrub and is native of the Levant. The resin it exudes is now the one most often used in perfumery. Liquid storax gives greater permanence to the odour of flowers extracted by maceration; it is also used in the imitation of other scents or to complement them. *L. styraciflora*, the Sweet gum or Gum storax of N. America, also supplies its balsamic resin to perfumery. The tree may reach a height of 40 ft (12 m). The palmately lobed leaves emit a balsamic fragrance before they fall which is retained until they wither. It bears small greenish flowers in small inflorescences in spring. It is the satinwood of cabinet makers. The tree was first mentioned by the Spanish botanist, Hernandez, who in 1650 described the resin as "like liquid amber". The resin, with rose water and witch hazel, of the same order, is a vauluable astringent, tightening the skin and preventing wrinkles.

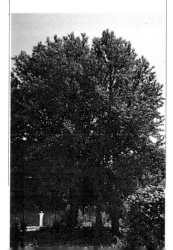

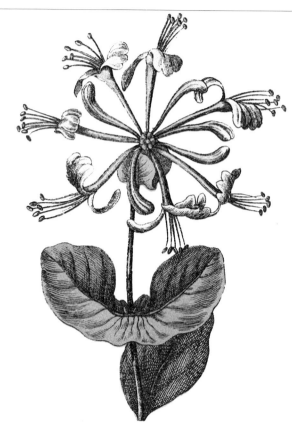

A genus of more than 200 species of shrubs or climbing plants, evergreen or deciduous and distributed in most parts of the world, including Europe and Asia – Malaysia and the Philippine Islands – also N. and S. America. Some species bear highly scented flowers, especially at night, like *L. caprifolium* which attracts hawk moths, the long tubular flowers being accessible only to the longest tongued insects. The genus was named by Linnaeus in honour of Adam Lonicer, the German naturalist, born at Marburg in 1528. The English and Italian honeysuckles are erect growing plants of open woodlands and hedgerows with twining stems, which pull the plants up to the sunlight for, as Shakespeare observed, it is only when "ripen'd by the sun" that the flowers emit their rich aromatic clove-like perfume at eventide. The plants have ovate leaves and bloom June–September, the flowers borne in terminal heads. They are creamy-yellow, shaded red on the outside and are followed by globular crimson berries. *L. caprifolium* is distinguished from *L. periclymenum* in having the uppermost leaves united at the base, whilst the flowers are of paler colouring. From the flowers of both species, collected at eventide, a lotion is made which cleanses the skin of impurities and leaves it soft and clear.

LYCOPERSICUM ESCULENTUM

TOMATO
Love apple

Solanaceae

95 C. + S. America
Temperate Zones

LYSIMACHIA VULGARIS

YELLOW LOOSESTRIFE
Willow-wort

Primulaceae

96 S. Europe

LYTHRUM SALICARIA

PURPLE LOOSESTRIFE
Spiked loosestrife

Lythraceae

97 Europe, Asia
N. America

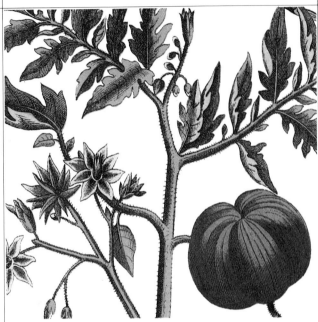

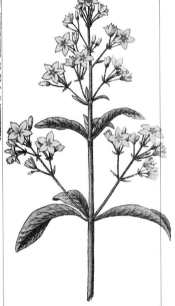

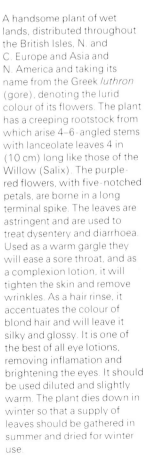

Native of Pacific S. America, it was introduced into Europe early in the 17th century by Spanish conquerors returning from Peru and was first grown by the Moors, hence its original name of Pomi dei Mori. The name was corrupted by the French to Pomme d'amour, or in English, love apples. The ripe fruits are rich in vitamins A, B and C and mineral salts, necessary for the proper functioning of the body. The B vitamins are needed for the correct functioning of the thyroid gland which secretes hormones to give the body vitality and prevents premature ageing, which no external beauty preparations can correct. The fruit has more culinary uses than any other food, for which purpose it is cultivated in large quantities throughout the world (in greenhouses in a cold climate). The pulp can be used as a refreshing and cleansing face pack, to remove pimples and blackheads and to reduce large pores. Rest the head on a towel before applying to the face. Leave on for 20 minutes, then remove with a cloth and wash the face in warm water. This natural and relatively inexpensive facial treatment will leave the skin smooth and clear of blemishes. In nature, the plant grows in sandy soil and fruits in summer. It forms a branching stem with large pinnate leaves, divided into 2–4 pairs of opposite leaflets. From the leaf axils, white flowers are produced in panicles of 20 or more throughout the summer months and are replaced by round juicy fruits 3–4 in (8–10 cm) in circumference. The fruits are green, turning red (or yellow) when ripe, a firm glossy skin enclosing pink flesh in which are embedded edible flat yellow seeds. The leaves and stems of the tomato plant are poisonous, which may partially account for the belief – which persisted until quite recent times – that the fruit itself was toxic.

Though in no way connected to Purple loosestrife, it has a similar distribution and also grows in damp ground, by the side of streams and ponds, increasing by its stolon-bearing rootstock. The ovate lance-shaped leaves are borne in whorls of 3 or 4, the underside being hairy, the uppersurface covered in black dots or glands. The stems are 3- or 4-angled, depending on the number of leaves in the whorls. The yellow flowers appear in July and August and are borne in panicled cymes from the axils of the upper leaves. Each small flower forms a cup and is pollinated only by a bee, *Macropsis labiata*, which visits no other plant. Pliny said the plant was named in honour of King Lysimachus of Sicily who discovered its many properties, it being a valuable vulnerary, stemming the flow of blood from wounds. The distilled water of the flowers and leaves will remove spots from the skin and tighten it, removing wrinkles.

A handsome plant of wet lands, distributed throughout the British Isles, N. and C. Europe and Asia and N. America and taking its name from the Greek *luthron* (gore), denoting the lurid colour of its flowers. The plant has a creeping rootstock from which arise 4–6-angled stems with lanceolate leaves 4 in (10 cm) long like those of the Willow (Salix). The purple-red flowers, with five-notched petals, are borne in a long terminal spike. The leaves are astringent and are used to treat dysentery and diarrhoea. Used as a warm gargle they will ease a sore throat, and as a complexion lotion, it will tighten the skin and remove wrinkles. As a hair rinse, it accentuates the colour of blond hair and will leave it silky and glossy. It is one of the best of all eye lotions, removing inflamation and brightening the eyes. It should be used diluted and slightly warm. The plant dies down in winter so that a supply of leaves should be gathered in summer and dried for winter use.

MALUS SYLVESTRIS

APPLE
Crab Apple

Rosaceae

98 *N. Temperate Zones*

MELALEUCA LEUCADENDRON

CAJUPUT
White Tea tree

Myrtaceae

99 Tropical Australia, S.E. Asia

MELILOTUS OFFICINALIS

MELILOT
Sweet clover

Leguminosae

100 Europe, Asia *Temperate Zones*

MELISSA OFFICINALIS

BALM
Common Balm

Labiatae

101 S.E. Europe, S.W. Asia *Temperate Zones*

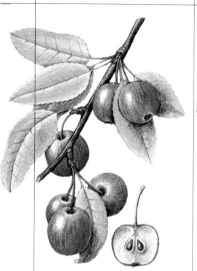

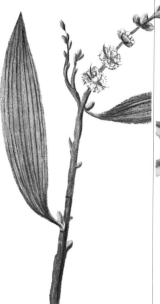

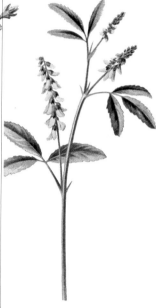

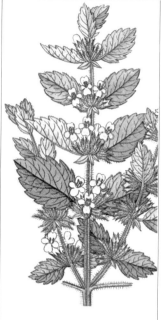

M. sylvestris is a smooth barked deciduous tree the most common of the 35 species distributed throughout northern temperate zones and believed to be a parent of *M. domestica*, the cultivated apple, most widely grown of all fruits. *M. sylvestris* is present in open woodlands and hedgerows and is a slow growing much branched tree with ovate short-stalked leaves and bears pinkish white flowers in large clusters. The flowers are followed by small yellow fruits (apples) which take on reddish tints as they ripen. Crab or cider apple juice with malt vinegar, makes a capital hair rinse and eating an apple a day will keep the teeth free from tartar and the enamel white and glistening. Apples contain large amounts of phosphorus which fortifies the nervous system and is vital for strong and healthy teeth, a most important asset in the quest for beauty.

A genus of about 100 species, native of tropical Australia and the islands of S.E. Asia, they are, for the most part, trees with a long trunk and ascending branches covered with thick flaking grey bark. The alternate lanceolate leaves are also greyish with short footstalks and with deep longitudinal veins. They are extremely aromatic, an essential oil being obtained from the leaves and twigs which has the scent of rosemary. Cajuput oil is greenish yellow. It is a stimulant and is used externally with 2 parts olive or almond oil to improve the complexion. Rubbed on sunburnt skin, the oil is especially efficacious in removing any soreness caused by over-exposure to the sun. Oil of rosemary is sometimes used as an adulterant. The small flowers are white and borne in long axillary spikes. *M. viridifolia*, which makes a small tree with bright green lanceolate leaves, yields a pale yellow oil known as Essence de Niaouli which is similar to Cajuput oil.

The melilots, of which there are several closely related species, were at one time widely grown as a fodder crop: now the clovers have taken their place but they persist throughout Europe and Asia, to be found around the sides of fields, by the roadside and on waste ground. Since earliest times they have been appreciated for their sweet perfume, all parts of the plant being scented. This is due to the presence of coumarin (as in newly mown hay) which increases in strength as the plant is dried. From the fresh and dried plant, a toilet water is made. The plant takes its name from the Greek *melissa* (honey) and *lotos* (a plant) for the small yellow flowers, borne in erect 1-sided racemes, are much visited by honey bees. *M. officinalis* is an erect, much branched slightly woody plant, its leaves divided into three pale green linear leaflets.

It is a hardy and leafy plant with branching woody stems and bright green wrinkled heart-shaped leaves which release a lemon-like fragrance when pressed. The plant takes its botanical name from the Greek *melissa* (honey), for the white flowers, borne in whorls in the leaf axils, are a principal source of nectar for bees in summer. The leaves are included in salads and a handful immersed in boiling water, provide a health-giving "tea". Balm oil is used in perfumery and to make toilet water. It was (with angelica) the principal ingredient of Carmelite water, used as a toilet water by cultured men and women of mediaeval Europe. It was rubbed over the body after bathing, whilst a handful of fresh leaves in a muslin bag immersed in the bath will impart a refreshing lemony scent to the water. Balm is a hedgerow plant, flourishing in semi-shade and growing well in any soil.

MENTHA PIPERITA
MENTHA SPICATA

PEPPERMINT
SPEARMINT

Labiatae

102 S. Europe
Temperate Zones

MICHELIA CHAMPACA

CHAMPAC
Michelia

Magnoliaceae

103 S.E. Asia, India, China

MORINGA OLEIFERA

BENJAMIN
Oil of Ben

Moringaceae

104 N.E. Africa, India

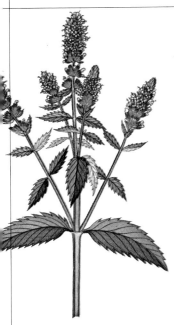

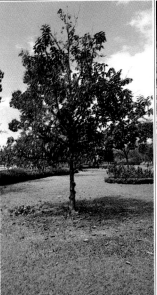

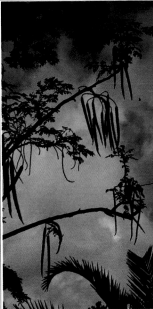

M. piperita is the most important of the mints. It is present in the British Isles in a few moist places, having been discovered in a field in 1700 and so named by John Rea because of its peppery smell. It may be a hybrid of *M. spicata* and *M. aquatica* and it occasionally appears in N. and C. Europe in damp places. It has stalked lanceolate leaves, serrated at the edges, and from the axils of the upper leaves bears reddish purple flowers in whorls. This mint may reach a height of 3–4 ft (1 m). There are two forms, "black" and "white", the former having purple stems and producing more oil by distillation though of an inferior quality. "White" peppermint has green stems and flowers borne in a blunt inflorescence. Turpentine is present in the plant but peppermint oil owes its value to the compound menthol which has a camphor-like smell. The oil improves with age and retains its strength for 10–12 years. It provides "coldness" to toilet preparations and is mixed with bay rum in after shave lotions. It also adds an invigorating fragrance to soaps and bath essences. The oil rubbed onto the teeth improves their whiteness, the reason for its inclusion in toothpastes. Owing to the numbing properties of menthol, chewing the leaves of peppermint provides a soothing relief to toothache. Spearmint, *M. spicata*, is present in dryer places and is found on banks and about hedgerows, its lanceolate leaves being brilliant green with a minty smell when pressed. The lilac flowers are borne in a spire-like inflorescence late in summer. The plant has more culinary uses than peppermint and has more limited use in toilet preparations. An infusion of the leaves taken hot is a warming beverage in cold weather and in a hot bath the leaves yield an invigorating fragrance whilst relaxing the muscles. The same may be said of Watermint, *M. aquatica*, which is found by streams and ponds and in ditches. It grows 3 ft (about 90 cm) tall with ovate leaves downy on both sides and with an orange fragrance which they release in a warm bath.

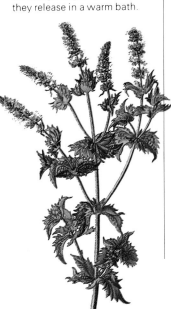

A genus of 50 species, differing from Magnolia in that the flowers are axillary, not terminal, being to the Old World what Magnolia is to the New World. Michelia is present in the warmer parts of Asia, especially India and China with *M. champaca* yielding a fragrant oil from which the most popular of Eastern perfumes is made, known as Champac. *M. champaca* is native of the lowlands of C. India where it grows on sandy wastelands. It makes a small evergreen shrub with dark green oval leaves, in the axils of which it bears lemon-yellow flowers. It is from these flowers, which are rather like small magnolia blossoms, that the powerful penetrating perfume is made. Hindu women decorate their hair with the ornamental blossoms, which leave behind their fragrance. The oil, used for dressing the hair, retains its sweet scent, long after the delicate flowers themselves have wilted.

A single genus of which there are 12 species, the seeds of which produce oil of Ben or Benjamin which is tasteless, colourless and odourless and does not turn rancid however long it is kept. It is therefore used in hair oil, suntan lotion and face cream which may be kept for some time. The ancient Egyptians were the first to appreciate its qualities for it was included in the celebrated solidified perfume Kyphi which was used on the body and burnt as incense. The moringas are tall trees with a thick trunk covered in a cork-like bark with deciduous alternate pinnate leaves covered with glandular dots. The honey-scented flowers are white and are borne in axillary panicles. They are followed by the fruits which are pod-like capsules often 16 in (40 cm) long and containing quite large seeds separated by spongy tissue. The seeds are used freshly gathered for the extraction of oil and yield up to 40% essential oil.

MUSA SAPIENTUM

BANANA
Plantain Fruit

Musae

105 W. + Tropical Africa, S. America, W. Indies

MYRICA CERIFERA

WAX MYRTLE
Candleberry

Myricaceae

106 N. America

MYRISTICA FRAGRANS

NUTMEG
Mace

Myristicaceae

107 S.E. Asia *Tropical + Warm Zones*

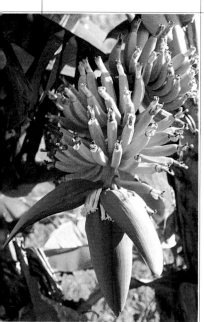

One of a genus of 60 or more species, native of the tropics of the old world. It is a plant of rain forests where it grows to a great height, though the dwarf or cavendish banana grows only 7–8 ft (2 m) tall. The plants have large spirally arranged leaves, the stems composed of overlapping leaf stalks. The flower bud which forms at the base of the plant, grows up inside the stem and droops down from the top, the females on the lower part of the inflorescence, the males on the upper part. Each cluster forms a hand or bunch of fingers each developing into a bunch of bananas arranged in circular rows. A single stalk may be composed of 300–400 berries (the bananas), each 6–10 in (15–25 cm) long and about 2 in (5 cm) in circumference filled with fibrous pulp. Unripe fruits have a green skin which turns bright yellow when ripe, the inner pulp being creamy-white. The pulp used in face masks will leave the skin soft and smooth and take away impurities.

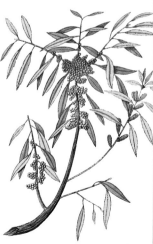

A genus of 30 species, these are plants of moist open places such as marshlands and bogs. *M. cerifera* makes a small tree 6–7 ft (2 m) tall, its numerous branches covered in grey bark. It has shining lance-shaped leaves covered in resinous dots and blooms in May, the greenish flowers being followed by small round black berries covered with white wax. All parts of the plant are fragrant, the leaves releasing a resinous smell when handled. The bark too, is fragrant and when dried and pounded is mixed with other powders to put in sachet bags to place amongst clothes. The wax persists on the berries for several years. It is removed and made into wax cakes to solidify and is known as myrtle wax. When softened, it makes an efficient lather shaving cream for it contains an acid resembling saponin and has a balsamic scent. It is also used to solidify beauty preparations and is made into candles.

It has a smooth grey bark containing a yellow juice which turns red when in contact with the air. It forms a conical crown and has elliptical alternate leaves about 4 in (10 cm) long and terminating in a point. They are dark green, aromatic and glossy above. The small yellow flowers are covered in pubescence and are like Lily of the valley. The fruit is a smooth coated globose drupe, the inner part, the hard endocarp, being the nutmeg, the fleshy outer covering, the arillus, providing the spice known as mace. The arillus is at first vivid red but when dry turns yellowish brown. The seed, the nutmeg, is hard and white with brown veins. When the mace is removed, it is dried separately, and the nutmegs dried over a charcoal fire, taking six weeks. When dry, they have a delicious fragrance and when grated, are used to flavour junkets and custards. From the nuts, a volatile oil is obtained by distillation. It contains the active principle myristicin which accounts for the distinctive fragrance. It is blended with sandalwood and lavender to make toilet soaps and the powder of the ground nuts is mixed with orris and other ingredients and put in sachets to place amongst clothes and bedding. "Nutmeg butter" is obtained by crushing the nuts and treating with steam. It is orange-yellow, soft but solid and is used in skin ointments and in perfumery.

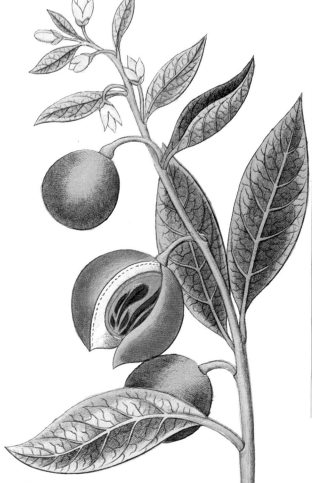

MYROXYLON PERUIFERUM

BALSAM OF PERU
Peruvian balsam

Leguminosae

108 S. America

NARCISSUS ODORUS

JONQUIL
Narcissus

Amaryllidaceae

109 S. Europe

NASTURTIUM AQUATICUM

WATERCRESS
Bittercress

Cruciferae

110 *Temperate Zones*

NEPETA CATARA

CATMINT
Catnip

Labiatae

111 Asia, Europe

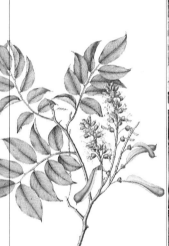

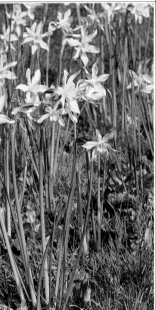

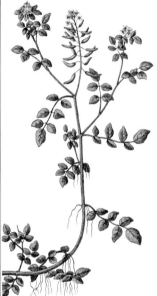

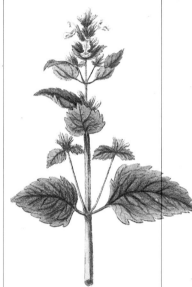

A genus of only two species, having no connection with Peru and present only in dense coastal forests of El Salvador, the strip of land being known as the Balsam coast. Balsam of Tolu, *M. pereirea*, is found with it. Both bear resins which have the odour of vanilla with undertones of cinnamon. All the exports from S. America, e.g. vanilla, heliotrope, and the balsams, have a similarity of odour, blending perfectly to make "bouquets" and sachet powders. The balsams give permanence to alcoholic perfumes and are included in hair tonics. They also give a creamy lather and pleasant perfume to toilet soaps. Like all the balsamic resins, they have medicinal value. *M. peruiferum* is a handsome tree of pyramidal form and every part is fragrant, even the calyces of the small white flowers which yield the finest balsam. The long narrow leaves are covered in oil glands and release a balsamic scent when pressed.

One of a genus of 60 species, *N. odorus* being one of the Jonquil group of rushleaf daffodils, distinguished from others by their deep green cylindrical and hollow leaves. Their heavily scented flowers which have undertones of orange, are used in perfumery. The plant is rare in the wild and may be a natural hybrid of *N. jonquilla* which is abundant in alpine meadows in Spain and Portugal and along the N.W. African coast. Its fragrance, like that of *N. odorus*, is so powerful that in a confined space it may cause headaches and nausea. Both plants bear their golden-yellow cup-shaped flowers in clusters of 4–6 on 8 in (20 cm) stems and there are double varieties of both species. The name of the genus may be derived from that of the classical youth who met his death vainly trying to embrace his image reflected in water; or from the Greek *narkao* (to be numb), from the narcotic properties of the plant.

An aquatic plant with hollow stems, to be found in fresh running water, streams and ponds, increasing by creeping underground stems, grows just above the water level. It is evergreen and greenish brown with pinnatifid leaves and heart-shaped leaflets. It bears panicles of small white flowers in July and August followed by cylindrical seed pods. The plant is so rich in iron and other mineral salts that if exposed to the sun for only a short time, the plant turns purple-brown. For its health-giving properties, being rich in vitamin C, it has been appreciated since earliest times. An infusion of the plant taken when cold will purify the blood and clear the skin of blemishes. As Culpeper said, when applied to the face at night, it will act in the same way and remove any roughness from the skin, leaving it smooth and white. The juice of the plant is included in the modern foam bath gels manufactured by Roger & Gallet of Paris.

It is distributed throughout the British Isles and temperate Europe and Asia, being less common in northern altitudes. It is a leafy plant with grey-green heart-shaped leaves covered in down, white on the underside, so that the whole plant has a hoary appearance. The pinky-red flowers are borne in whorls at the ends of the branched stems and bloom from June until September. The whole plant has an aromatic minty smell which attracts cats who in summer will lie upon the plants for hours, hence its common name. The plant dies down in winter. It is effective in removing dandruff from the scalp, the decoction being rubbed well into the head, whilst a catmint rinse will impart a healthy gloss to the hair. It is a plant of dry banks and the sides of woods and fields, growing well in gravelly soil of a chalky nature. The flowering 'tops' infused in boiling water is carminative if a wineglassful is taken at bedtime and is sleep inducing. It will also relieve headaches.

NEPETA GLECHOMA

GROUND IVY
Gill-by-the-ground

Labiatae

112   N. + C. Europe

NIGELLA SATIVA

NUTMEG PLANT
Roman coriander

Ranunculaceae

113   Mediterranean
     Warm Temperate Zones

OLEA EUROPAEA

OLIVE
Oliver

Oleaceae

114   S. Europe, N. Africa,
     S.W. Asia
     S. Africa, W.-N. America,
     Australia

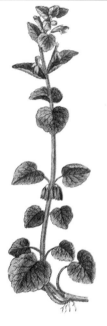

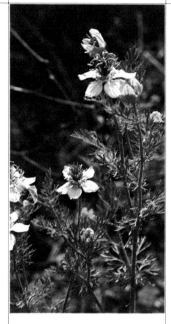

Native of the Near East, the plant has been grown in Mediterranean countries since early in history for the oil obtained from the fruit is the purest of all vegetable fats being widely used in cooking, especially for salad dressings, also medicinally and for maintaining the body in top condition by massaging it into the skin. It guards against dry skin. The oil mixed with alcohol is a valuable tonic for hair when massaged into the scalp and it is included in many facial creams. Unripe olives for use as hors d'oeuvres are steeped in a solution of lime water and wood ashes for several days to reduce their bitterness before being bottled in salt solution. The green virgin oil is obtained by crushing the ripe fruits in hessian bags in tubs of water and collecting the oil from the surface by skimming. The oil, which is almost tasteless, is non-drying and, because of its purity, was the symbol of all that is good in the Bible, the tree representing peace and goodwill. For the same reason, victors at the Olympic games were crowned with its branches. *O. europaea* makes a small twisted tree with pale green bark and thorny twigs. The lanceolate leaves are about 2 in (5 cm) long, dark green above, grey on the underside. The fruit is a small purple drupe with a thick bony stone surrounded by the flesh which has a high oil content.

It is a soft, hairy plant with creeping stems and rooting at the nodes. The heart-shaped bluntly toothed leaves are sage-green in colour and marked with purple and white. They are aromatic, with a resinous smell and before the introduction of hops were used to clarify and flavour ale to which they imparted a pleasantly bitter taste. The purple-blue flowers are borne in 3s or 4s at the leaf axils during the early weeks of summer, the lower lip being spotted deeper purple. The plant takes its botanical name from Nepet in Tuscany where it abounds. It is usually found in woodlands and hedgerows, growing in semi-shade and, as it is evergreen, can be used all year fresh or dried. It is anti-scorbutic and an infusion of the whole herb makes a wholesome tonic drink known as gill tea, which clears the blood of impurities, keeping the skin free from pimples. It is also used by the French herbalist, Maurice Mességué, in a warm foot bath to relieve asthma.

Its seeds were eaten by women of ancient Egypt to plump and firm the breasts. The Romans believed they increased the flow of milk when feeding. It has an erect branching stem and deeply cut grey-green leaves of fern-like appearance. The flowers are deep blue, about 1 in (1·5 cm) across, the whole plant resembling *N. damascena*, also native of the Near East and known in English gardens as Love-in-a-mist because of the misty blue-green appearance from a distance. The flowers are followed by toothed seed pods filled with small black seeds which, when dry, emit a spicy aroma, like nutmeg (absent in *N. damascena*) for which they are used as a substitute in cooking. They have a pungent taste. A decoction of the seeds rubbed on the breasts will bring about firmness and the finely ground seeds rubbed into the hair will rid it of ticks and lice.

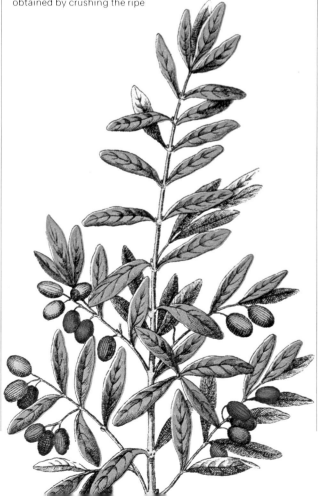

ORIGANUM MARJORANA

MARJORAM
Sweet marjoram

Labiatae

115 S. Europe, W. Asia, N. Africa
Warm Temperate Zones

PANDANUS ODORATISSIMUS

PANDANG
Screw-pine

Pandanaceae

116 *Warm Temperate Zones*

PARIETARIA OFFICINALIS

PELLITORY-OF-THE-WALL
Sneezewort

Urticaceae

117 S. Europe

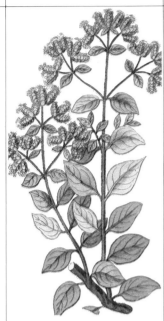

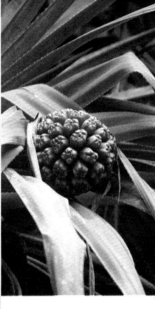

It is distributed throughout the British Isles and most of Europe, usually growing on old walls and stoney ground in full sun. A many branched plant with elliptic hairy long stalked leaves, its reddish stems and small green stalkless flowers are borne in the leaf axils. If touched, the filaments spring upwards, releasing pollen which "causes one to sneeze exceedingly", noted one old writer. Snuffs were made from the dried and powdered leaves, with those of ground-ivy and chamomile, which would cause sneezing and clear the head when in a close atmosphere. The plant takes its name from the Latin *paries* (a wall) and is a valuable diuretic. A decoction of the leaves mixed with oil of rosemary and massaged into the scalp is said to promote the growth of hair and relieve inflammation caused by shingles. It will also remove soreness from the face and hands if gently rubbed in at night. The distilled water sweetened with a little honey will clear the blood of impurities and the skin of blemishes.

O. marjorana, a plant of woody habit, has small ovate leaves and bears tiny rosy red flowers with purple bracts, in terminal cymes throughout summer. They are much visited by bees. It is known as sweet marjoram, for in warm parts it secretes a sweetly resinous oil from its stems. It is therefore much used to make toilet waters, perhaps mixed with rose water, to bathe the face after washing, whilst a handful in a muslin bag placed in a warm bath will perfume the water and relax muscles. The oil obtained from the distillation of the fresh shoots, forms a deliciously scented embrocation to rub into the body after bathing, whilst if massaged into the scalp, it gives dry hair a gloss and prevents it falling. An infusion, used with sage or rosemary and rubbed into the scalp has the same effect. *O. vulgare* may be used in a similar way to sweet majoram but its scent is not nearly so pronounced.

A genus of about 600 species, native of the tropics and warm parts of the old world, being plants of the coast and marsh-lands, their stems being supported by aerial or flying-buttress-like roots which grow down from the stem to the ground. The pandanus is one of the most primitive of plants and known as the screw-pine, from the screw-like formation of the leaves as they develop from the main stem in spirals. The leaves are long and narrow, terminating in a sharp point. They are thorny at the margins and appear in tufts at the end of the branches. The flowers are arranged in large inflorescences enclosed in spaths, the male flowers appearing above the females and arranged in a dense cylindrical spike. They open first, their pollen carried by the wind onto the females below. The male flowers of *P. odoratissimus* are the most heavily scented and produce a perfume much used by Hindu women for toilet purposes.

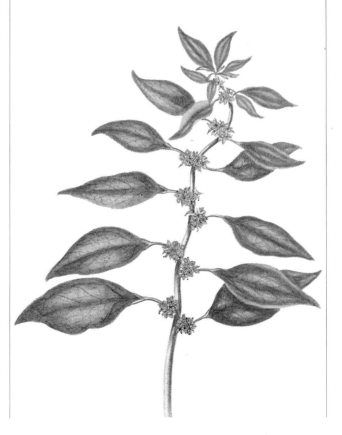

PELARGONIUM CAPITATUM

SCENTED-LEAF GERANIUM

Geraniaceae

118 S. Africa
Warm Temperate Zones

PERSEA AMERICANA

AVOCADO
Avocado pear

Lauraceae

119 Tropical America, Asia
Tropical Zones

PIMENTA ACRIS

BAY RUM
American myrtle

Myrtaceae

120 Tropical Africa, W. Indies

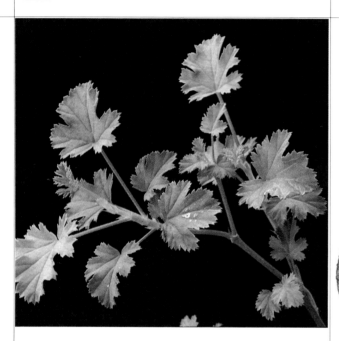

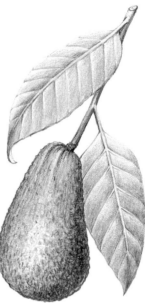

A genus of smooth or downy herbs or sub-shrubs of more than 170 species, with opposite toothed or lobed leaves. Many species carry the fragrance of roses, orange, lemon or nutmeg, amongst many other scents, when the leaves are pressed. Most species are native of S. Africa, especially Cape Province, where they grow amongst rocky outcrops in the full glare of the sunlight and protected from too rapid transpiration of moisture by the dense hairs which cover the leaves of most species. The flowers, are borne in large heads and in many species are brilliantly coloured, those with scented leaves flourishing in semi-shade and requiring little attention through the years. *P. capitatum* is that most widely used in cosmetics and perfumery. It is an erect woody plant, the leaves and stems being covered in short glandular hairs. The pale green leaves are 3–5-lobed, deeply toothed and wrinkled. The pale pink flowers, veined with purple, are borne in dense heads all year. The rose perfume of the leaves is due to an alcohol, geraniol, the substance predominating in rose flowers, combined with other substances. Geraniol is purest in the rose-scented geranium. The plant grows along the N. African coast and from it is made the "otto of roses" sold in Algerian bazaars and exported to all parts to use in the manufacture of soaps and to adulterate the true rose perfume. Its juice is included in face creams as an alternative to cucumber. Another rose-leaf geranium is *P. radula rosea*, a plant of compact habit, its narrow leaves having straight lobes. The small crinkled leaves of *P. citriodorum* smell strongly of lemon verbena, as do those of *P. crispum variegatum*, a plant of spire-like habit, its small crisped leaves being edged with gold. All can be used in pot-pourris and several leaves placed in a muslin bag will impart their perfume to a warm bath.

A genus of about 150 species originally grown in swamplands, hence its name of Alligator pear. But it is in no way connected with the wild pear, being of the Magnolia and Bay laurel family, though the fruit (a drupe) with a single seed or stone enclosed in aromatic flesh is almost pear-shaped. The fruits may weigh as much as 3 lb (1·4 kg) and are covered in a smooth, thin green skin. The stone is surrounded by soft butter-like flesh which is rich in vitamins A and E and contains up to 20% fat. The fruits have direct and indirect uses as an aid to beauty. Avocado oil is included in extra-emollient skin creams. The tree is similar to the bay in habit and has glossy laurel-like leaves 6 in (5 cm) long, terminating in a point and about 2 in (5 cm) wide at the broadest part. The small flowers are borne in a large terminal inflorescence.

One of a genus of 60 species, native of tropical America and the West Indies, only one of which, *Myrtus communis*, is present in Europe. A handsome tree of pyramid form, with slender branches and opposite short-stalked glossy leaves 3 in (7·5 cm) long with prominent veins. On the underside are the oil glands which release a sweet resinous scent in the wind. The oil is, at first, colourless but upon exposure to air soon takes on a yellow tint before turning dark brown, and assuming its agreeable fragrance. The flowers are small and arranged in threes. The fruit is a globular pea-sized berry, smooth and black when ripe, with the same aromatic smell as the leaves. The oil may be mixed with pimento, before adding alcohol and water in equal parts and Jamaica rum, in the preparation of the bay rum hair tonic which is used in shampoos and massaged into the scalp. Mixed with rosemary water it is even more effective. Bay rum is also used to make a refreshing toilet soap.

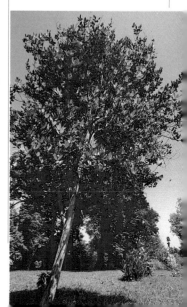

PIMENTA OFFICINALIS

ALLSPICE
Pimenta

Myrtaceae

121 S. America, West Indies
*Tropical Zones
of the New World*

PINUS SYLVESTRIS

PINE
Pine-apple tree

Pinaceae

122 Europe, N. + W. Asia
Temperate Zones

PISTACIA LENTISCUS

PISTACIA
Mastic

Anacardiaceae

123 S. Europe

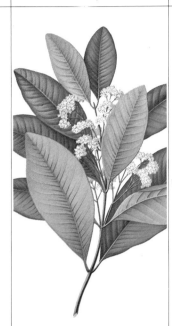

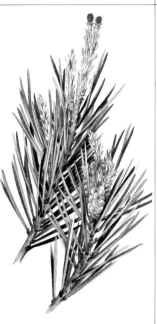

A slender evergreen tree with highly aromatic smooth pale grey bark and leaves. It makes a widely branched crown with opposite oval dark green leaves which are smooth and leathery and about 6 in (15 cm) long, like those of the laurel. They have a prominent mid-rib and are covered with pellucid dots (oil glands) which release a resinous perfume when pressed. The small greenish white flowers are borne in panicles at the ends of the branches and in summer release their perfume over a considerable distance. They are followed by shining succulent berries of pea-size with the remains of the calyx persisting. They are harvested when still green and unripe, for as they ripen they lose their aromatic property. They yield on distillation about 4% volatile oil composed mostly of Eugenol, similar to oil of cloves and used to impart a carnation fragrance to the less expensive toilet soaps and perfumes.

A large genus of coniferous trees with straight cylindrical trunks branching at the top. It takes its name from the pineapple-shaped cones which are placed in casks to flavour wine and ale and the fresh seeds used by "comfit makers and cooks". The blue-green leaves are sheathed in pairs and are slightly twisted. The male flowers ripen early in summer, the pollen reaching the reddish purple females in billowing clouds, but fertilisation does not take place for a further 12 months and the cones ripen the following year. The timber is used for furniture making and for building boats. From the resin, pitch is obtained and applied to boats to make them waterproof, and oil of turpentine, used in varnishes and oil paints. From the distillation of pine wood by steam pressure, pine oil, with a scent like that of juniper oil, is obtained and is used to impart its refreshing scent to bath essence. It is also used in the manufacture of brown soaps which have the distinctive pine fragrance.

A genus of five trees or shrubs, yielding a resinous gum from incisions made in the bark. *P. lentiscus* is the Mastic tree of the island of Chios from which is collected the gum known as mastic, used in medicine and to make the liqueur, mastiche, a celebrated drink since earliest times and which the Greeks make from grapes. The tree reaches a height of about 20 ft (6 m) with pinnate leaves, from the axils of which it bears, in spring, scented flowers of palest green resembling catkins. The gum is also chewed. *P. terebinthus*, the Turpentine tree of Cyprus and Asia Minor, is a small deciduous tree which grows on rocky ground in full sun with leaves resembling those of the ash. The leaves when young are enhanced with a red hue, like walnut leaves and in the same way they are resinous. From the reddish bark a resinous gum, collected by making incisions, appears as pale yellow drops. It is collected into cakes and used as a base in modern perfumery.

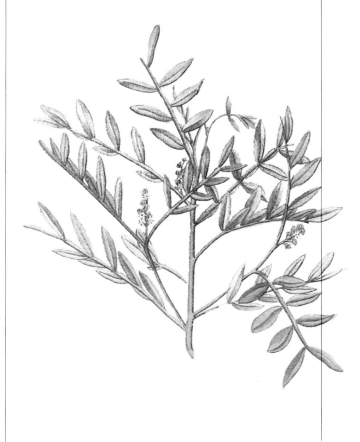

PLANTAGO MAJOR	PLUMERIA RUBRA	POGOSTEMON PATCHOULI

PLANTAGO MAJOR

COMMON PLANTAIN
Waybroad

Plantaginaceae
124 N. + C. Europe, N. America

PLUMERIA RUBRA

FRANGIPANI

Apocynaceae
125 S. America

POGOSTEMON PATCHOULI

PATCHOULI

Labiatae
126 S.E. Asia, India

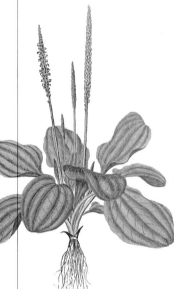

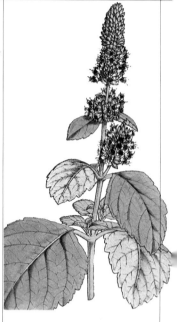

A small genus of ornamental trees native of Mexico, Peru, Equador, Martinique and islands of the West Indies, two species of which are associated with the famous frangipani perfume. The genus was named by Tournefort in honour of the Franciscan monk and French botanist, Father Charles Plumier (1664–1706), but the perfume owes its origin to a famous Roman family. The Marquis de Frangipani, Marshal of the army of Louis XIII of France during the regency of Mary of Medici, created the perfume bearing his name. It is obtained from *P. alba* and *P. rubra*, the former growing 16 ft (5 m) tall with brittle leaves 12 in (30 cm) long, curling inwards and growing in tufts at the end of the branches. The flowers are pure white and funnel-shaped, growing at the branch ends, in clusters. The plant was first brought to the attention of Europeans by Mercutio Frangipani, a botanist who accompanied Columbus in 1492. Found with it on the islands of Jamaica and Martinique is *P. rubra*, known also as Red jasmine. The tree rarely exceeds a height of 18–20 ft (6 m), the oblong leaves having downy peduncles. The crimson flowers, yellow at the centre, have oval petals and like the Red Rose, they retain their scent after drying and are used in scent bags and pot-pourris.

A genus of more than 200 species distributed over the north temperate regions of the world, usually found by the wayside and on waste land. The ovate leaves are conspicuously 5–10 ribbed and contract at the base into a long channelled footstalk arising from the rootstock, down which every drop of moisture can be directed to the roots. The tiny purplish green flowers, which have purple anthers, are borne in a rat's-tail-like spike 10 in (25 cm) long and are wind pollinated. The fresh leaves, when applied to a rash caused by nettle stings or where the skin has been burnt or scalded, will give instant relief. The action is even more rapid when the juice is squeezed from the footstalks and rubbed onto the skin. The juice of the leaves after they have been boiled in milk for 5 minutes, when applied to the face, will leave the skin smooth and free of any soreness caused by hot sun or wind.

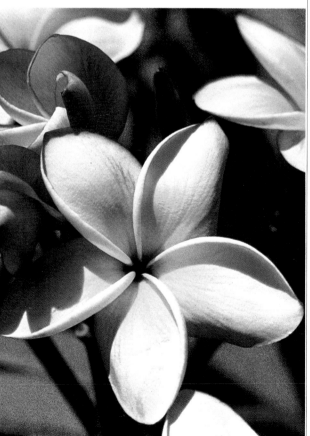

A genus of 40 species of herbs resembling lemon balm in appearance with quadrangular stems and crinkled lance-shaped nettle-like leaves, serrated at the edges and terminating in a point. The purple flowers are borne in the leaf axils. The plant grows on rocky hillsides and wasteland, in sandy soil and full sun which brings out its perfume to the full. In its original state its greenish yellow essential oil has an unpleasant goat-like smell but when mixed with otto of roses and dissolved in rectified spirit, it is more pleasing, though typically eastern in its heaviness. The perfume is the most popular of all with eastern women and has many uses. It first became popular in the West early in the 19th century when the Paisley weavers of Scotland made shawls to Indian designs which were exported to Europe and elsewhere, but, unless impregnated with the patchouli fragrance, like the shawls worn by Indian women, it was impossible to sell them anywhere.

POLEMONIUM COERULEUM

JACOB'S LADDER
Greek valerian

Polemoniaceae

127 N. Europe, Asia

POLIANTHES TUBEROSA

TUBEROSE

Amaryllidaceae

128 S. America

POLYGONATUM MULTIFLORUM

SOLOMON'S SEAL

Hiliacea

129 N. Europe, Asia
North Temperate Zones

POPULUS BALSAMIFERA

BALSAM POPLAR
Tacamahac

Salicaceae

130 N. Asia, N. Europe, N. America

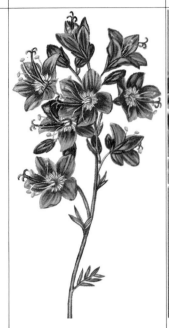

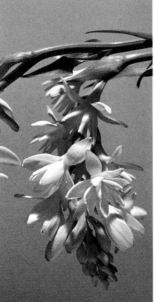

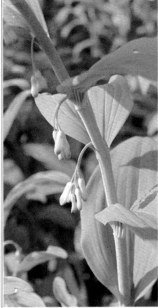

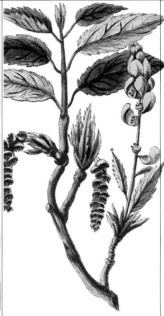

A genus of 50 species. It is a plant of upright rather than spreading habit with tufts of bright green pinnate leaves divided into 11–12 opposite segments each about 1 in (2·5 cm) long, which open like a ladder with small brilliant mid-blue flowers with conspicuous yellow stamens about 1 in (2·5 cm) across. They are borne in sprays at the top of 20 in (50 cm) stems, hence its country name, Ladder-to-heaven. It takes its botanical name, which it gives to the Order, from the Greek *polemos* (war), for Pliny said that the discovery of the plant there led to the Trojan War. It blooms from the end of May to the end of July. There is an ever rarer white flowered form, Album. After flowering, the plant can be cut down to almost ground level and if boiled in olive oil for an hour or so, will colour the oil black. It makes a valuable hair dressing for men with dry hair and will colour any greying hairs jet black, like walnut oil.

A genus of a single species (also a Mexican plant), bearing possibly the most powerful scent of all flowers, and widely used in perfumery. It grows in hedgerows and open woodlands and forms a dahlia-like tuber from which arise linear leaves of emerald green, spotted on the underside with purple, whilst the flower spike reaches to a height of more than 3 ft (1 m). At the end is borne a raceme of pure white funnel-shaped flowers, of wax-like texture, which open flat and star-like. The perfume is intoxicating and, indoors, is heavy and sickly almost to the point of unpleasantness, like white lilies. Perfume is extracted from the flowers during darkness, because its fragrance is more powerful at night. Though so powerful, essence of tuberose is extremely volatile and requires a fixative such as tincture of storax or vanilla essence to give it permanence.

A small genus native to the British Isles, North and Central Europe and Asia where it grows in open woodlands and hedgerows, increasing by rhizomatous roots which become knotted together. It is said that the juice from the freshly dug roots when applied to wounds, would seal or heal them quickly whilst the round marks on the roots resemble a seal and are like a six-pointed star. This gave rise to the belief that they represented the seal of King Solomon. The common Solomon's seal has round arching stems and alternate elliptical leaves which are dark green and ribbed. From the leaf axils, bell-shaped flowers of greenish white which hang down in twos and threes appear in early summer. They are similar to those of Lily of the valley and the plant enjoys similar conditions, semi-shade and a cool leafy soil. The scented Solomon's Seal, *P. odoratum*, bears fragrant flowers which impart a sweet scent to toilet water.

A genus of 35 species of deciduous trees, several yielding a fragrant resin from the unopened leaf buds, of which the most fragrant is the Balsam poplar of N. America. It makes a large spreading tree with brown, pubescent wood and has smooth heart-shaped leaves tapering to a point, with hairy footstalks. Before the leaf buds, which are protected by outer scales, begin to open, they are covered with extremely sticky balsamic resin. The substance is used in the manufacture of soaps and as a fixative for perfumes. The female flowers, which appear early in spring before the leaves unfold, are borne in pendulous catkins and have pink stigmas. Pollination is by wind. *P. niger*, the Black poplar, is native of N. Europe and has deeply furrowed black bark and widely spreading branches with twigs covered in grey down when young. The tree is found in damp open woodlands and by river banks, for it requires moisture at its roots.

POTENTILLA TORMENTILLA

TORMENTIL
Cinquefoil

Rosaceae

131 Europe, N.W. Asia, N. Asia, N.E.-N. America

PRIMULA VERIS

COWSLIP
Fairy cups

Primulaceae

132 C. Europe
Temperate Zones

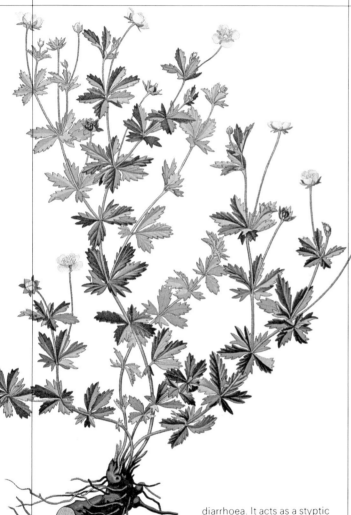

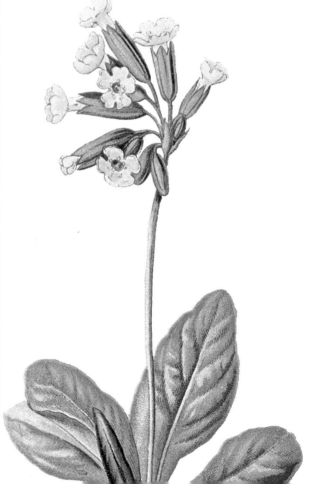

One of the loveliest of wild flowers, it is distributed throughout the British Isles and N. and C. Europe, growing in open meadows and on grassy banks, usually over limestone formations. With burnet and clover, its presence denoted good husbandry. It has deeply channelled obovate leaves, down which moisture can reach the roots before evaporation. The leaves are hairy on the underside. The drooping bell-shaped flowers appear in April and are borne in 6–8 umbels with short, downy peduncles. They are yellow, with an orange-red spot at the base of each petal and are sweetly scented like aniseed, due to anethol present in the stems and roots. The plant takes its name cowslip from the Anglo-Saxon *cusloppe* meaning a cow's breath, for to some its scent resembles the breath of a cow. From the flowers cowslip wine is made and a tea which, when taken at night, will ensure sound sleep. A cold infusion, applied to the face will cleanse and improve the complexion and an ointment made by macerating the flowers in lard or olive oil, in the words of a writer of the time of Elizabeth I of England, "taketh away spots and wrinkles of the skin, and doth add beauty exceedingly". The leaves eaten in a salad are a valuable spring tonic.

A genus of more than 500 species, taking their name from the Latin *potens* (powerful), from the valuable medicinal qualities of certain species. The Common tormentil, a small erect shrubby plant, is native of heaths and dry banks, and has a red woody rhizomatous root, containing a high percentage of tannin, a decoction of which will stem the flow of blood from internal wounds and is an astringent in cases of diarrhoea. It acts as a styptic for external skin sores and can heal skin blemishes. The rhizome-like roots are about 2 in (5 cm) long and of finger thickness, tapering at one end. They have a resinous smell. The plant resembles the strawberry, the leaves, held on long stalks, being divided into three or five oval toothed leaflets; the stem leaves being stalkless with three leaflets. The yellow flowers are borne in corymbose cymes, ¾ in (about 2 cm) across with four petals arranged like the cross of Jerusalem. As the season advances, the stems become weaker and trail along the ground.

PRIMULA VULGARIS

PRIMROSE

Primulaceae

133 N. + C. Europe

PRUNUS ARMENIACA

APRICOT
Apricock

Rosaceae

134 S. Europe, S. America
Warm Temperate Zones

PRUNUS PERSICA

PEACH
Persian apple

Rosaceae

135 S. Europe, S. America, Australia

Widely distributed throughout the British Isles and N. Europe in deciduous woodlands and hedgerows, usually growing in semi-shade, it has deeply wrinkled lanceolate leaves, downy on the underside. The flowers are borne on short peduncles and are pale yellow, about 1 in (2·5 cm) across. It blooms in spring, hence its name from the Latin *primus* (first). For its hardiness and earliness to bloom it has always been the best loved of all wild flowers, the poets of old referring to the fragile quality of its flowers which are sweet to the taste and included with the young leaves, in spring salads. They clear the blood of impurities and the skin of blemishes. The juice from the leaves in a little warm water and applied to the skin will remove spots and pimples from the face. Culpeper said that primrose ointment was "as fine a salve to heal wounds (and a sore skin) as any I know" and the English Poet Laureate, Alfred Austin, described how to make a skin salve from the flowers. Both the roots and flowers contain a fragrant oil and from the flowers in spring, an astringent toilet water is made to apply to the face at bedtime. Plants in the wild give rise to many different forms including those with double blooms and the Jack-in-the-Green, where the flowers are backed by a ruff of small green leaves.

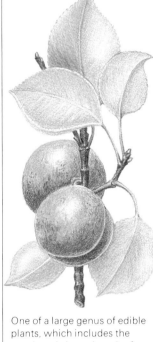

One of a large genus of edible plants, which includes the peach and almond, each of which has an important part to play in the world of beauty. It makes a small twiggy round-headed tree with oval leaves pointed at the apex and in early spring bears white flowers tinted with red. The plant takes its name apricot, from the Latin, praecox, early flowering. It is distributed about the temperate regions of the old world, from Armenia (the Balkans) from which it takes its botanical name, to C. China. The fruit is a drupe with a downy golden yellow skin, tinted red on the sunny side and measuring about 2 in (5 cm) across. Orange-yellow flesh surrounds the kernel or stone which is similar to the bitter almond and yields an essential oil used in confectionery. The fruit used fresh or dry and put through a blender, makes an effective and nourishing face mask, leaving the skin clear and soft.

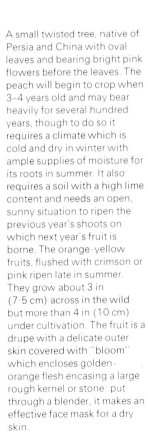

A small twisted tree, native of Persia and China with oval leaves and bearing bright pink flowers before the leaves. The peach will begin to crop when 3–4 years old and may bear heavily for several hundred years, though to do so it requires a climate which is cold and dry in winter with ample supplies of moisture for its roots in summer. It also requires a soil with a high lime content and needs an open, sunny situation to ripen the previous year's shoots on which next year's fruit is borne. The orange-yellow fruits, flushed with crimson or pink ripen late in summer. They grow about 3 in (7·5 cm) across in the wild but more than 4 in (10 cm) under cultivation. The fruit is a drupe with a delicate outer skin covered with "bloom" which encloses golden-orange flesh encasing a large rough kernel or stone: put through a blender, it makes an effective face mask for a dry skin.

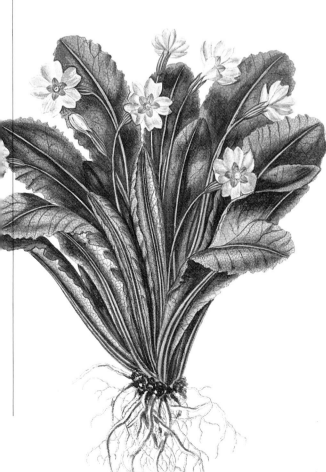

PRUNUS SPINOSA

BLACKTHORN
Sloe

Rosaceae

136 Europe, N. Africa, W. Asia
N. America

PYRUS CYDONIA

QUINCE

Rosaceae

137 C. Asia, S. Europe

QUERCUS ROBUR

OAK
Common oak

Fagaceae

138 N. + S. America, Asia,
N. Africa
Warm Temperate Zones

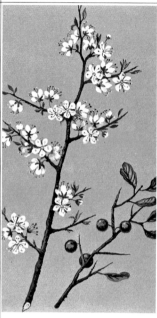

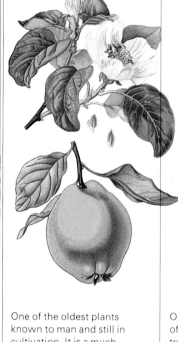

It is distributed throughout the British Isles and N. and C. Europe, occasionally as a small tree, more often as a dense twiggy shrub, found in open woodlands and hedgerows. It forms its flower buds during the previous summer so that they open in March, before the leaves appear. The flowers are white and are borne all along the black spiny branches, each lateral ending in a long thorn, to be followed by large, fleshy black fruits, like damsons, which are used for preserves and to make sloe gin. The syrup from sloes is an astringent medicine: It is massaged into the gums, causing firmness and so preventing the teeth from becoming loose. And rubbed onto the teeth, it can remove tartar and improve their whiteness, giving them a sparkle. An infusion of the leaves in warm water and used as a mouthwash has much the same effect. Blackthorn leaves appear in April and are small and elliptic. They are used fresh or dry.

One of the oldest plants known to man and still in cultivation. It is a much-branched twisted twiggy tree with entire dark green leaves and bearing large pink or white flowers which are self fertile. The fruit is the size of a small apple with a unique fragrance but away from its native lands it is too acid to be eaten raw though making delicious preserves. The tree is found in damp woodlands, requiring a moist soil and it is long living. The almost black seeds, flattened on both sides, are like apple pips and when soaked in water for 10–15 minutes, they form a thick mucilage. Their ability to do so is unique amongst plants. The mucilage has demulcent properties taken internally and is used in skin creams. It acts as an efficient suspending agent, mixed with rose water, to add to toilet preparations for use in baths and in skin lotions. Mixed with gum arabic, it makes an effective cream mascara.

One of more than 450 species of evergreen or deciduous trees distributed throughout N. and S. America, temperate Europe and Asia and N. Africa, with *Q. robur*, native of Europe, N. Africa and Asia Minor. It is a long-living tree with deeply furrowed grey bark and eventually making a broad head of rugged branches. It is a deciduous slow growing tree, prominent in woodlands and hedgerows, its close-grained timber being highly durable and used in house construction and boat building. The leaves are sessile with shallow lobes and its fruits (acorns) are borne one to several on slender bright green stalks and are held in a cup-shaped scaly involucre. The green acorns which ripen in autumn, yield a nourishing flour after drying and peeling. The bark is used as a substitute for quinine to allay a fever, whilst it is highly astringent, an infusion being taken for diarrhoea and dysentery. When rubbed onto the gums, it strengthens them and a decoction of the bark or galls applied to the face and neck removes wrinkles. Galls are present on the leaves and shoots are formed by the gall-wasp which lays its eggs on the leaves the larvae feeding on the tissues and secreting a fluid which results in the formation of a round mass, like a marble but perforated. The best galls are known as Aleppo galls containing 50% gallotannic acid. They are employed in tanning and in ink making. They make a dye to colour hair black and make an internal or external astringent and a healing ointment.

RANUNCULUS FICARIA

LESSER CELANDINE
Smallwort

Ranunculaceae

139 N. + C. Europe

RESEDA ODORATA

MIGNONETTE
Little darling

Resedaceae

140 N. Africa, W. Asia, S. Europe

RICINUS COMMUNIS

CASTOR OIL PLANT

Euphorbiaceae

141 Africa, S. Asia *Torrid + Warm Temperate Zones*

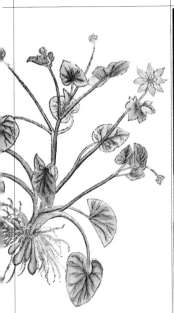

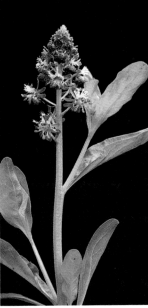

It is one of the world's most important economic plants, having valuable medicinal uses and being a lubricant. It is also used in the cosmetics industry. Mixed with lanolin it makes a lip salve and, with beeswax and lanolin, an effective eyebrow pencil. It is also widely used in hair lacquers. The plant has become naturalised in the Near East and along the N. African coast as well as in those parts of Europe bordering the Mediterranean. It is grown as a decorative indoor pot plant throughout the world, its sturdy hollow stems being smooth and cylindrical. The drooping alternate leaves, about 8 in (20 cm) across, have long footstalks and are deeply cut into 9–10 segments. They are of a blue-green colour. In warm climes the plants flower and seed. The flowers are borne in a terminal spike. They have no corolla but a red calyx and are followed by capsules 1 in (2·5 cm) long containing large oval seeds with a brown glossy coat. The seeds contain a poisonous principle and the oil is extracted by expression; it is termed "cold drawn" as heat would cause the poison to dissolve. The oil is obtained by macerating the crushed seed in alcohol, after removing the seed coats by winnowing. One drop of ointment in the eye can remove inflammation and brighten the eye.

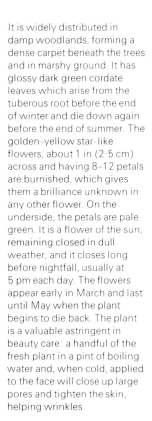

It is widely distributed in damp woodlands, forming a dense carpet beneath the trees and in marshy ground. It has glossy dark green cordate leaves which arise from the tuberous root before the end of winter and die down again before the end of summer. The golden-yellow star-like flowers, about 1 in (2·5 cm) across and having 8–12 petals are burnished, which gives them a brilliance unknown in any other flower. On the underside, the petals are pale green. It is a flower of the sun, remaining closed in dull weather, and it closes long before nightfall, usually at 5 pm each day. The flowers appear early in March and last until May when the plant begins to die back. The plant is a valuable astringent in beauty care: a handful of the fresh plant in a pint of boiling water and, when cold, applied to the face will close up large pores and tighten the skin, helping wrinkles.

A genus of 60 species. *R. odorata* is a loose, straggling plant growing amongst rocky outcrops in N. Africa, especially Egypt where it is a common weed. It was named mignonette, little darling, by the French who were the first European people to grow it. They planted it in small pots placed on their balconies where, in summer, the fragrance of the flowers would counteract the unpleasant smells of the streets. *R. odorata* has small alternate leaves and bears its inconspicuous brownish yellow flowers in a short raceme or spike in mid-summer. The fruit is a capsule open at the top and containing many small kidney-shaped seeds. The flowers have a violet-like perfume and are amongst the most difficult of flowers from which to extract an essential oil. Mignonette yields only 0·002% of oil yet so powerful is its scent that it is used in perfumery at a strength of only 1 part in 500 parts of alcohol. The perfume is obtained by enfleurage, no heat being used.

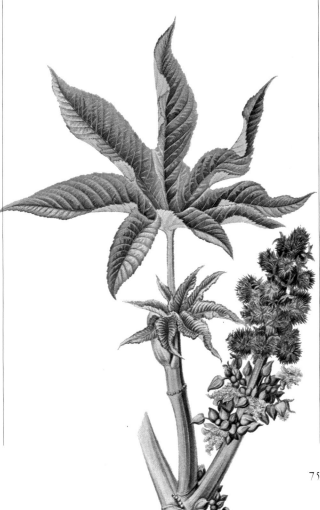

ROSA DAMASCENA	ROSA GALLICA OFFICINALIS	ROSMARINUS OFFICINALIS
DAMASK ROSE	RED ROSE Gallic rose	ROSEMARY
Rosaceae **142** Near East	Rosaceae **143** Near East	Labiatae **144** S. Europe, N. Africa, S.W. Asia *Warm Temperate Zones*

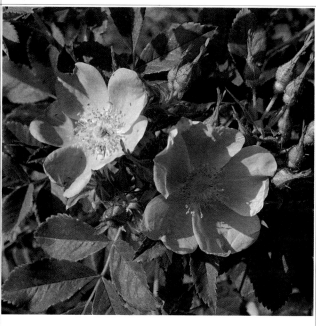

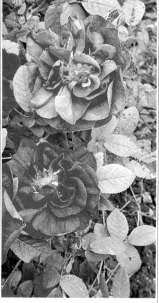

It is a shrubby plant with stalkless linear leaves, hoary on the underside and with pale blue flowers which appear in short axillary racemes almost the whole year round. The leaves and stems release an aromatic resinous smell when handled, due to its essential oil which is stored in goblet-shaped cells, invisible to the naked eye just beneath the leaf surface. The scent is released in a warm breeze and also in hot sunshine. The plant grows on waste ground in dry sandy soil, usually in sight of the sea, hence its name from the Latin *ros-marinus*, dew of the sea. It will eventually make a large spreading bush, as wide as it grows tall and its flowers are

Like the Red rose (*R. gallica*) of which it may be a natural hybrid, it is one of the oldest plants known to man still in cultivation. In the valleys of N. Bulgaria where the world's finest otto is produced, in Rose Valley at Kazanlik, it is grown by the million for export to the perfumers of Paris and elsewhere, for it is present in almost every known perfume. Its natural home is lost in obscurity but it is believed to be the Near East, where it is present on barren hillsides from the Black Sea to Kashmir, including Iraq and Iran. One legend has it that the rose was borne from a drop of sweat that fell from the brow of Mohammed. It gave its name to the town of Damascus several thousand years ago and to the silk material made there in the colour of the flower. Syria means "land of the rose". From the Near East, its culture spread to Greece and Italy and the Mediterranean islands. The flowers are depicted on the walls of the Palace of Knossos in Crete dating from 2000 BC whilst the Autumn

Damask which blooms twice yearly (*R. damascena bifera*) was mentioned by Virgil in the Georgics and is depicted in the mosaics at Pompeii. Herodotus mentions the Damask rose as having 60 petals and a scent surpassing all others. It has pale pink flowers and is one of the few flowers to have its essential oil unharmed by distillation. It takes about 250 lb (110 kg) of rose petals to produce an ounce of attar or otto, the flowers being gathered at daybreak, before the sun causes evaporation of the essential oil from the petals. Geraniol is the chief substance of the oil and is present also in the pelargonium, lavender, lemon grass and neroli from which the oil is used as an adulterant for otto of roses. Rose water, obtained by distillation, is a valuable astringent and relieves tired eyes. Along with almond oil, spermaceti and wax, it makes a soothing cold cream.

Its origin is lost in antiquity, though it was cultivated by the Greeks and Romans, early in their history, for the fragrance of its petals which increase in perfume as they dry. The dried petals were sold from barrels in apothecary's shops, hence its name of Apothecary's Rose. The flower was used to adorn the shields of Persian Warriors several thousand years BC and was introduced by Roman legions wherever they went, reaching Gaul in N. France 2000 years ago and, later, the British Isles. That the plant is able to survive in the most arid conditions accounts for it being possibly the oldest plant known to man still in cultivation. It is a plant of erect, shrubby habit, almost free of thorns and with alternate pinnate leaves and reddish flowers borne singly and in corymbs during late summer. Rose water to sooth a sore skin is one of the most effective of modern complexion lotions, being astringent and healing. Diluted, it is soothing to the eyes.

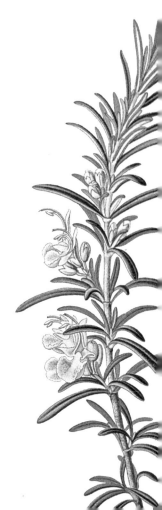

SALVIA OFFICINALIS	SALVIA SCLAREA
SAGE Red Sage	CLARY Bright eyes
Labiatae	Labiatae
145 S. Europe *Temperate Zones*	**146** Near East, W. Asia, S. Europe

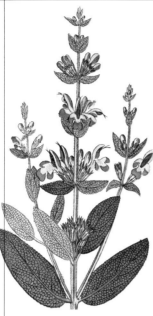

much visited by bees. The scent is invigorating and in Banck's Herbal (1525) one is advised to "smell it oft and it shall keep thee youngly". As the stems remain green for a long time, when cut from the plant it was given to mourners at funerals as a token of remembrance and it was also worn as a headdress by brides. The tops, placed in a muslin bag and in a warm bath, will scent the water and tone the body and an infusion of the tops, taken when cold, will act as a tonic and sweeten the breath. It makes a valuable hair rinse and when massaged into the scalp, is said to prevent hair falling and keep it glossy. Spirit of rosemary is also used as a hair restorer.

It is found on wasteland, in full sun and in a sandy soil when it is fully perennial. In earlier times it was given pride of place amongst all aromatic plants and there is a saying translated from an Anglo-Saxon manuscript which reads: "why should man die when he can have sage?" For this reason it took its name from the Latin *salvia*, salvation. The red-stemmed variety, purpurea is the best for all purposes whilst *S. nutilans*, the Pineapple-scented sage, imparts its rich fruity scent to pot-pourris. The common sage is one of the best of all plants for darkening and toning the hair. An infusion of the fresh leaves or tops is used. *S. officinalis* is a plant of shrubby habit, eventually making a bush as wide as it grows tall. The square stems are covered in down whilst the wrinkled, oval leaves are also downy, which gives the plant a greyish look.

This member of the sage family is a glandular plant with square stems, tinted purple, and hairy ovate dark-green leaves, wrinkled and serrated at the edges. The flowers are violet-blue with three white marks on the lower lip. The calyx is glandular with long white hairs at the base. Flowering time is June–September. The leaves emit a pleasing pineapple scent and produce a bright green essential oil used for fixing perfumes as an alternative to animal fixatives. When dry, they are placed in sachets to put amongst clothes and are also used in pot-pourris. The water distilled from the leaves and flowers and used warm to bathe the eyes will give them a sparkle, like eyebright, and soothe away soreness. It also makes a soothing toilet water for fair skins. One or two drops of the mucilage produced after steeping a half ounce of seed in a little water for 24 hours, will remove the most stubborn intrusion from the eye. Applied to an infected blackhead, will draw it and quickly heal the skin. So useful is the plant for the eyes that in Italy where it grows in abundance, it is known as "Oculus Christi", its botanical name being from the Latin *clarus*, clear. The tops, placed in a warm bath will relieve tired limbs and tone the body.

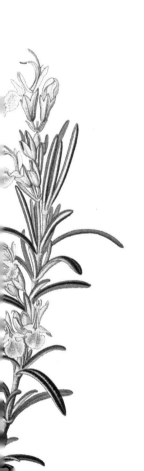

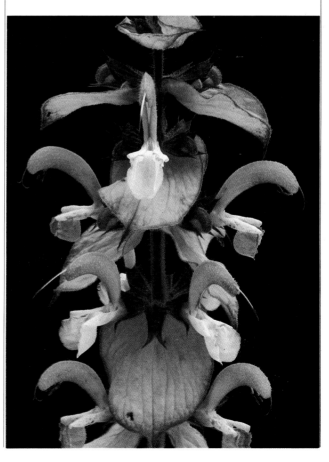

SAMBUCUS NIGRA

ELDER

Sambucaceae

147 Europe
W. Asia, N. America

SANICULA EUROPAEA

SANICLE

Umbelliferae

148 Europe, W. Asia

SANTALUM ALBUM

SANDALWOOD
Sandal

Santalaceae

149 S.E. Asia, India

A genus of 40 species. *S. nigra* has furrowed bark with a foetid smell and dark green pinnate leaves of similar smell, though the flowers, which are borne in early summer in large flat umbels, have a pleasant muscatel scent which they retain when dry. They are replaced by small green fruits which turn deep purple when ripe at the end of summer. Elderflower water has many uses in beauty and toilet preparations. An infusion in hot water and allowed to cool, makes a pleasant after shave lotion for men and is an astringent. Mixed with cucumber juice it keeps the skin white and free from blemishes. Elderflower water is also known as *eau de sureau* and is especially useful to use on oily skins after cleansing the face at night. For a skin cleanser, elder flower cream, which contains an emollient, is useful for an oily skin. The flowers are used fresh and when dry. They are collected when fully open and placed in heaps when they heat slightly. The corollas become loose and if put through a sieve, they come away from the stems cleanly and are spread out in an airy room to complete their drying. They retain their fragrance. Another way to preserve them is to place the open flower trusses in a wooden tub or container and to salt them in layers. This will keep them in a fresh condition for several months. The salt is washed away before the flowers are used.

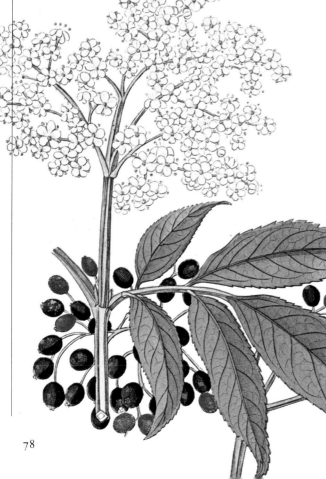

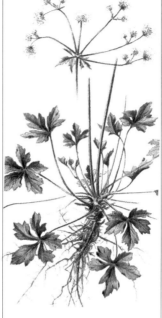

One of a small genus present in damp deciduous woodlands often in dense shade. Its name is derived from the Latin *sano* (I heal) from its skin healing properties. *S. europaea* is a slender glabrous plant with glossy green 3–5 lobed leaves with serrate edges. The basal leaves form a rosette and it is these which are most effective in curing dysentery and diarrhoea and checking internal bleeding. The plant is also a blood purifyer, clearing the skin of blemishes. Externally the plant is used for skin rashes and soreness. It blooms during June and July, its flowers of dull pinkish white being borne in small round umbels at the top of reddish stems. The fruit is covered with hooked prickles causing them to adhere to clothing. The plant should be collected in early summer when fresh and the leaves dried for use in winter.

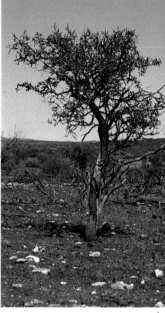

A genus of 25 species, of which *S. album* supplies its highly fragrant wood to burn as incense in eastern temples and on funeral pyres. *S. album* is native of S.E. India, Malaysia and the island of Timor where it grows in dense moist forests. It is a parasitic tree, attaching its roots to those of other trees and, although eventually reaching a height of 40 ft (12 m), it is one of the slowest growing of all trees. It has opposite, oval leaves terminating in a point whilst the flowers are composed of four stamens only, arising from the calyx. The yellow wood yields, by distillation, a highly fragrant oil. It is colourless and enters into the composition of many perfumes as "sandal". It is the base for all "green" and "woody" perfumes and is the chief ingredient of the Indian perfume, Abir. The essential oil of sandalwood is also obtained from *S. yasi*, native of the Fiji Isles. Its oil is mixed with coconut oil and used by the women to rub into the hair.

SASSAFRAS OFFICINALE

SASSAFRAS
Safras

Lauraceae

150 E.-N. America

SEDUM ROSEA

ROSE-ROOT

Crassulaceae

151 C. Asia, N. + C. Europe

SESAMUM INDICUM

SESAME

Pedaliaceae

152 S. Asia, C. Africa
*Tropical Zones
of the Old World*

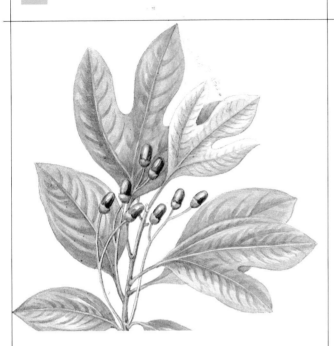

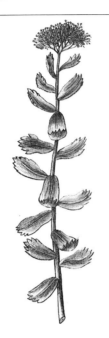

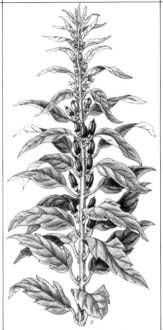

A genus of three species of woodland trees, *S. officinale* being native of E.-N. America, the others of China and Formosa. *S. officinale* is a tree or shrub, usually about 18ft (5·5 m) tall but in Florida may attain a height of 100 ft (30 m) with many cylindrical branches covered with deeply furrowed greyish bark which is highly aromatic, the root bark being the most aromatic of all. From the young shoots a health-giving beer is brewed. The alternate leaves with petioles about 1 in (2·5 cm) long are remarkable for the variety of form on the same tree, those opening first being oval, those opening later being lobed, the last to open having three lobes. The greenish yellow flowers are borne in drooping racemes at the same time as the leaves. They are followed by pea-like oval fruits of deep purple, held erect on a red peduncle. It is from the ripe fruits that the best oil of sassafras is extracted by distillation and is used in modern perfumery. The oil obtained from the bark and roots is used to scent toilet soaps and to make the less expensive perfumes. The external bark of the roots is spongy like cork and of a dull grey colour whilst the inner bark is reddish brown or cinnamon colour and is rich in essential oil. The roots are lifted in winter when the sap is down; 1000 lb (440 kg) of root chips will yield a gallon of crude oil under steam pressure. It is pale yellow, containing 90% safrol, a staple compound with a pleasant odour like that of cinnamon and bergamot mixed together. It is present in the essential oil of *Cinamomum Camphora* and is identical with the body shikimol, the chief constituent of the Star anise, *Illicum religiosum*. By treating it with permanganate of potash, safrol yields piperonylic acid, known in perfumery as heliotropin, used to imitate the scent of wild heliotrope. The American Indians used the powder obtained from dried sassafras leaves to thicken soup.

A grey-green succulent with broad flat leaves overlapping up the erect stems. The obovate leaves are rounded at the base, toothed at the apex, the lower leaves being almost scale-like. The greenish yellow flowers have purple anthers and are borne in a terminal inflorescence throughout summer. The plant is scentless, but the rhizomatous root when dry has the scent of roses which it imparts to toilet water. It is astringent and is rubbed onto the face after washing. It softens the skin, removes wrinkles and closes large pores. Rose-root water is sprinkled over clothes and linen to impart its rose scent which is not lasting. The plant grows on cliffs and rocky ground exposed to the sun and usually close to the sea. The thick fleshy leaves store moisture for a long time so that it will survive with the minimum of soil over its roots. If hung up in a room to keep away insects, the plant retains its freshness for many weeks.

A genus of 16 species, of which *S. indicum* is the most common. Early in history, the Egyptians, Greeks and Romans used the oil for culinary and cosmetic purposes. *S. indicum* is a plant of upright shrubby habit with opposite leaves arranged spirally. They are lance-shaped, ending in a point and bright green. The funnel-shaped flowers are pinkish white and borne singly in the axils of the leaves. They are scented and from them a perfumed toilet water is made by distillation. The fruit is a nut or capsule about 1 in (2·5 cm) long, with hooks or thorns, which attach themselves to the coats of browsing animals. The fruit is divided into four chambers, each containing many small egg-shaped seeds which when pressed release a pale yellow odourless oil used in cooking, in the manufacture of margarines, in sauces and in cosmetics. The seeds are included in face creams and natural sun-tan lotions.

SOLANUM TUBEROSUM	SOLIDAGO VIRGAUREA	SONCHUS OLERACEUS
POTATO	GOLDEN ROD	SOWTHISTLE
Solanaceae	Compositae	Compositae
153 S. America *Temperate Zones*	**154** Europe, N. Asia, N. America	**155** N. Asia, C. Europe

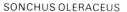

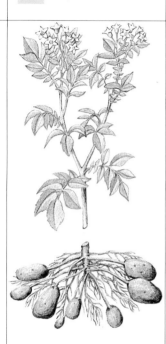

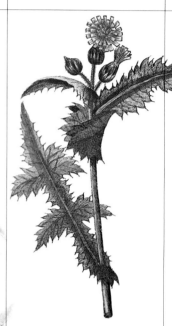

A genus of 1200 species of mostly poisonous plants, with *S. tuberosum* now the staple food of most western countries. From the "eyes" in the tubers which grow to 6 in (15 cm) or more in length, being oval or round, arise bright green stems of finger thickness which carry large lobed leaves and bear white bell-shaped flowers followed by black, many-seeded berries. With the exception of the tubers, all parts are poisonous. Potatoes are rich in protein and in potash and phosphoric acid. They contain vitamins of the B complex and vitamin C as citric acid. The tubers are lifted in autumn, when the foliage dies down and is removed. They must be stored in the dark or they will turn from yellow or crimson to green and take on poisonous properties. If washed and peeled and then sliced and rubbed onto the face and neck, left for an hour before washing off, they will leave the skin soft and white.

This common flower, which blooms freely throughout N. America, Europe and Asia, takes its name from the Latin *solidare* (to unite or make whole) for its power, known even in antiquity, to heal wounds. Apothecaries sold the dried leaves from their shops to make an infusion which, taken internally, stemmed the flow of blood from open wounds, whilst, externally, applied as a lotion, both the fresh and dry leaves were used as an effective treatment for skin made sore by wind and sun exposure. Today the flowers, which contain tannins, saponins and pigments, are sometimes used in pharmaceutical treatments for intestinal and kidney inflammations. The plant grows in deciduous woodlands and hedgerows, also about mountainous heathlands, where it grows to only half its normal height. It is an erect plant with rough angular stems and narrow, sharply pointed serrated leaves. It blooms from August to September, the bright golden-yellow flowers being borne in large terminal panicles. When the flowering is over, the calyx holds a crown of hairs (pappus), which later carry the small fruits on the wind. The flowering tips of the branches are used in teas and pharmaceutical preparations. Another species, the Canadian goldenrod, is taller 2–7 ft (60–200 cm), has 1-sided spikes, in a branched cluster, of numerous yellow flower heads $\frac{1}{2}$ in (3–5 mm), and spreads widely in Europe.

A widely distributed genus known to the Anglo-Saxons as *suwe-distel* (later sowthistle) or sprout thistle, for the young milky shoots of early summer were cooked as a nourishing vegetable. It is also known as turn-sole for the flowers always follow the sun in its orbit. The milky juice from the stems, mixed with a little warm water, is a rejuvenating skin cleanser, especially for acid skins. Countrywomen add an eggcupful of juice to a pint of warmed rain water and apply it to the face at night. It is an erect, much-branched plant of grey appearance, its hollow stems being filled with milky juice which is more plentiful in older plants. The oblong leaves are prickly, the upper leaves being stem-clasping and covered in soft spikes in place of prickles. The pale yellow flowers, which bloom in July and August, are borne in terminal heads, the pappus resembling that of the dandelion.

STELLARIA MEDIA

CHICKWEED

Caryophyllaceae

156 *Temperate Zones*

STYRAX BENZOIN

BENZOIN

Styracaceae

157 S.E. Asia

SYRINGA VULGARIS

LILAC

Oleaceae

158 Near East, China, S. Europe

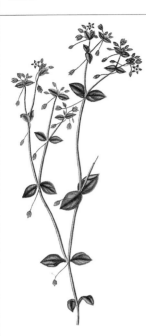

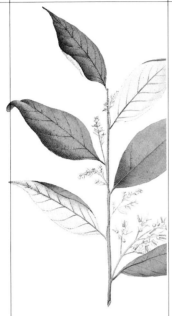

A genus of 30 species, native of S.E. Europe, W. Asia and China, which have decorated gardens since early in history. Small trees or shrubs of twiggy growth, they are found in mountainous woodlands and bear their flowers of white or purple in large conical panicles 6–8 in (15–20 cm) long early in summer. The plants are usually found growing in a chalky subsoil and are of erect habit whilst making an abundance of twiggy growth. The flowers are borne at the ends of the new seasons shoots and are powerfully scented. The buds are enclosed by scales in winter, which release a sticky substance as the buds elongate in spring. The heart-shaped leaves, about 4 in (10 cm) long, are smooth and held on 1 in (2·5 cm) foot-stalks. The name Lilac is the Persian word for "flower" and it was from that country the plant first reached Europe. Indol is present in the flowers, as in privet, of the same family. It is an alcohol closely related to methyl indol or scatol, the active principle of civet, and if inhaled in excess may cause nausea and depression. Gerard described the scent as "troubling the head in a strange manner exciting sexual instincts". The perfume is extracted by enfleur-age and treating the pomatum with rectified spirit. The scent is similar to tuberose, for which it is often used as an adulterant.

Probably the commonest of all weeds, for it is distributed over the entire world including the Arctic Circle and has been used as an antiscorbutic since earliest times. It forms weak, much branched stems, pale green and juicy, which trail over the ground for some distance. It is present on waste ground and by the side of fields, in ditches and by the roadside, suppressing other plants growing near it with its dense growth. The small succulent leaves are oval, pale green and glabrous, whilst the small white flowers which form in the axils of the upper leaves are star-like. They appear all summer and are followed by small seed capsules. An infusion of the plant added to hot olive oil, lard or goose grease and allowed to set will take away soreness from the skin when gently rubbed in. A "tea" made from chickweed, ground ivy and wood sage will keep the skin clear of impurities and firm the flesh.

A genus of 130 species, yielding a fragrant gum resin, collected from incisions made in the bark, which is used medicinally and in cosmetics. The main source of benzoic acid which prevents fats turning rancid and is odour-less, is that obtained from *S. benzoin*. The plant grows to 18 ft (5·5 m) tall and is topped for its resin when seven years old. For the next 12 years, it will yield about 3 lb (1·5 kg) of resin annually. It is reddish brown with a balsamic scent due to the presence of cinnamic acid. It is soluble in alcohol and used in perfumery to give permanence to an odour. *S. officinale* is the storax of the Middle East which is obtained from the outer and inner bark of the tree, that from the inner bark being used in perfumery in the same way as benzoin. It is a small shrubby tree present on rocky hillsides. The oval leaves are 2 in (5 cm) long, hoary on the underside, and it bears fragrant white flowers in short racemes.

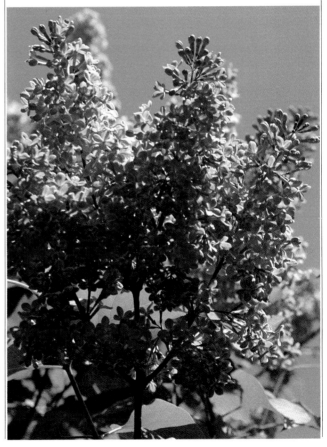

TANACETUM BALSAMITA	TANACETUM VULGARE	TARAXACUM OFFICINALE	THYMUS VULGARIS
COSTMARY	TANSY	DANDELION Priest's crown	THYME
Compositae **159** Near East, C. Asia	Compositae **160** Europe, Asia *N. America*	Compositae **161** *Temperate Zones*	Labiatae **162** S. Europe *Warm Temperate Zones*

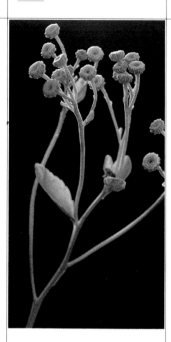

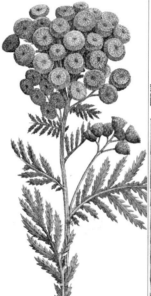

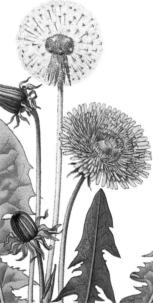

It is native of S. Europe, N. Africa, the Near East and Mediterranean islands and is a shrubby plant growing on rocky ground in full sunlight, which brings out its pungent aroma to the full. It has wiry stems and small oblong ovate leaves, dark green above, grey on the underside, and during the latter weeks of summer it bears purple flowers in conical clusters which are much visited by bees. The honey of thyme-frequenting bees is used in many beauty preparations, for it is especially soothing and healing. When burnt, thyme can rid a home of fleas and other flying insects, and the dried leaves placed in muslin bags, along with those of cotton lavender, and put amongst clothes will keep away moths. Sprigs of fresh thyme can be hung to dry in closets with much the same effect. Essence of thyme is used in soaps and cosmetics. Thymol is the chief principle but borneol and linalol are also present to give thyme products a pleasanter smell. Thymol is such a powerful antiseptic that it is used as a base in many deodorants and also in the treatment of throat infections and colds. With rosemary, an infusion to use as a hair rinse will darken the hair and keep it soft and silky as well as free the scalp of dandruff.

Native of the Near East and C. Asia where it grows on waste ground, in full sunlight and in dry sandy soil. It is closely related to tansy and feverfew but differs in that its dark green leaves are entire, being finely toothed at the margins. Late in summer it bears small yellow flowers in loose clusters. The plant has a creeping rootstock. Its name is derived from the Latin *costus amarus* (a bitter shrub), though the plant was dedicated to St. Mary Magdalene, being also called Maudlin. Writers of old have described the custom of tying together small bundles of costmary and lavender to place amongst clothing and bedding. It was also used to impart its sweet balsamic fragrance to ale and wine. To clear the face of blemishes a cold cream is made from an infusion of the leaves in warm olive oil, with a little beeswax to set it when cool, and the leaves placed in buttermilk for several hours and applied to the skin will have the same effect.

It is widespread in hedgerows and on waste ground and has a creeping rootstock and an erect angular stem. The dark green fern-like leaves, 6 in (15 cm) long, are divided into numerous pairs of deeply pinnatifid leaflets which emit a camphor-like smell when handled, the essential oil being enclosed in glandular dots. Late in summer, the plant is conspicuous by its flat-topped heads of small, round pale yellow flowers, like gold buttons. The essential oil has a minty smell. It contains an aldehyde which, with bisulphate of sodium, forms a crystalline compound known as tanacetone. The plant takes its name from the Greek *athanaton* (immortal), for the flowers remain fresh for many months. In mediaeval times, the leaves were placed in beds and strewn over floors as their camphor smell kept away flies and fleas. Tansy leaves have long been popular for improving the complexion.

It is usually considered an obnoxious weed of lawns and pastureland though it is one of nature's most wonderful assets in the quest for health and beauty. The plant forms a thick dark brown tap root which is white within and contains a milky juice as does the leafless flower stem at the end of which is borne, from spring until autumn, a single bloom with bright yellow ray florets which are an attraction to bees. From the tap root, the long toothed leaves (like the teeth of a lion) radiate to form a rosette almost flat on the ground by which every drop of moisture is directed to the root. Thus, the plant is able to flourish in arid conditions and in areas of low rainfall, plants are grown to replace lettuce, to include the young leaves in salads and sandwiches. From the cleaned roots and those of horseradish, an effective skin lotion is prepared whilst a decoction taken twice daily (a wineglassful) will clear the skin of eczema and eruptions.

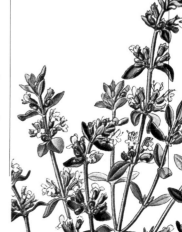

TILIA EUROPAEA	TRIFOLIUM PRATENSE	TRITICUM VULGARE	ULMUS FULVA
LIME TREE	RED CLOVER Trefoil	WHEAT Corn	RED ELM
Tiliaceae **163** N. Europe	Leguminosae **164** C. Asia, N. + C. Europe	Gramineae **165** Mediterranean, W. Asia *Temperate Zones*	Urticaceae **166** N. America

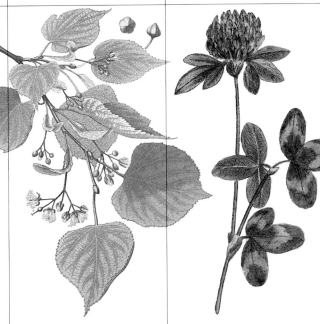

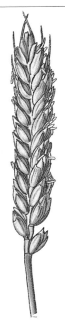

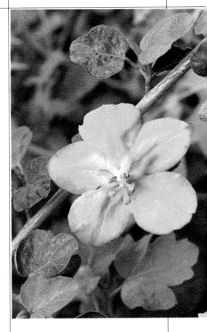

A genus of 50 species, all are deciduous woodland and hedgerow trees. But their compact habit makes a number of the species ideal for street planting including *T. europaea*, the Common lime, which is that most often seen in the British Isles and N. Europe. It has smooth bark and pale green heart-shaped leaves and bears, in mid-summer, from the leaf axils, scented creamy-white flowers in small cymes. The flowers ferment unless quickly dried, when they will keep indefinitely if stored in wooden containers. A distillation of the flowers makes a soothing complexion lotion, removing soreness from the skin and leaving it soft and smooth. It is more effective if mixed with equal parts of rose water, and with alcohol, it makes a soothing after shave. *T. americana* is the N. American lime with large coarsely toothed leaves. Its flowers are used in the same way and from its bark a sugary maple-like syrup, used for sweetening, is obtained.

A downy plant, it is one of the principle crops for milking cows, whether fresh or dried as hay. The ternate dark green leaves are divided into three leaflets, each with a white crescent on the upper surface and stipules terminating in a long bristle. The flowers, which are purple-pink, are borne in terminal heads, the secretion of honey being greater than with white clover. It is a plant of well drained meadows, flowering in May and is known to country children as "honeysuckles" for the honey is easily sucked out. It is the high honey content which makes a lotion of red clover so soothing when applied to a sore skin caused by winds or over exposure to the sun. Red clover grows more upright than the white and the honey of both is of a pale amber colour with a delicate aroma. It is widely used in beauty treatment.

A genus of 20 species, wheat grains have been found in Egyptian tombs of 2000 BC and in pre-historic lake dwellings in Switzerland. Wheat is grown in all parts of the warm and temperate world for making bread. The plant has a hollow stem and an unbranched flower spike which becomes an ear of corn (seeds) and changes from green to golden-brown as it ripens. The wheats vary in the denseness of the spikes and in the presence or absence of awns. *T. compositum* is a bearded wheat which bears seven ears to each stalk. White bread, in which the outer portion of the grain and the embryo (germ) have been removed, is less nourishing but more popular than brown bread in which all parts of the grain are included. The embryo or wheat germ is sold as a dietary supplement. The oil extracted from it, mixed with witch hazel, is a natural skin tonic; or wheat germ meal with yoghurt in equal parts can be used.

It is a small twiggy tree with long toothed leaves covered on both sides with silky hairs, likewise the leaf buds, stems and branches. The tree generally grows in self-sown plantations. It is the inner bark or bast that is used in illness and in cosmetics. When 10 years old the tree is stripped naked of its bark from which the inner bark is removed in lengths of 2 ft (60 cm) and about 6 in (15 cm) wide. It is reddish brown and fibrous, and when dried and powdered should be of a greyish colour. It is highly mucilaginous so that a pinch in a cup of water will form a thick jelly. It is taken hot internally or, to remove skin blemishes, is used warm, spread over the face and left for two hours before washing off. It will also take inflammation from skin made sore by sun or cold wind. Used with marshmallow and lard (or olive oil) it makes a soothing face cream.

URTICA DIOICA

STINGING NETTLE

Urticaceae

167 Europe, Asia
Temperate Zones

VANILLA PLANIFOLIA

VANILLA

Orchidaceae

168 S. America
Tropical Zones

VERBASCUM THAPSUS

MULLEIN

Scrophulariaceae

169 Europe, W. Asia

It is found throughout the temperate regions of Europe and Asia, including Japan and, with the dandelion, is the most widespread of all weeds of waste ground. It is an unbranched plant with ovate toothed leaves, from the axils of which it bears tiny greenish white flowers throughout summer. The whole plant is covered with stiff hairs, at the base of which, contained in minute vesicles, is an acrid substance (formic acid) which the plant releases into the skin when touched, causing a rash and pain. The plant has numerous medicinal uses, most important being its ability to reduce blood pressure and to enhance one's appearance. An infusion of the tops sweetened with honey will, taken internally, purify the blood and clear the complexion, whilst it may be used externally for the same purpose when applied to the face with pads. An infusion also makes an excellent hair tonic, preventing the hair from falling out and leaving it soft and glossy. To stimulate hair growth, use a stiff brush to apply nettle juice to the roots.

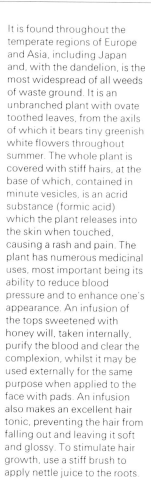

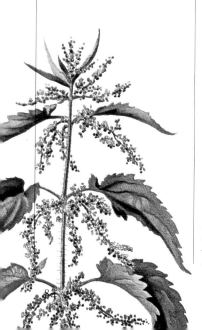

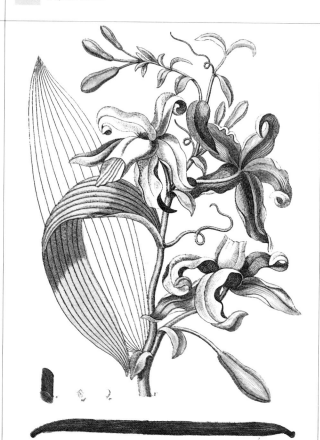

A genus of 90 species of epiphytic plants, native of tropical forests of Mexico and Brazil where it attaches itself to tall trees by aerial roots and pulls itself up to the sunlight, often to a considerable height. Its greenish yellow orchid-like flowers, which appear in a dense inflorescence, diffuse a soft sweet perfume and are followed by clindrical pods or beans as they are called, for they resemble runner beans, about 8 in (20 cm) long and containing small beans enclosed in black pulp. For centuries the pods have been in demand for confectionery and in perfumery. The pods are harvested in autumn, just before they are fully ripe. After a process of cooking and drying, they are dark brown, wrinkled and usually covered on the outside in needle-like crystals of the odoriferous principle vanillin, a condition known as "frosted". They are sliced like runner beans and placed in alcohol for 4–5 weeks, to make a tincture. After the tincture or essence has been extracted, it is strained and is then ready to use in floral "bouquets", in which no one odour pre-dominates. It was included by François Coty in his L'Aimant perfume, introduced in 1927, which has remained one of the all-time classic perfumes of the world. *V. planifolia* forms a smooth stem often as thick as a man's thigh and has thick fleshy leaves up to 8 in (20 cm) long, terminating in a point. From the leaf nodes the aerial roots are formed by which the plant clings to its host. A plant yields pods in its fourth year.

A genus of more than 200 species, distributed throughout Europe and the British Isles, W. and C. Asia and N. Africa, it grows on waste ground in full sun and in sandy soil. In its first year it forms a grey rosette from the centre of which, in its second year, arises a thick woolly stem up to 9 ft (about 3 m) tall, the top half bearing numerous dull yellow flowers in a dense inflorescence. Each flower measures 1 in (2·5 cm) across and they bloom June–August. The plant is enhanced by its broad lanceolate leaves, densely covered in white hairs, hence its botanical name from the Latin *barbascum* (bearded). If the stems are dipped in grease (tallow) they will burn slowly with an iridescent light, hence its country name of candle wick. While country folk would put the fresh leaves in their shoes to protect the feet from the uneven surface of the roads. In Italy, the women make an infusion of the flowers to tint the hair a rich golden colour as shown in paintings by Titian. Throughout Europe, until recent times, mullein water was as highly regarded as that of rosemary as a hair restorer and for toning. The flowers, boiled in milk for five minutes, with a little honey added, makes a soothing complexion milk. The saponins and volatile oil of mullein make it a suitable expectorant, while its mucilage is used to treat mouth inflammations.

VERBENA OFFICINALIS	VERONICA BECCABUNGA	VIOLA ODORATA
VERVAIN Sacred herb	**BROOKLIME** Limpwort	**VIOLET**
Verbenaceae	Scrophulariaceae	Violaceae
170 S. + C. Europe, C. Asia	**171** N. Europe, W. + N. Asia *North Temperate Zones*	**172** S. Europe *Temperate Zones*

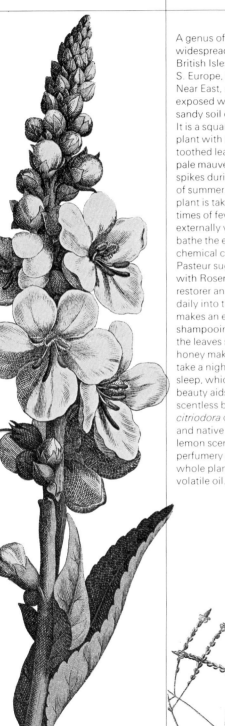

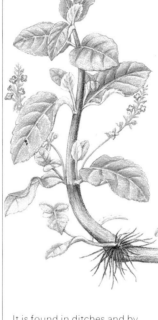

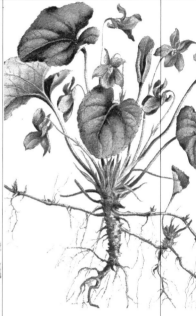

A genus of 80 species, it is widespread throughout the British Isles and C. and S. Europe, C. Asia and the Near East, usually growing on exposed waste ground and in sandy soil of a chalky nature. It is a square stemmed, hairy plant with opposite unstalked toothed leaves and bearing pale mauve flowers in elegant spikes during the latter weeks of summer. A decoction of the plant is taken internally in times of fever and used externally when warm to bathe the eyes. Due to its chemical composition, Louis Pasteur suggested using it with Rosemary as a hair restorer and tonic, massaged daily into the scalp and it makes an excellent rinse after shampooing. An infusion of the leaves sweetened with honey makes a pleasant tea to take a night to ensure sound sleep, which is the best of all beauty aids. The plant is scentless but *Aloysia citriodora* of the same order and native of S. America has a lemon scent which is used in perfumery and soaps. The whole plant abounds in volatile oil.

It is found in ditches and by the side of ponds and streams usually growing in muddy ground. The plant takes its popular name from the Anglo-Saxon word *lime*, meaning mud or slime, which was then used for building; when the calcareous stone used in mortar for binding together bricks and stones came to be used, it took the same name. The plant has succulent hollow stems which creep about the mud, rooting at the nodes. It has a glossy appearance with small oval leaves, leathery to the touch and bearing dark blue flowers during May and June in opposite clusters in the axils of the leaves. The plant is rich in vitamin C. Before citrus fruits were imported into England, it was sold in London's streets for sailors to take to sea to prevent scurvy. A wineglassful taken daily of an infusion of the whole plant, will keep the skin smooth and clear of blemishes and used externally, will act in the same way.

A genus distributed throughout the N. temperate regions, the plants seek the shade and coolness of hedgerows and woodlands and a cool moist leafy soil. The plant has a short rootstock and sends out long runners which root at the leaf nodes to form new plants. The heart-shaped leaves are deep green and held on long footstalks whilst the purple-blue flowers are spurred and have four upper oblong petals and two side petals. The plants are inconspicuous, the flowers mostly hidden by the evergreen foliage and cleistogamic, i.e. those which appear first, early in spring, do not set seed. Seed is set by the smaller blooms which appear later. Plants begin to flower with the first warm rays of February sunshine when they are most fragrant, but although their perfume exceeds that of most flowers, it quickly fades when inhaled. This is due to the chemical composition containing aketona, ionine, from which the word violet is derived.

Tintoretto's *Susanna and the Elders* is a splendid encomium to woman's beauty and the dangers inherent in it. While bathing in her husband's garden, the beautiful and pious Susanna was seen by two lascivious elders who made advances to her. Rejecting her adulterous suitors, Susanna became the target of their libelous accusation that she had indeed committed adultery. On her way to her death, she was saved by the wise cross-examination of her accusers by Daniel. In this story from the book of Daniel, beauty is clearly a liability.

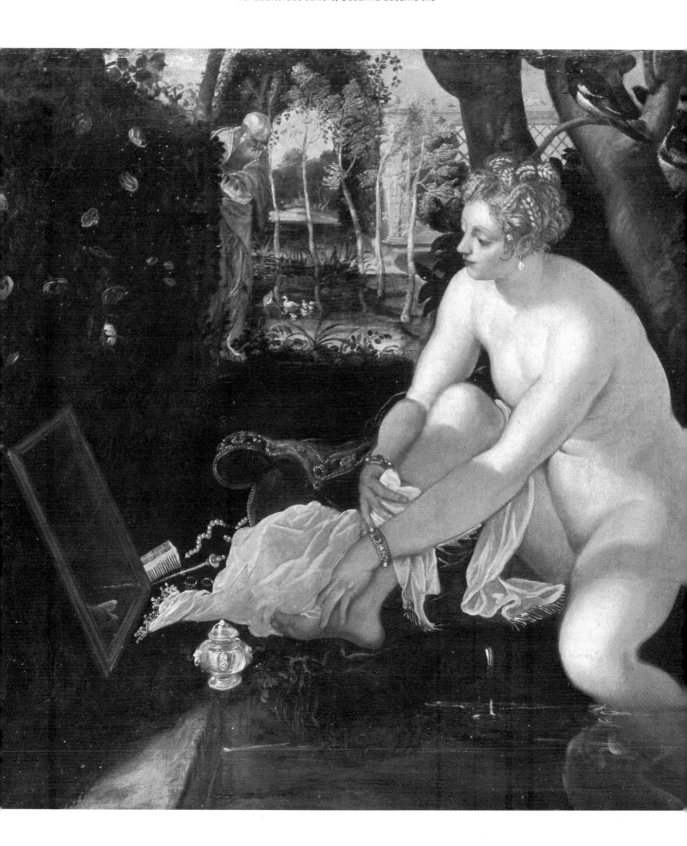

Paradise lost: In quest of beauty

Since man and woman first appeared on earth in the Garden of Eden, it has been the desire of every female to harness every aid to beauty and allurement in her efforts to please and attract the opposite sex, in the same way that a flower uses its scent or colour to attract pollinating birds and insects for the continuity of the species.

The first people known to us who used perfumes and cosmetics for personal adornment were the early Egyptians whose refined tastes and habits made it necessary for them to import large quantities of fragrant gums and resins, roots and barks from as far away as N India in the east and S Arabia in the south. The caravan trains laden with these refineries were endless and were a source of great wealth to those exporting countries.

Perfume and unguent flasks dating from more than 2000 BC and discovered in archaeological diggings point to the lavish use of perfumes and cosmetics in ancient Egypt. In the magnificent temple built by Queen Hatshepsut at Thebes in about 1500 BC and carved from the mountain face, is a painting still in its brilliant colours which shows a lady of high rank going through the daily routine of her toilet. She is attended by four maidens, one of whom pours fragrant oils over her hair and body whilst another massages it into her shoulders. It is said that of all eastern women, those of Thebes and others who inhabited the Nile banks in upper Egypt were the most beautiful. They applied paint and powder to the face, including the dried leaves of henna to rub onto the cheeks to give a

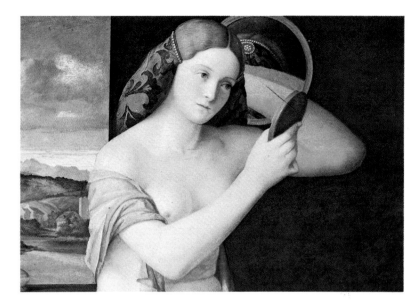

Coming to kiss her lips, (such grace I found)
Me seemed I smelt a garden of swete flowers:
That dainty odours from them threw around
For damsels fit to deck their lovers bowers.
Her lips did smell like unto Gillyflowers,
Her ruddy cheeks like unto Roses red:
Her snowy brows like budded Bellamours,
Her lovely eyes like Pinks but newly spread.
Her goodly bosom like a strawberry bed,
Her neck like a bunch of Columbines:
Her breasts like lillies, ere their leaves be shed,
Her nipples like young blossm'd Jessamines.
Such fragrant flowers do give most odorous smell.
But her sweet odour did them all excel.

Edmund Spenser, *Sonnet To his Wife*

rosy tint and to wash the hair to make it a dark red colour as popular with early Egyptian women as it is today with women everywhere. It is used in exactly the same way in modern beauty salons the world over by mixing the powdered leaves into a

Bellini's magnificent *Young Girl at a Mirror* seems to be a monument to beauty unadorned. Perhaps the radiant complexion of this young woman owes its beauty entirely to her youth. Perhaps she was exceptionally adept in the use of natural cosmetics.

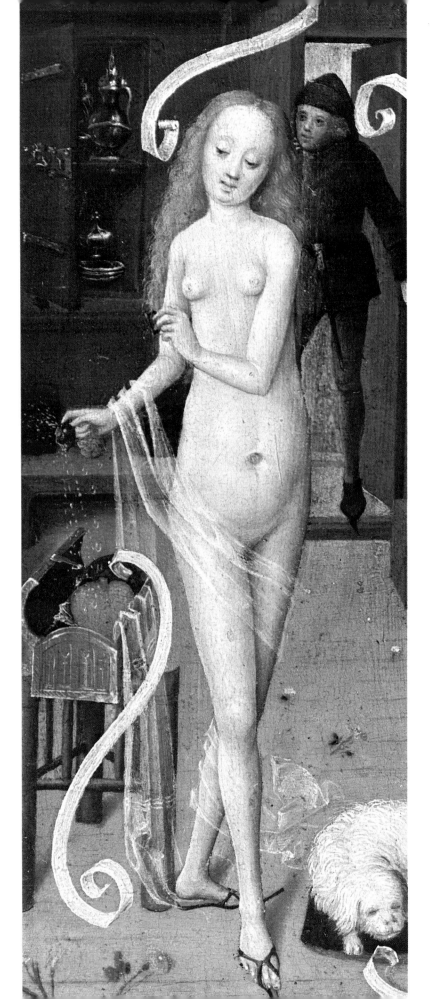

paste and allowing it to remain on the head for an hour or more before washing off. Henna is a vegetable colouring agent and coats the hair without penetration and so does not harm it. It also colours greying hair just as the aging Mohammed used it to colour his greying beard. The Persian poet Sheik Sadi of Shiraz delightfully ridiculed the vogue amongst older women of his time, who, as today, used everything at their disposal to prevent their hair greying and giving away their age, when there were so many other things that did so and which they could not hide:

... thy hair with silver bent
May cheat us now; yet little mother;
 say
Canst thou make straight thy back
 which time has bent

But fashions change and two thousand years later, in the years leading up to the French Revolution, ladies of fashion used scented powders on the hair, following a fashion of a lady of the Court of Louis XIV, and believed to be Madame du Barry, whose hair had turned prematurely grey and who wished to set a new idea by introducing to court procedure an order that all should follow her example. To make the powder stick, the hair was first covered with macassar oil before buckwheat flour and then scented powder was applied with bellows. Later, wigs made of hair of different shades were used by both men and women, especially by those who through age had lost their hair, or whose hair lacked lustre, so they no longer attracted the opposite sex.

Hair styles changed but little through the centuries, Egyptian women wearing the hair long and worked into small plaits or curls. In the Brooklyn Museum, New York, is a statue of an Egyptian lady of about 1500 BC, her long plaits covering the back of her head and shoulders. A popular style with actresses of the Hollywood movies of the 1920s and 30s, who employed a private hairdresser to attend to their coiffure just as wealthy Egyptians did 4000 years ago, as seen on a stone carving at Deir-el-Bahari, which shows a lady attended by her coiffeuse who is massaging perfumed oil into her scalp before setting her hair into the latest style.

The eyes perhaps received more attention than any other part of the body apart from the hair, belladonna being used to inflate the pupils, to give the eyes greater prominence. Nothing has changed but today Eyebright is used instead for it is less harsh on the eyes whilst achieving the same results and it is in great demand throughout the western world.

Powders for whitening the face were used by Assyrian women 1000 years BC. Herodotus has told of powdered pumice, as used in modern talcum powders, being used on the face and body and which gave to the skin a delicate smoothness. The men painted their faces with white lead which the women were later to copy, mixing it with white of egg and leaving it on overnight as a face mask, a dangerous practice which later spread to Europe by way of Athens and Rome and continued until the end of the 18th century, often resulting in disfigurement and

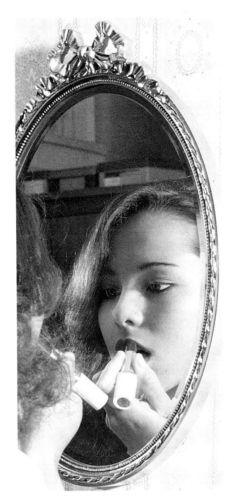

As the Flemish painting (opposite) by an anonymous artist illustrates, beauty has the power to bewitch.

"Mirror, mirror on the wall/ Who's the fairest of them all?" The question has been posed for ages, and for ages women have been looking for the mirror that will answer only "you". The young woman at the left is making up in her mirror just as a Greek woman might have made up in front of the polished bronze mirror (below) five centuries before Christ.

death by poisoning.

Anything at all which would improve the complexion was tried in the search for beauty and allurement, even by men. It is said that Astyages, king of the Medes in about 500 BC, wore a wig of flowing ringlets, darkened his eyes with mascara and coloured his face red by the regular use of henna, whilst Ashurbanipal, king of the Assyrians, had his hair styled like his wife's and adopted female dress, a practice followed today by some men of London and New York.

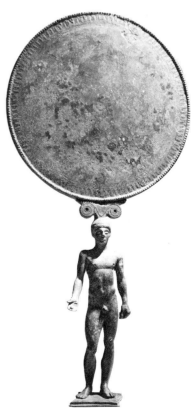

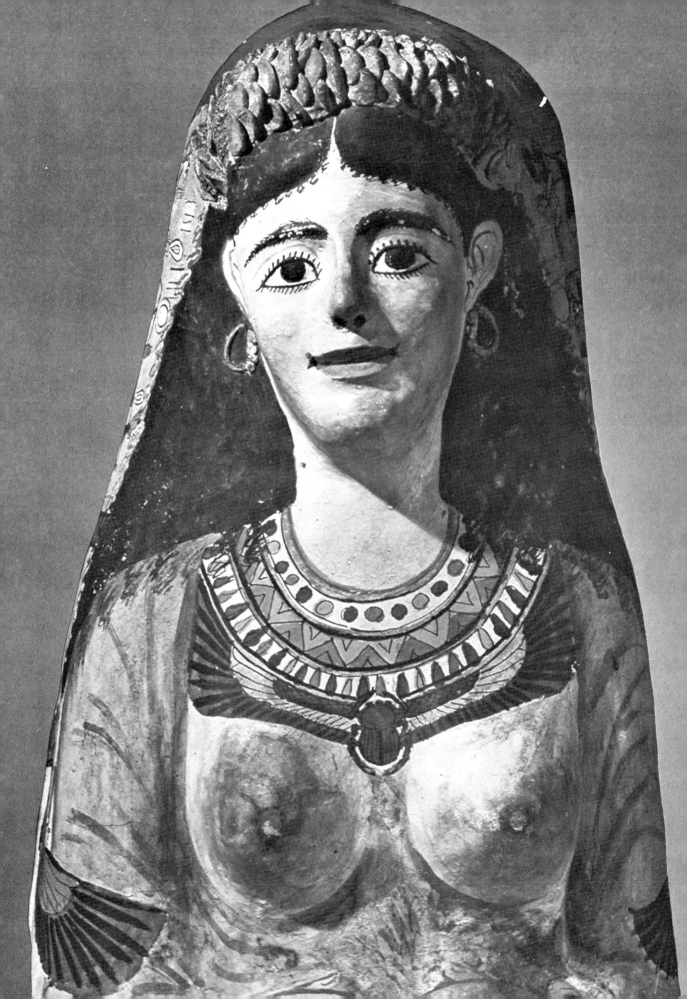

Adornment in the ancient world

The early Egyptians were the first people to take an interest in perfumes and cosmetics. They had acquired a love of cosmetics from earlier people, those of the Mesolithic period who roamed the valley of the Nile some ten to five thousand years before Christ and who painted and anointed their dead not only to sweeten the body but to make it more presentable shading to which modern beauticians devote such attention was made from lapis lazuli. They used ochre to colour the cheeks; carmine for the lips, the same materials they used for their pottery and unguent jars. By about 2000 BC, the Egyptians had come to appreciate all manner of perfumes and cosmetics and began their importation in large quantities.

The noble Egyptian woman, whose death mask is depicted on the opposite page, is made up with the utmost care for her journey in the nether world.

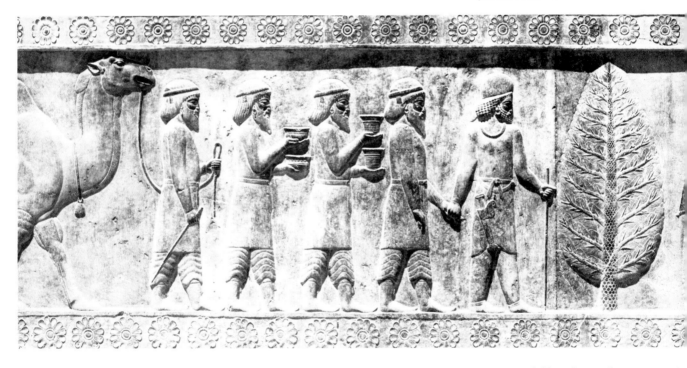

in the next world. On the walls of the tomb of Khum-Lotep at Beni Hassan is a painting dating from 5000 BC, or earlier, which shows guests bringing with them eye paint as a gift for a distinguished person who had died. Various preparations were used for the eyes, which the Egyptians considered to be the most important part of the body. Only minerals were used – black antimony for the eyebrows, kohl for the eyelids, and the green Ointments were generally used to renew the youth of the departed and to maintain appearances in the after-world, in other words, to render the body as attractive in death as in life. For use in the next world, perfumes and unguents were buried with the dead, the fragrant oils to rub into the flesh to maintain its elasticity. This is evidence that the Egyptians went to great lengths to preserve the body and to beautify the features so that

Above, a relief from Persepolis, 6th to 5th century BC, shows a caravan of perfume merchants. Incense or some form of burning aromatic wood has been part of religious observance since earliest recorded history. Precious oils have likewise played their part in the rites of worship.

91

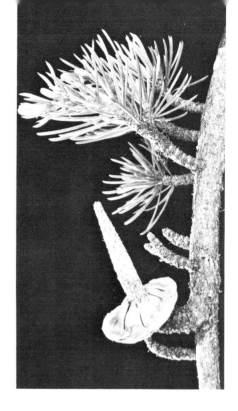

Right, a pine cone of cedar of Lebanon. Cedar had almost mystical properties to the ancient world. Its wood was thought to be indestructible, and was used as incense in religious worship, while the oil was used as a body rub, and is still an ingredient in many expensive cosmetics and perfumes.

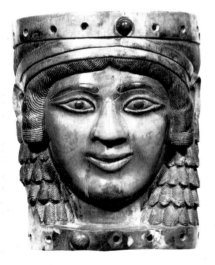

Above, a relief of Ishtar the goddess of War and Love, the potheosis of Vengeful Beauty.

Opposite page, a bas relief of one of the great beauties of all times, Cleopatra. She was queen of Egypt from 40–30 BC when the kingdom, conquered by her countryman Alexander, had already fallen to the Romans. It was through her exquisite beauty, augmented by her lavish use of perfume, that she seduced Mark Antony in the vain hope of recovering her lost territories.

they would endure for all time.

Genesis mentions that the gums and resins were carried into Egypt by Ishmaelite traders who went "from Gilead with their camels, bearing spices and balm and myrrh". Ancient Ishmaelia was then the centre of the important caravan routes which traded spices and aromatics and was situated in the most southerly part of Palestine. It later became the kingdoms of Edom and Moab, now under Jordanian sovereignty.

Jericho was the principal trading post for aromatics, many of which arrived by camel and donkey train from Babylon on the Euphrates. One of the most highly prized substances was spikenard, from the valleys of the West Himalayas, which the caravans would stop to collect at Mari, birthplace of Abraham and the most important city of the East until overrun by the Babylonians in 1700 BC.

From Mari, the caravans would turn westwards, crossing the Syrian Desert by way of the oasis at Palmyra, still important as a watering place for tribesmen and for the oil pipeline that runs through it. From Palmyra the caravans would turn southwards to Damascus. From here, the traders would follow the green valley of the Jordan as far south as Jericho on the northerly shores of the Dead Sea and there unload their precious cargo for the Ishmaelite traders to collect and carry into Egypt by way of Canaan. "Land of Purple" it was called after a dye obtained there from the shellfish Murex, which took on its deep purple colouring only when out of the water, was one of the most important articles of commerce. No caravan train would make the journey into

Egypt without taking a quantity, for it was used to dye the robes of the Egyptian kings and queens, from which time purple became the symbol of royalty the world over.

Here too, in that part of Canaan to the north of the Sea of Galilee, were situated the dense cedar forests of Mount Lebanon, the wood being used by the Egyptians for coffins as they believed that since it was imperishable it would preserve forever anyone enclosed therein. The fragrant wood was also burnt as incense, whilst cedarwood oil was used to rub over the body after bathing to give it elasticity, and was included in many of the most expensive cosmetics and unguents in 1950 BC. It was in order to safeguard the forests and ensure supplies, that Sesostris I had brought Canaan under Egyptian control, setting up a consular office at Tyre, then the most flourishing port of the ancient world.

Ishmaelia was also the terminus of another important spice route taken by the caravans bringing frankincense and myrrh from S Arabia, from the territory of Shacba, now the Yemen, and which was known as the

Incense Road. Here, "in fortunate Arabia", wrote Dionysius, "you can always smell the sweet perfume of marvellous spices, whether it be incense or myrrh", for both grew plentifully in the spice kingdoms of Minaea and Shaeba. Almost daily, the caravans, consisting of large numbers of the finest camels, travelled along the tortuous coastal road of the Red Sea and before reaching Ishmaelia, would have covered more than a thousand miles. It was a journey of great hardship but the cargo was of extreme value, for the spices were much in demand by the Egyptians and also the Assyrians who were used to good living and were prepared to pay well for it.

EGYPTIAN WOMEN AND THEIR TOILET

Both men and women of high rank considered perfume and cosmetics essential accessories though the men only used them for festive occasions. But the women improved their appearance with all manner of cosmetics: indeed, the women of Thebes had toilet boxes and dressing cases filled with bottles and jars containing everything imaginable for beautifying the body.

In the British Museum in London is a beauty box of 1400 BC belonging to Queen Thuthu, which had been buried with her and was removed from her tomb at Thebes. It still contains pumice stone to remove rough skin from her knees and elbows and eye pencils of wood and ivory with which to apply kohl and antimony. With the pencils is a

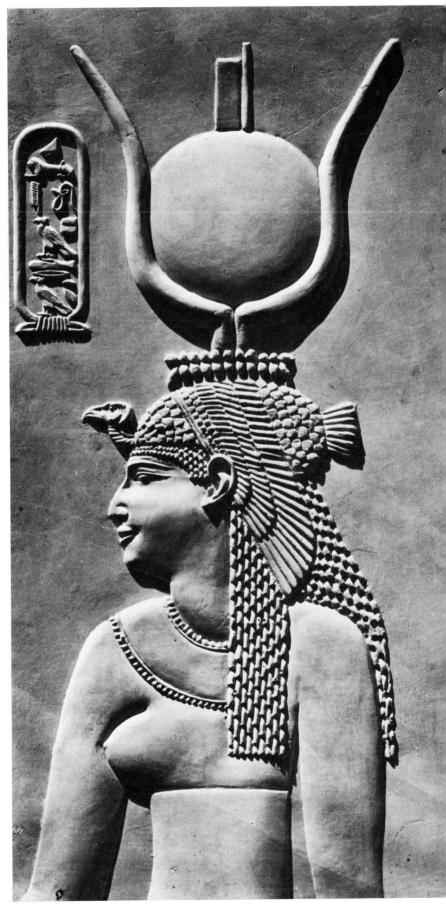

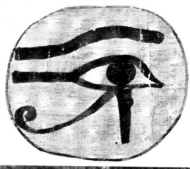

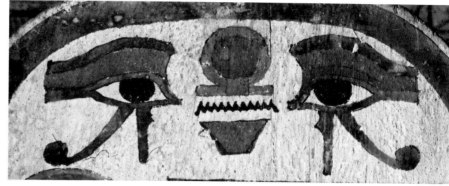

The symbol of the Egyptian sun god Ra-Horus combines images of the sun and the eye. Right, two solar eye symbols with the symbol of eternity between them.

Kohl, used to accentuate the beauty of the eyes for which Egyptian women were famous, was found in the beauty box of every woman of Thebes as it is in modern beauty cases, for "kohl" means something to "brighten the eyes" and any preparation that did so was named "kohl".

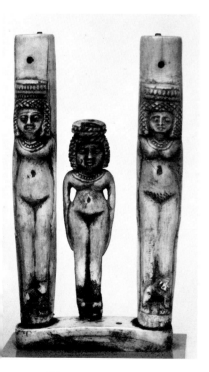

bronze dish used for mixing and putting out the ingredients for shading the eyes. And there are three empty cosmetic pots which might perhaps have contained dried henna leaves to rub on the cheeks for creating a rosy tint and to stain the toe and finger nails red; some women would use henna to give their normally black hair an auburn tint. There would be scented oils made from almonds to massage into the various parts of the body and quince cream for the complexion. There would be talcum powders made from orris root, sandalwood and the roots of lemon grass which grew on the sand-dunes everywhere and olive oil to rub into the hair.

When the tomb of Queen Hetepheres, mother of the Pharoah who built the Pyramids was opened, it was found that she had been provided with thirty alabaster cosmetic jars which contained various unguents to use on all parts of the body in the after-life and with them was a toilet box of cedarwood, which the ancients believed to be imperishable, containing eight other jars.

Cedar was used to make the chest found in the tomb of Tutankhamun and in it was a mirrorbox for use in the after-life.

In the glorious temple of Hatshepsut at Thebes, carved out of the mountain face, there is a painting which shows a lady of high rank going through the daily routine of her toilet. She is attended by four maids, two of whom pour fragrant oil over her body whilst a third massages a shoulder with one hand and with the other, holds a lotus flower for her to smell. A fourth maiden holds a polished copper mirror before her, the metal having been introduced into Egypt by Ammenemes III in about 1800 BC.

The blue-flowered lotus or water lily of the Nile was held to be sacred on account of its blue colour representing the heavens and for its soft delicate perfume. It was the flower of the handsome young Memphis god, Nefertum. In the Book of the Dead discovered in the tomb of King Tutankhamun in the Valley of the Kings, he is shown arising in all his beauty from a blue lotus bud, its long elegant petals pointing to the heavens.

Egyptian women copied the lotus lily for the arrangement of their hair in one of the more popular styles of the New Kingdom period. The hair

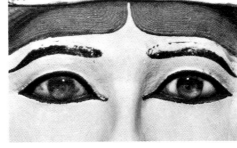

The eyes of Egyptian Princess Nefertiti, known for her adherence to monotheism as well as for her great beauty.

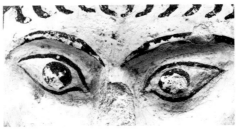

The female eyes from a painted limestone head. The bust is Mycenean, from the 14th to 13th century BC.

was worn long and was worked into small plaits or curls, the well-to-do employing a private hairdresser to attend to the daily ritual. A stone carving at Der-el-Bahari shows one such lady attended by her coiffeuse. She holds in one hand the familiar circular copper mirror with its decorated ivory handle, and in the other she holds a bowl of fragrant oil with which an attendant close-by massages her scalp and sets her hair in the latest style. Wigs were often used and arranged in a similar manner, with the long curls flowing down to the waist.

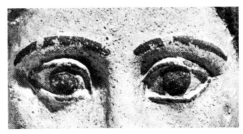

Eyes of a maenad, late 6th century BC of Etruscan provenance.

Huge quantities of aromatics were consumed for every occasion. Food and drinks were perfumed and their fragrance filled the air of every abode. Women bathed in scented water and both men and women used scented unguents to rub into their bodies. Pastilles were eaten to sweeten the breath, and the women of Thebes, said to be the most attractive of the Near East, applied paints and powders to the face. Kohl, a black powder made from antimony, was applied to the eyes to increase the size and brilliance of the pupils. It is still used as a basic ingredient of mascaras. The attractive green-shading on the eyelids was made from powdered lapis lazuli, whilst bangles and necklaces of beads made from scented woods and gums covered the neck and arms.

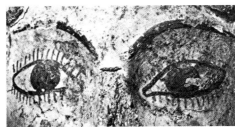

The eyes of a Roman woman.

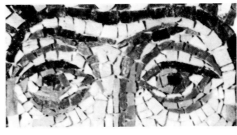

The penetrating gaze of the Empress Theodora is captured in mosaic in Ravenna.

The cosmetics and scented unguents were made in the laboratories of the temples where most of the aromatics brought into the country were stored and were in the care of the priests. They were stored in large jars made of onyx and alabaster to pre-

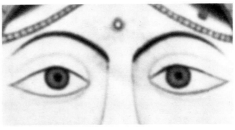

The mystical allure of oriental eyes is evident in this tantra painting. They are the eyes of the Goddess of Speech.

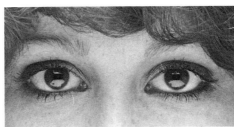

Well made-up eyes are, to our day, a powerful means of allurement.

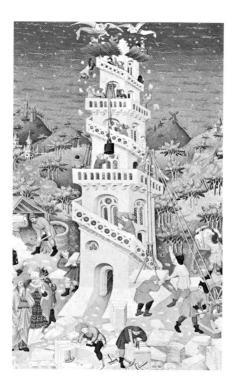

Herodotus, who visited most countries of the Near East during the Hellenistic period around 300 BC, has told in great detail of the temple erected at Babylon in honour of Baal, consisting of seven towers raised one upon another and believed to have been the biblical Tower of Babel. The "tower" was composed of seven squares, the sides of the base being 290 feet long and according to Herodotus, in the uppermost part was an ornate couch occupied by a woman lavishly attired and redolent with perfumes and covered with cosmetics and chosen by the god for his own pleasure.

To the Assyrians, care of the hair and beard was of greatest importance and both sexes used large amounts of fragrant oils and pomades to massage into the scalp and would then spend hours plaiting the curls which fell on their shoulders and the men their beards. The wealthy had gold thread interwoven in their hair and beards.

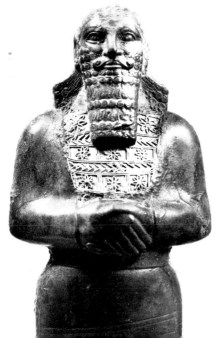

vent their evaporation. One of these laboratories can be identified in the great temple at Edfu on the left bank of the Nile, sixty miles south of Luxor. It was built by Ptolemy III in 237 BC and dedicated to Horus, god of the sky, who was the son of Isis and Osiris. On the walls of a room there in almost complete darkness, where the aromatics were stored away from the direct rays of the sun, are numerous inscriptions which reveal the manner in which unguents and perfumes and ritual oils were made, the most subtle perfumes taking up to six months to concoct and mature.

At Heliopsis, city of the sun, where the fiery orb was worshipped under the name of Re, incense was burnt thrice daily: resinous gums with the rising of the deity; myrrh when in the meridian; and a concotion of sixteen herbs and resins at the setting. This was known as Kyphi or Kyphri and was the most expensive of all offerings. Plutarch said that it was composed of "those things that delight most in the night", from which it would appear that it was also burnt at the setting of the sun in the homes of the wealthy.

PERFUMES OF ANCIENT EGYPT

Democrates, who visited Egypt when Cleopatra ruled as queen, declared that at this time the Egyptians were masters in the art of perfumery and cosmetics. It was during this period in Egypt's history the Egyptians became familiar with the art of floral extraction as depicted on the walls at Edfu. A relief there shows perfume being distilled from flowers of the Madonna Lily, and a floral perfume, green in colour, was to be obtained from the flowers of henna or camphire. It was known as Cyprinum and was heavy and lasting. It was Cleopatra's favourite perfume and was used to drench the sails of the royal barges on the Nile during festive occasions.

Another of the royal perfumes was the unguent Medesium composed of oil of ben, cinnamon and myrrh. Cinnamon was found in the valleys of Sikkim and Nepal and the fragrant bark would have been transported by donkey or mule, together with the hairy roots of spikenard, to meet the caravan trains which left Babylon for Mari. The same substances were used to make the unguent known as metopium which in addition contained honey, wine and almond oil. It was rubbed onto the feet and legs and made an excellent complexion cream, keeping the skin soft and smooth. Since 202 BC when the Roman armies defeated Hannibal at Carthage to become undisputed leaders of the

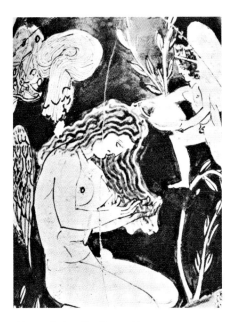

Above, Aphrodite, the goddess of love and beauty, is having her sumptuous locks anointed with precious oil in this detail from a Greek amphora.

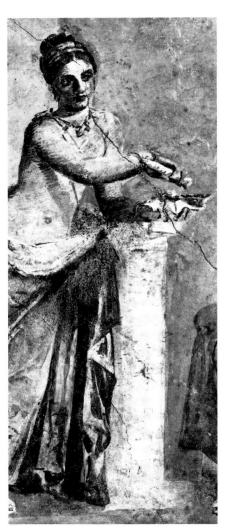

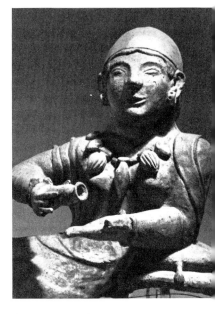

Above centre, a Roman matron prepares for the bath. For the Romans bathing was more than simply a matter of hygiene or physical fitness; it was a veritable social and cultural event.

Above right, the Etruscans were especially adept at the decorative arts, no less so when it came to decorating their own faces.

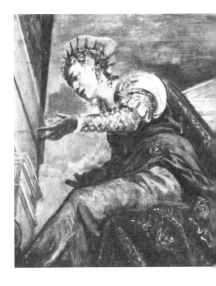

Mediterranean, they began to import large quantities of aromatics into Italy for their personal requirements. In their use, they outdid the Greeks who had begun to appreciate the aromatics of the East shortly after Alexander's campaigns had opened the way for their importation. Though the East supplied the Athenians with valuable gums and resins from Arabia and Babylon, they added to the fragrant plants already in use there which abounded in southern Europe. Amongst these were lavender and rosemary, thyme and marjoram which were used to maintain the hair in a healthy condition and when dried and mixed with orris root, were ground into talcum powders and applied to clothing and to the body after washing.

PERFUMES AND COSMETICS OF ANCIENT GREECE AND ROME

The Greeks ascribed a divine origin to scented flowers and leaves. In Greek mythology, the invention of perfumes is attributed to the gods, and according to ancient beliefs, men derived their knowledge of them from Aeone, a nymph of Venus. It was believed that if the Olympian gods were to honour anyone with a visit, they would leave behind a sweet perfume as a token of their divinity. The Greeks began to use aromatics on a lavish scale following Alexander's conquests of the Near East which he had completed by 330 BC. According to Theophrastus, who was living at that time, aromatics reached Athens by way of the

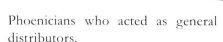

The skill and precious materials lavished on the accoutrements of cosmetics throughout the ancient world are proof of the value with which they were held. Shown on these pages is a variety of make-up spoons and containers from ancient Egypt.

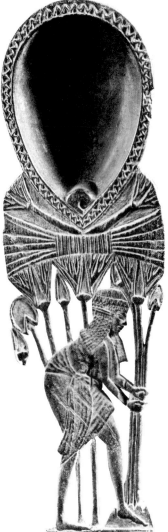

Phoenicians who acted as general distributors.

The name of a perfume usually took that of its maker. Thus Megaleion was the invention of Megallus, a renowned maker of perfumes and cosmetics in Athens at the time of Alexander, who asked high prices for his products. Amongst the ingredients used in his preparations were the celebrated oil of balanos famous for its rejuvenating qualities; and myrrh, cassia, cinnamon and various resins.

Another of the popular perfumes of Athens was susinum which Pliny, in his *Natural History*, tells was made from lilies. He gives its composition as follows: oil of ben, an odourless oil obtained from the seeds of the Moringa tree, which did not turn rancid however long it was kept; otto or attar of roses, cinnamon, myrrh and saffron. Another favourite perfume was crocinum which was made almost entirely from saffron and oil of ben. Megaleion also possessed healing properties and warriors from

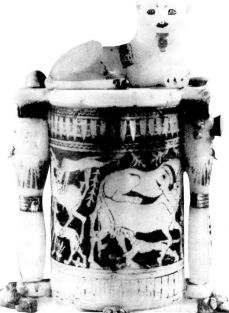

wealthy families would rub it into wounds received in battle.

Because many of the Grecian perfumes contained similar ingredients, their inventors coloured them so that they would be more easily distinguished. Megallus used alkanet root to colour his perfume pink and from the plant made a rouge to apply to the cheeks, whilst rose perfumes were tinted red, the colour of the red rose.

Antiphanes mentions another expensive perfume known as "Egyptian", made from a recipe imported during Alexander's conquests from Egypt where it had been one of the more fashionable perfumes during the reign of Tutankhamen. It contained cinnamon and myrrh and was said to keep its strength longer than any other with the possible exception of iris, the chief ingredient of which was orris root. Theophrastus, who wrote a treatise on perfumes and cosmetics during Alexander's time and who has been described as the Father of Botany for he had a knowledge of plants unrivalled in his time, told that a perfumer known to him in Athens, kept "Egyptian" in his shop for eight years and "Iris" for twenty, at the end of which time they were "better than when freshly made". Theophrastus mentions that perfumed powders were sprinkled about the bed and came into contact with the skin at night. "In this way", he wrote, "the perfume gets a better hold and is more lasting. And men use it thus instead of applying it to their body directly". He was familiar with most plants used in perfumery and considered that "the most fragrant came from Asia and the sunny regions", meaning Egypt and

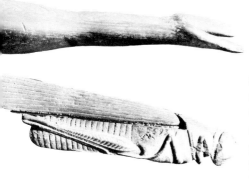

Arabia. "From Europe", he wrote, "came none except the iris (orris)".

What the Egyptians developed, the Athenians perfected. The high reputation of the perfumers of Athens is referred to in the writings of Athenaeus. "From Argos", he wrote, "come the best cauldrons; from Phlius, the best wine; from Corinth, tapestry; from Sicily, cheese. The best eels come from Boeotia but the best perfumes are made in Athens". Though the philosophers condemned their use as effeminate, perfumes and cosmetics came to be more and more used by both men and women.

GREEK MAIDENS AND THEIR TOILET

In the Metamorphoses, Ovid has described the toilet preparations of a Greek maiden of the time: "her hair is smoothed with a comb; now she decks herself with rosemary (perhaps meaning rosemary water which is one of the best of hair conditioners); sometimes she wears white lilies; she washes her face twice daily in springs which trickle from the top of Pegasean woods; and twice she dips her body in the stream".

During Alexander's time, Greek women rolled their hair and tied it into a knot at the back of the head, in a style known as "korymbos", a golden clasp being used for ornamentation. In the "strophos" style, the hair was allowed to fall upon the shoulders in ringlets but in some parts of Greece, the hair was allowed to grow long only during mourning. In the "mitra" style, the hair was held in place by a perfumed and powdered cloth band tied round the head, fragrant oils were massaged into the hair which in a sun-drenched land, prevented the hair becoming dry and falling out.

The powder of Medea rested on her skill as a perfumer and on her ability to turn grey hair black by employing a vegetable dye. She also was known to take men into her home who were suffering from rheumatic pains. After removing their clothes, they would stand in a cauldron filled with water placed over a charcoal fire, while the ensuing steam eased their stiff and tired muscles.

As there was an element of danger in it, she became notorious for her practices and magical powers of improving one's health and appearance, though all she did was to invent the so-called Turkish bath which was later to be superseded by the sauna. A new fashion was to bathe their faces in rose water and paint their cheeks with red colouring obtained from a root called poederos, similar to alkanet which was used by northern women. Greek maidens would use it to paint their lips red and with an ivory bodkin would apply the scented soot of gum labdanum or antimony to their eyelids. After throwing the gum, which would most likely have been collected in Crete or Cyprus, onto a charcoal fire,

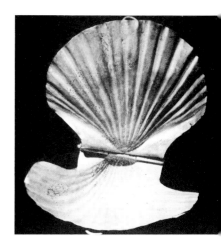

The seated woman doing her hair is probably a bride. She holds a mirror in her hand and there is a perfume jar hanging behind her. The Greeks inherited from the Egyptians the taste for perfumes and brought it to perfection.

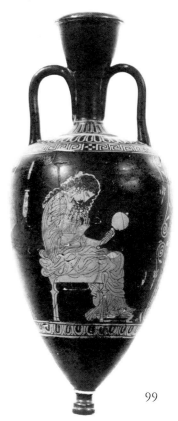

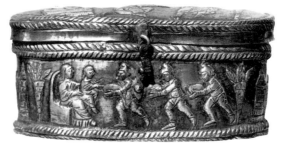

Above, a silver Byzantine cosmetic box of the 5th century AD with embossed the offerings of the Three Kings. Below, a double-potted make-up jar of Etruscan provenance.

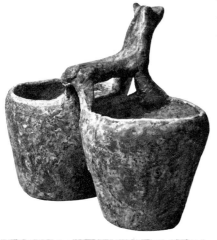

they would collect the ascending smoke as soot on a plate held above the flame. They would apply it by closing one eye, taking the lashes between finger and thumb, and rubbing.

Modern mascara, which contains wax instead of gum to make it adhere to the lashes is applied in exactly the same way.

PERFUMES AND COSMETICS OF ANCIENT ROME

The perfumes and cosmetics so popular with the Greeks soon became fashionable in Rome. However, it was only after the Roman conquest of Egypt, N Africa and the Near East, and also of their own country, with the annexation of the provinces of southern Italy then held

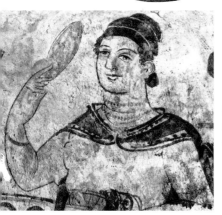

Above, a woman looking at herself in a hand-held mirror from an Osco-Campanian tomb painting and, right, the back of an Etruscan mirror, showing Paris's judgement.

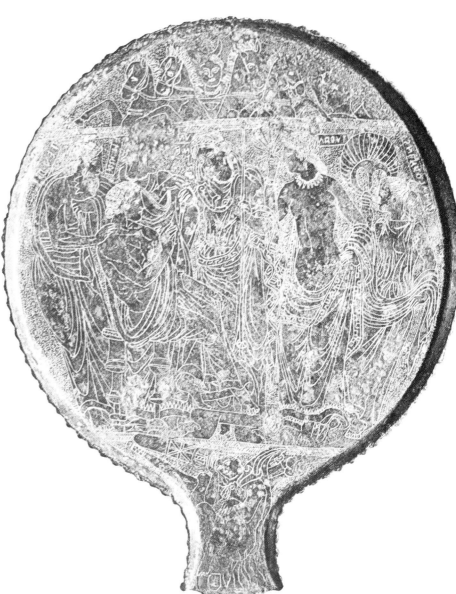

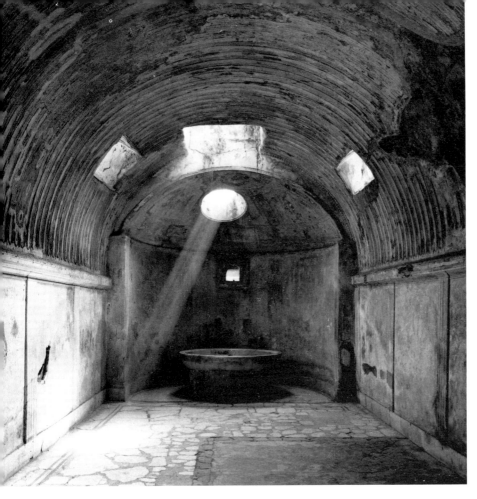

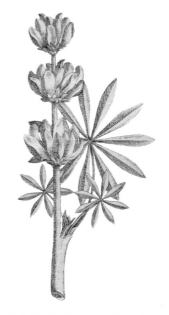

by the Greeks in the name of Magna Graecia, that perfumes and cosmetics came into daily use. Capua became the centre of the industry; it is said that the main street there was occupied solely by perfumers and makers of cosmetics. Here, as in Athens, the well-to-do would meet each morning to try the various preparations and discuss the affairs of the day.

Pliny has told of various cosmetics in use at the time. The Romans dyed their hair black with St. John's wort, myrtle and walnut husks, walnut oil being such an excellent preparation that it is still in use at modern hair salons. Myrtle and juniper berries were prescribed for baldness whilst fragrant plants were macerated in bear's grease and rubbed into the hair to prevent it becoming dry and falling out.

It was the custom of Roman women to darken their eyes with kohl, whilst rouge, obtained from alkanet root, or carmine, was rubbed onto the cheeks. To colour the hair blond, either quince or lemon juice mixed with the distilled water of privet flowers, was popular. Indeed, so great was the use of cosmetics in ancient Rome that Ovid wrote a treatise on their uses including some interesting preparations. Although only a fragment of the work remains, it is still in daily use. He borrowed the word he used to describe the adornment of the body, *kosmetikos*, from the Greek. It means a person "skilled in personal decoration". To remove blemishes from the skin, Ovid suggests the Egyptian treatment of steeping lupin seeds in water and applying it to the face and other affected parts. But for a more drastic cure, he advises pounding lupin seeds which have been roasted with broad beans and orris root and making it into a paste after mixing it with honey.

Left, the Calidarium of the Thermae, the public baths of Pompei. The Lupinus, above and the Myrtle (below) were two plants the Romans used respectively to remove blemishes from the skin and as a treatment against baldness.

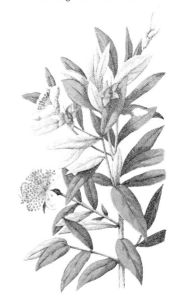

A NATURAL BEAUTY
CHEST
The plants on the opposite
page and following are
grouped according to their
application. The Lexicon of
plants, on page 25, lists all the
plants mentioned for use in
this book alphabetically,
according to their Latin name.
A Key to the Lexicon, giving
the common names of the
plants with the Latin names
beside them is provided on
pages 28–29.

In about 450 BC, Ticinus Menias, a native of Sicily, introduced the practice of shaving, establishing a chain of barber shops in Rome, one being near the temple of Hercules. Here, the elite of Rome called for a daily shave which was performed with a razor made of sharpened bronze. Afterwards, the sore face would be covered with hot towels and then massaged with scented unguents. The hair was then washed and treated with perfumed pomade, susinon being the most popular. It was made to a Greek prescription which included saffron and calamus. Nardinum, made from myrrh and spikenard, was also popular. Horace mentioned that an onyx jar of the ointment was worth the value of a cadus of wine.

BATHING AND TOILET PREPARATIONS

In his golden palace, the ruins of which are to be seen near the Colosseum in Rome, Nero installed warm baths. Fed by Mediterranean waters and perfumed with bay and rosemary leaves, the baths had concealed pipes which sprinkled scented waters on the emperor and his friends as they sat at table.

The Romans were the world's greatest bathers, not only appreciating the cleansing powers of warm water but also its health-giving qualities. The baths or *thermae* of ancient Rome became the centre of the city's social life. The finest were erected by the Emperor Caracalla in about AD 220 and were large enough to accommodate 2000 bathers, each of whom was provided with a seat of

polished marble. Before entering the warm spring baths, the bathers, having undressed and handed over their clothes to the care of the *capsarii*, would wash in the cold water of the *frigidarium*, then would go to the *unctuarium* to receive a massage of cheap scented oil. It was here too, that the bathers returned after their warm bath, to be scraped with a *strigil* and again massaged with oil, these duties being perfomed by the *aliptor*. The bather would then go into a separate room, a kind of gymnasium, to do simple exercises to tone up the muscles, and would leave completely refreshed and with a sense of well being.

Though there was a separate room for women, few bathed in public, preferring the privacy of the home where the wealthy were attended by numerous slaves known as *cosmatae*, who were in turn overseen by the *ornatrix*, the mistress of the toilet. Each performed a given task in order, beginning with the hair which was styled and dyed if necessary and then treated with fragrant oils. The face was then massaged with more oils, the cheeks rouged, the eyes shaded with kohl. Finally the neck and shoulders were massaged with fragrant oils and the rest of the body washed in rose water.

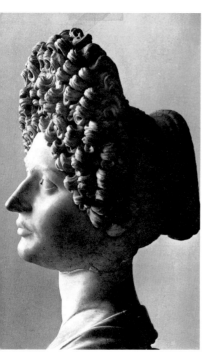

A bust of Titus' daughter, indicating the fashion among Roman women to curl their hair in tight coils. This fashion returned in the French Empire style of the 19th century.

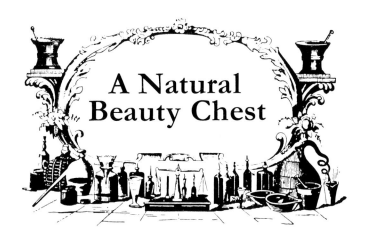

A Natural Beauty Chest

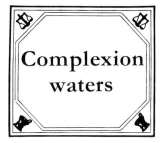

Complexion waters

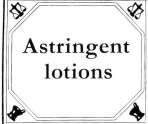

Astringent lotions

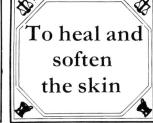

To heal and soften the skin

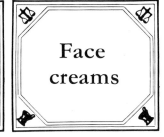

Face creams

Complexion waters	Astringent lotions	To heal and soften the skin	Face creams
23 BIRCH	157 BENZOIN	87 BAY	9 ALMOND
171 BROOKLIME	36 CORNFLOWER	99 CAJUPUT	119 AVOCADO
34 CARAWAY	147 ELDER	38 CARRAGEEN MOSS	104 BENJAMIN
146 CLARY	154 GOLDEN ROD	35 CEDARWOOD	49 CARNAUBA WAX
159 COSTMARY	112 GROUND IVY	156 CHICKWEED	47 COCONUT PALM
132 COWSLIP	77 HOP	78 COMMON ST. JOHN'S WORT	124 COMMON PLANTAIN
17 CUCKOO-PINT	60 HORSETAIL		159 COSTMARY
39 FEVERFEW	5 LADY'S MANTLE	6 GARLIC	132 COWSLIP
69 FUMITORY	139 LESSER CELANDINE	20 GUM TRAGACANTH	52 CUCUMBER
154 GOLDEN ROD	48 LILY OF THE VALLEY	55 HOUND'S TONGUE	46 HORSERADISH
112 GROUND IVY	91 MADONNA LILY	8 MARSHMALLOW	91 MADONNA LILY
46 HORSERADISH	153 POTATO	117 PELLITORY-OF-THE-WALL	28 MARIGOLD
60 HORSETAIL	133 PRIMROSE	90 PRIVET	8 MARSHMALLOW
48 LILY OF THE VALEY	144 ROSEMARY	164 RED CLOVER	114 OLIVE
163 LIME TREE	151 ROSE-ROOT	148 SANICLE	133 PRIMROSE
115 MARJORAM	167 STINGING NETTLE	15 SOUTHERNWOOD	137 QUINCE
65 MEADOWSWEET	37 SWEET FERN	74 SUNFLOWER	166 RED ELM
117 PELLITORY-OF-THE-WALL	92 TOAD FLAX	2 SWEET FLAG	118 SCENTED-LEAF GERANIUM
97 PURPLE LOOSESTRIFE	83 WALNUT	160 TANSY	152 SESAME
29 RAMPION	73 WITCH HAZEL	85 WILD LETTUCE	92 TOADFLAX
10 SCARLET PIMPERNEL	96 YELLOW LOOSESTRIFE		131 TORMENTIL
129 SOLOMON'S SEAL	50 CORIANDER		172 VIOLET
155 SOWTHISTLE			106 WAX MYRTLE
160 TANSY			165 WHEAT
110 WATERCRESS			73 WITCH HAZEL
18 WOODRUFF			96 YELLOW LOOSESTRIFE
86 YELLOW ARCHANGEL			

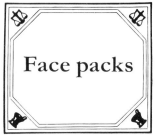

Face packs

76 BARLEY
56 CARROT
21 OAT
166 RED ELM
68 SEA KELP
67 STRAWBERRY
95 TOMATO
165 WHEAT

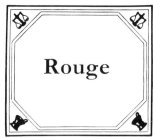

Rouge

11 ALKANET
33 SAFFLOWER

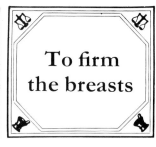

To firm the breasts

5 LADY'S MANTLE
113 NUTMEG PLANT

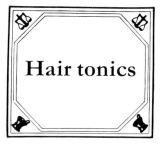

Hair tonics

14 ARNICA
120 BAY RUM
27 BOX
41 CASSIA
13 CHAMOMILE
47 COCONUT PALM
55 HOUND'S TONGUE
88 LAVENDER
45 LEMON
115 MARJORAM
114 OLIVE
116 PANDANG
117 PELLITORY-OF-THE-WALL
144 ROSEMARY
15 SOUTHERNWOOD
167 STINGING NETTLE
170 VERVAIN
16 WORMWOOD

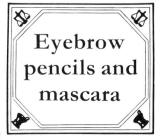

Eyebrow pencils and mascara

141 CASTOR OIL PLANT
20 GUM TRAGACANTH
149 SANDALWOOD

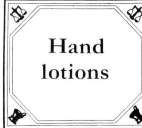

Hand lotions

38 CARRAGEEN MOSS
117 PELLITORY-OF-THE-WALL
74 SUNFLOWER

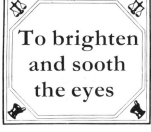

To brighten and sooth the eyes

4 AGRIMONY
145 CLARY
124 COMMON PLANTAIN
36 CORNFLOWER
147 ELDER
64 EYEBRIGHT
66 FENNEL
112 GROUND IVY
28 MARIGOLD
8 MARSHMALLOW
65 MEADOWSWEET
100 MELILOT
97 PURPLE LOOSESTRIFE
40 SUCCORY
131 TORMENTIL
170 VERVAIN

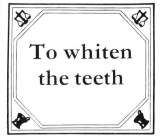

To whiten the teeth

136 BLACKTHORN
102 MINT
123 PISTACIA
67 STRAWBERRY

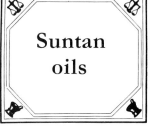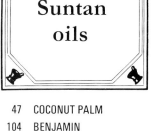

Suntan oils

47 COCONUT PALM
104 BENJAMIN
152 SESAME

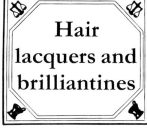

Hair lacquers and brilliantines

104 BENJAMIN
49 CARNAUBA WAX
141 CASTOR OIL PLANT
103 CHAMPAC
47 COCONUT PALM
149 SANDALWOOD
79 STAR ANISE
30 YLANG-YLANG

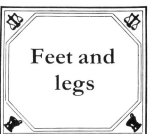

Feet and legs

14 ARNICA
87 BAY
115 MARJORAM
51 SAFFRON

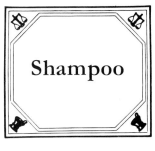

Shampoo

120 BAY RUM
34 CARAWAY
13 CHAMOMILE
47 COCONUT PALM
115 MARJORAM

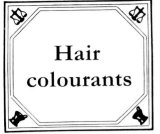

Hair colourants

- 89 HENNA
- 169 MULLEIN
- 97 PURPLE LOOSESTRIFE
- 51 SAFFRON
- 145 SAGE
- 162 THYME
- 83 WALNUT

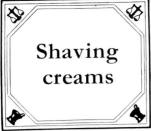

Shaving creams

- 106 WAX MYRTLE

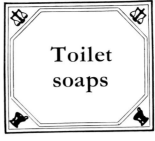

Toilet soaps

- 121 ALLSPICE
- 108 BALSAM OF PERU
- 130 BALSAM POPLAR
- 87 BAY
- 25 BOLDO
- 34 CARAWAY
- 54 CITRONELLA
- 63 CLOVE
- 102 MINT
- 22 MYRRH
- 107 NUTMEG
- 122 PINE
- 130 SASSAFRAS
- 118 SCENTED-LEAF GERANIUM
- 79 STAR ANISE
- 71 WINTERGREEN
- 18 WOODRUFF

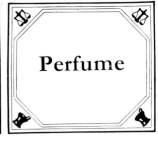

Perfume

- 1 ACACIA
- 121 ALLSPICE
- 108 BALSAM OF PERU
- 130 BALSAM POPLAR
- 157 BENZOIN
- 23 BIRCH
- 25 BOLDO
- 99 CAJUPUT
- 32 CANELLA
- 57 CARNATION
- 41 CASSIA
- 103 CHAMPAC
- 54 CITRONELLA
- 142 DAMASK ROSE
- 31 ELEMI
- 125 FRANGIPANI
- 26 FRANKINCENSE
- 75 HELIOTROPE
- 82 JASMINE
- 109 JONQUIL
- 42 LABDANUM
- 88 LAVENDER
- 62 LEMON GUM TREE
- 158 LILAC
- 140 MIGNONETTE
- 22 MYRRH
- 44 NEROLI
- 31 ORRIS
- 116 PANDANG
- 123 PISTACIA
- 149 SANDALWOOD
- 150 SASSAFRAS
- 93 SWEET GUM
- 58 TONQUIN
- 128 TUBEROSE
- 168 VANILLA
- 172 VIOLET
- 30 YLANG-YLANG

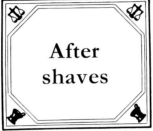

After shaves

- 50 CORIANDER
- 147 ELDER
- 102 MINT
- 122 PINE
- 166 RED ELM
- 144 ROSEMARY

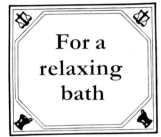

For a relaxing bath

- 101 BALM
- 87 BAY
- 145 CLARY
- 3 HORSE CHESTNUT
- 115 MARJORAM
- 102 WATERMINT, PEPPERMINT SPEARMINT
- 122 PINE
- 137 QUINCE
- 144 ROSEMARY
- 110 WATERCRESS

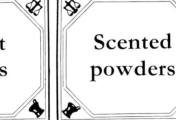

Toilet waters

- 12 ANGELICA
- 101 BALM
- 50 CORIANDER
- 159 COSTMARY
- 115 MARJORAM
- 100 MELILOT
- 44 NEROLI
- 90 PRIVET
- 143 RED ROSE
- 144 ROSEMARY
- 151 ROSE-ROOT
- 51 SAFFRON
- 129 SOLOMON'S SEAL
- 2 SWEET FLAG

Scented powders

- 25 BOLDO
- 32 CANELLA
- 35 CEDARWOOD
- 63 CLOVE
- 7 GALANGA
- 113 NUTMEG PLANT
- 81 ORRIS
- 126 PATCHOULI
- 2 SWEET FLAG
- 58 TONQUIN
- 53 ZEDOARY

Body lotions and deodorants

- 14 ARNICA
- 140 MIGNONETTE
- 169 MULLEIN
- 144 ROSEMARY
- 162 THYME

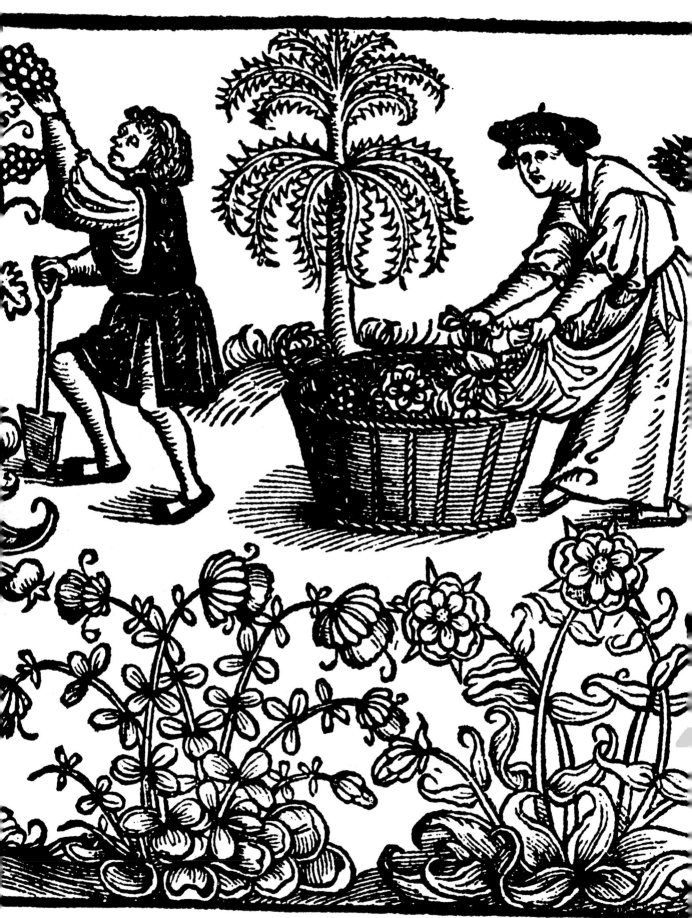

Nature's beauty parlour

Reference Section II
A closer look at the plants for cosmetics and natural health. The following pages present a breakdown of the 172 plants examined in this book: the specific parts that are used, with the contents (active principles) and effects as beauty aids. The reader learns how and when to harvest, gather and store the plants. The following abbreviations are used:

 wax/gum

 fruit/berry

 leaf

 flower

 wood

 whole plant

 seaweed

 nut

 bark

 seeds

 rind

 stem

 tuber

roots

bulb

The synoptic table in the preceding pages allows you to find immediately the plants for a specific cosmetic use.

Opposite, Garden scene. Woodcut from the title page of *The grete herball*, London 1526. Right, Early Middle Age woodcut showing a convent's herb garden.

Make-up has had a multitude of uses throughout history. Men used it as a form of disguise to frighten off enemies, or perhaps to search for wives; women used it to frighten away illness and, later, to attract members of the opposite sex. Throughout history, too, plants and natural preparations obtained from the soil have provided all that is necessary to beautify the features and to protect the skin against drying wind and sun.

For example, the cucumber, native of the Near East and the avocado of the New World provide the skin with nourishment in the form of vitamins.

From earliest times, roots such as orris root, dried and ground to a fine powder, were used in dusting and face powders. The tuberous root of kapurkadri is also dried to use in dusting powders. The roots of rhatany are included in dentifrice powders.

The extracts of nuts and seeds are included in complexion milks and face creams. Almonds have been used from earliest times in Eastern beauty preparations; for along with olive oil there is nothing more soothing to the skin nor a better source of essential foods for the complexion. So that they will keep longer without turning rancid, a few drops of alcoholic tincture of benzoin, obtained from the resin of the shrub styrax benzoin, should be added to creams.

Oil extracted from the large fruits of the coconut palm is included in shampoos and soaps, also in face creams, for it is soothing and nourishing. Sesame seed and oil is used in sun-tan lotions for it provides excellent protection from the sun's harmful rays.

To colour and condition the hair, the dried and powdered leaves of henna have been used since earliest times, to give the hair a deep auburn tint. Henna is still used in modern hair salons as a dye and conditioner. As a colouring agent, it coats the hair without penetration and is safer to use than chemical dyes. Walnuts, sage and box leaves are natural dyes to colour the hair black, whilst mullein and purple loosestrife will impart a glamorous golden tint to the hair and leave it smooth and silky.

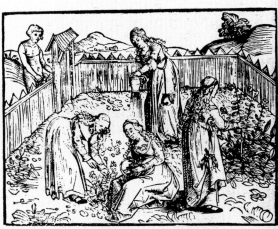

For the eyes, clary and eyebright, weeds of hedgerow and waste ground, are used in modern eye lotions and gels, to impart a sparkle to tired eyes and to take away inflammation.

Plant	Part used	Components and effects	Harvesting and further processing
AGRIMONY 4		Cleanses the blood and clears skin blemishes.	The fresh flowers and leaves are gathered between May and late August.
ALKANET 11		The red dye extracted from the roots is used in rouges.	The plant is lifted at the end of summer and a red dye extracted from the cleaned roots with spirits of wine.
ALLSPICE 121		Its essential oil, which has a clove-like smell, is used with other oils to make eastern perfume.	The berries (fruits) are gathered late in summer whilst green and unripe, their drying completed in an open shed or airy room. From them, an extract is obtained for use in "bouquets", after treating with rectified spirit.
ALMOND 9		The juice and meal of the nuts is healing and soothing to the skin and is included in face creams and emulsions.	It blooms early, the nuts being gathered from mid-summer until autumn. When expressed the nuts yield a pale yellow, odourless oil and when pounded in water yield a milky juice.
ANGELICA 12		The root is distilled and used to make the celebrated carmelite water. The seeds are burnt over a low fire to fumigate apartments.	From cuts made in the stems early in summer, a resinous liquid is obtained to use in soaps and as a perfumed fixative. From the ripe seeds, collected late in summer, a fragrant toilet water is obtained.
ANNATTO 24		The pulp surrounding the seeds makes an orange-red dye used to colour lipsticks.	The fruit capsules are removed late in summer and autumn and placed in vats (or bowls) of water, when the orange coloured pulp rises to the surface.
APPLE 98		The juice with malt vinegar makes an excellent hair rinse, imparting a golden tint to fair hair.	Fruits are gathered late summer and in autumn and are peeled and cored and put through a blender to extract the juice. The fruits will store for several months in a dark, airy room and the juice will keep several weeks under refrigeration.
APRICOT 134		The fruit, put through a blender, makes a nourishing face mask for a dry skin.	It blooms early and the ripe fruit is ready to gather mid-summer to early autumn.
ARNICA 14		The root yields tincture of arnica. A few drops in warm water will relieve tired and sore feet.	The roots are lifted in late summer and after cleaning and slicing are treated with rectified spirit of tincture of arnica.
AVOCADO 119		Known for its high vitamin E content, the pulp is now used in the best skin foods.	The pear-shaped fruits are harvested as they ripen almost the whole year. After removing the stone (drupe) put through a blender or squeeze out the oil.
BALM 101		Used in toilet waters, relaxing baths and pot-pourri, it is the main ingredient of Carmelite water.	Fresh leaves are gathered between early June and late summer and placed in a still or kettle to distill.
BALSAM OF PERU 108		It has no connection with Peru being found in the wild only on the Balsam Coast of El Salvador. It gives a pleasant smell and creamy lather to soap. Balsam of Tolu is obtained from another species. It has a vanilla scent and gives permanence to alcoholic perfumes.	The resin is collected late summer from incisions made in the trunk so as to remove strips of bark. Cotton rags are inserted to collect the resin and are then placed in large jars, boiling water being poured over them. Resin rises to the surface and is collected.
BALSAM POPLAR 130		The gum extracted from the buds with spirit of wine is used as a fixative for perfumes and to flavour toilet soap.	The resin is extracted from the buds with spirits of wine. They are removed in spring before they open and placed in a large jar. Shake daily for a month and collect the resinous tincture by straining.
BANANA 105		The near-ripe fruit is used as a face mask to rid the skin of blemishes and leave it soft and smooth.	After removing the yellow skin, pulp the pith and mix with yoghurt.

Plant	Part used	Components and effects	Harvesting and further processing
BARLEY 76		Uncooked barley (ground) used as a face pack, removes blemishes from the skin and as beer, makes an efficient setting lotion for the hair.	The green ears are cut in mid-summer. Ripe corn cut in late summer is ground into meal. It can be stored through winter.
BAY LAUREL 87		Used in relaxing baths and pot-pourri. The leaves in a warm bath relax and tone the body as they did for Roman legions.	The fresh leaves and berries are collected between mid-summer and late autumn when the oil is most prolific.
BENJAMIN 104		Its seeds yield oil of Ben used in pomades and hair oils as it is tasteless, odourless and does not go rancid with age.	The pods are gathered during the last six months of the year and the seeds extracted, to be used freshly gathered.
BENZOIN 157		Like Storax, it "holds" the flower perfumes, giving them permanence. It is the resin from the inner barks which is used.	The resin is collected by incisions made in the bark. Oil is also obtained by boiling the bark. It is odourless and soluble in alcohol.
BLACKTHORN 136		A decoction of the leaves rubbed on the gums firms them and tightens the teeth.	The fruit (sloes) is gathered in later summer and boiled in an equal amount of water. After straining, the syrup thickens and is used as a substitute for gum acacia.
BOLDO 25		From all parts of the tree fragrant oil is obtained and the berries are dried and used as scented beads by the women of Chile.	It is evergreen and the bark, twigs and leaves are collected throughout the year and dried in the sun; as are the pea-size fruits.
BOXWOOD 27		John Wesley, founder of the Methodist church, said a decoction of the leaves rubbed onto the scalp was the best of all hair restorers. Modern science has proved him right for the leaves contain 'buxine" which stimulates the hair nerves.	The freshly gathered evergreen leaves and wood shavings are boiled in water at any time of the year.
BROOKLIME 171		Clears the blood and skin of impurities.	The plant is used fresh in summer.
CAJUPUT 99		The aromatic oil obtained from the leaves and twigs is mixed with olive oil to improve the complexion.	The leaves and twigs are collected from October to June and the oil obtained by distillation.
CANDLEBERRY 106		A shrub of Louisiana and New Brunswick, the berries are covered with a white wax. It is removed by scalding and made into scented candles.	The berries are removed in late summer and placed in vats or bowls of boiling water to melt the wax which is skimmed off.
CANELLA 32		The dried and ground bark is used in talcum powders.	The trees are beaten with sticks during late summer to remove the grey bark which is dried in the shade. The undried bark is distilled.
CARAWAY 34		Used in scented soaps and in sachets to put amongst clothes.	Seeds are collected late in summer and distilled.
CARRAGEEN MOSS 38		The glutinous material from soaking the fronds is used in face packs and cleans and heals the skin. It makes a soothing hand cream.	It is a seaweed and is collected on the seashore. After washing, it is soaked for 2 hours in water, then boiled in milk to release its mucilage. The seaweed can be dried in the open and ground to a powder to use as required.
CARROT 56		The roots, after pulping, make a valuable face mask, ridding the skin of blemishes and leaving it soft and smooth.	The roots are lifted at the end of summer and after cleaning are put through a blender. The roots can be kept in boxes of peat or sand in a frost free room to use in winter.
CASSIE 1		From the bark and leaves a sweet-smelling oil is obtained (oil of cassie) which is massaged into the hair and keeps it dark and oily, preventing baldness. (Cassie oil is used in barber's shops everywhere).	The yellow flowers open in spring and early summer in long succession and the scent is extracted by enfleurage.

Plant	Part used	Components and effects	Harvesting and further processing
CASTOR OIL PLANT 141		The oil (with lanolin) makes an effective lip salve and with beeswax, an eyebrow pencil.	The seed capsules are collected late in summer, the seeds extracted and their coats removed by winnowing: the oil is extracted by crushing as the seeds contain a poisonous principle.
CATMINT 111		An infusion of the whole plant (not the root) clears the hair of dandruff and imparts a healthy gloss.	The "tops" are gathered in summer.
CEDARWOOD 35		Oil of cedarwood was used by ancient Egyptians for embalming and was burnt in the temples. Modern cedarwood perfume is extracted from the Virginian Juniper of N America and is used in soaps and fragrant bath oils. It is still called cedarwood.	Now rare and a "protected" plant in the Lebanon so that Red Cedar (Juniper virginiana) is used instead. The wood is cut up (with the bark) and the oil obtained by distillation in vats.
CENTUARY 61		The water takes away skin blemishes and is astringent.	The flowers and leaves are gathered from June until September and used fresh.
CHAMOMILE 13		Used as a tonic hair rinse.	Long in bloom, the flowers are collected from mid- to late-summer and are used fresh or dried. To dry, spread out on trays in an airy room, turning often.
CHAMPAC 103		The flowers yield perfume with a jasmine-like scent.	The flowers are gathered all summer and their fragrance obtained by maceration, the perfume being drawn from the pomade by rectified spirit.
CHERVIL 37		The water takes away skin blemishes and is astringent.	The "tops" and leaves are gathered fresh in summer.
CHICKWEED 156		The leaves macerated in olive oil and applied to the skin removes blemishes. A "tea" made from ground ivy, chickweed and wood sage will keep the skin free of spots.	The whole plant (not the roots) is gathered in summer.
CHICORY 40		From the blue flowers a water is distilled to soothe tired eyes and clear the skin of blemishes.	The entire plant is gathered when in bloom in mid-summer.
CINNAMON 41		Schimmel & Co. of Leipzig discovered the sweet-scented saffrol in the bark which is used in the east to fumigate clothes and bedding.	
CLARY 146		Clears the eyes and takes away soreness.	The flowers and leaves (the "tops") are gathered June until September. The seed will make a mucilage to use to remove intrusions from the eyes.
CLEAVERS 70		The roots yield a red dye which, mixed with powder, acts as rouge and give colour to the cheeks.	The entire plant is pulled up in summer and after washing, the roots are boiled to yield a red dye.
CLOVE 63		The ground cloves were included in most scented powders to place amongst clothes and bedding. The cloves were placed (with coriander, etc.) in pomaders to carry around to counteract unpleasant smells when there were no drains.	The flowers are gathered as unopened buds August until December and are dried in the sun. They then have a long life and when ground are included in sachet powders.
COCONUT PALM 47		The oil from the shell is used in shampoos and as a nourishing dressing for dry hair.	The large fruits (coconuts) are gathered by scaling the tall trees and from the shell, oil is extracted by distillation.
COMMON ST. JOHN'S WORT 78		An infusion of leaves and flowers in olive oil is excellent for skin burns.	

Plant	Part used	Components and effects	Harvesting and further processing
CORIANDER 50		An infusion of seed with honey and orange flower water makes excellent "after shave", worthy of attention of cosmetic firms. It is used in modern perfumery as it was by the ancients.	Seed is harvested late in summer and is dried before using, to bring out its perfume. The longer the seed is kept, the better the scent.
CORNFLOWER 36		From the petals a distilled water is obtained which is soothing to the eyes and acts as an astringent.	It blooms from July until September.
COSTMARY 159		Leaves boiled with adder's tongue in olive oil takes away spots and sores.	The fresh leaves are gathered in summer.
COWSLIP 132		Elizabethans made an ointment of flowers which, applied to the skin, took away spots and wrinkles.	The flowers appear early in summer and are macerated in refined lard or olive oil.
CUCKOO PINT 17		Root boiled in milk and applied to skin takes away spots and freckles.	Lift the roots late in summer before the plant dies down. Boil in water for 10 minutes and drain off the water, then add a litre of milk and simmer for another 10 minutes.
CUCUMBER 52		A chunk of cucumber with yoghurt in a blender, makes the best of all face creams.	Remove the fruits grown in summer outdoors when 6 inches (15 cm) long and after peeling, put through a blender.
DAMASK ROSE 142		From this rose, the world's finest rose perfumes are made.	The flowers, just as they are fully open are gathered early morning before the sun causes evaporation of the essential oil, which is obtained by distillation.
DANDELION 161		Blood purifyer – takes away skin blemishes. The milky juice removes warts.	Lift the roots late summer and clean before simmering in water for 20 minutes.
ELDER 147		Elder flower water (*eau de sureau*) with almond oil makes an excellent complexion cream; also a gell to give ease and a sparkle to the eyes; also a splendid "after shave".	The corymbs of flowers are gathered early in summer.
ELEMI 31		The resinous gum is used to fix sachet powders and perfumes and in toilet soaps.	From incisions in the bark at the end of summer a resinous gum is obtained. It is dried and powdered whilst its verbena-like perfume is drawn off by rectified spirit.
EUPHRASIA/ EYEBRIGHT 64		London cosmetic shops are enjoying a big demand as it really does brighten the eyes.	The entire fresh plant is collected in summer.
FENNEL 66		Oil of fennel is used in the best herbal soaps. Fennel water brightens the eyes.	The seeds are harvested late September and October. Store the seeds in the wooden containers to use all the year.
FEVERFEW 39		It was one of the ingredients of Gervase Markham's famous 17th century skin lotion, the first on the market commercially.	Use the whole plant when in bloom throughout summer.
FRANGIPANI 125		Discovered by the Marquis Frangipani on Antigua on Columbus's 1st voyage to America. The perfume contains Cascarilla bark. Esprite de Frangipani is a famous French perfume.	The crimson or white flowers are gathered in summer and spread out to dry on shelves in an airy room or shed to include in pot pourris for they long retain their fragrance when dry.
FRANKINCENSE 26		A fragrant "gum" of the Yemen, burnt as incense and used in perfumery.	The gum resin exudes from incisions in the trunk, which is covered in smooth bark, as round pale yellow drops which is collected by scraping and is moulded into cakes.

Plant	Part used	Components and effects	Harvesting and further processing
FUMITORY 69		The leaves contain alkaloid fumarin which makes the skin whiter and relieves burns caused by sun or wind.	The entire plant (except the roots) is collected when in bloom all through summer. The plant can be dried in an airy room and used through winter.
GALANGA 7		It is known to have been used in eastern perfumery as long ago as 1450.	The plants are lifted in autumn and the roots dried in the sun before being ground. The seed capsules are harvested at the same time and removed from the capsules for drying.
GARLIC 6		A blood purifyer, also the juice in lard clears the skin of any soreness.	The plants are lifted late in summer after the foliage has died down. The "cloves", after drying off the soil in the sun, can be placed in string bags and strung up in an airy room to use during winter.
GILLYFLOWER 57		Clove scented pinks are used in pot-pourris and in perfumes.	The flowers are at their best June-August, their clove-like perfume being obtained by maceration. The scent is drawn from the pomade by rectified spirit.
GOLDEN ROD 154		Its leaves macerated in oil or lard make an excellent skin healer.	It blooms in August and September. For winter use, gather the leaves and flowers late in summer and spread out on shelves in an airy room, turning often.
GREATER PLANTAIN 124		With Southernwood, blackcurrant leaves and elder flowers, it makes an excellent healing salve. The juice, diluted, gives the eyes a sparkle.	The leaves are gathered in summer when an infusion in milk and applied to the face will leave the skin clear and smooth. The juice squeezed from the fresh leaf stalks and diluted in water will give the eyes a sparkle.
GROUND IVY 112		Valuable blood purifyer and skin tonic.	To dry for winter use, gather the plant in summer when in bloom and spread out on shelves in an airy room, turning often.
GUM TRAGACANTH 20		The gum exudation yields a mucilage which is used as a base for liquid mascaras and face creams.	The gum exudes from the bark after incisions have been made in it and is made into cakes. It becomes hard when stored.
HELIOTROPE 75		Its extract has much of the scent of almonds. It is used in soaps and perfumes. From safrol, contained in the essential oil of the Camphor tree, Heliotropin is synthetically obtained.	The flowers are gathered throughout the summer for it is long in bloom and their scent is obtained by enfleurage whilst they are fresh.
HENNA 89		Colours hair dark red. With a cupful of hot red wine gives hair a lovely satin finish. With a few cloves, it colours the hair very deep auburn. Fresh leaves rubbed onto the cheeks colour them red. A perfume Cyprinum is made from the flowers.	The leaves are collected almost all the year and dried in the sun on trays. When quite dry they are ground to a powder and stored in wooden containers to use all the year.
HERB BENNET 72		Dried roots impart a clove-like scent to clothes kept in cupboard or chest. An infusion of the roots makes an effective skin lotion, removing wrinkles and tightening the skin.	The roots are dug in spring as the plant makes new growth. To dry, spread out the roots in a sunny room, turning often and store in cardboard boxes.
HOP 77		A hop pillow of dried flowers encourages sound sleep, always an aid to beauty. from the fresh flowers a scented otto is obtained.	The fragrant male flowers are collected in midsummer.
HORSE CHESTNUT 3		The juice extracted from the fruits (nuts) is used in bath oils to tone the flesh.	Collect the nuts in autumn, boil them for an hour and remove the outer skin. Put the nuts through a blender to extract the juice.
HORSERADISH 46		Sliced root boiled in milk and applied as a lotion will clear skin of pimples and spots.	The thong-like roots are lifted in autumn as the plant dies back and are chopped and put through a juicer. They are best used freshly lifted.

Plant	Part used	Components and effects	Harvesting and further processing
HORSETAIL 60		The distilled water from the stems will relieve the skin of soreness and remove blemishes.	Gather the stems in summer.
HOUND'S TONGUE 55		The juice from the leaves and stems in olive oil, prevents falling hair and heals a sore skin.	Gather the whole plant above ground when in bloom in mid-summer.
INDIGO 80		From the leaves and stems a yellow dye is extracted which turns purple-black upon oxidation and is used to intensify the colour of black hair.	The leaves are removed during summer or the whole plant is cut at soil level and dried in an airy room or shed. The leaves are ground to a powder and made into a paste with water.
JACOB'S LADDER 127		The whole plant boiled in olive oil colours the hair black and gives it a gloss.	From June until the end of summer, cut down the plant to just above soil level and simmer for almost an hour in olive oil which turns jet black.
JASMINE 82		They yield the most popular of eastern perfumes, and are present in hair and face creams. François Coty based his famous L'Aimant perfume on white jasmine. It is the dominant note in Lancome's Magie perfume.	The flowers are collected July-October, the scent being extracted by enfleurage and drawn off the pomade by rectified spirit.
JONQUIL 109		The heavy fragrance is extracted from the flowers and used with tuberose and balsam of tolu to give it permanence.	The flowers are removed in spring and the perfume obtained by maceration at 60°F, the scent being drawn from the pomade by rectified spirit.
LABDANUM 42		It produces a fragrant gum which is the base of many perfumes. (That from Crete is the best).	The resin is secreted from the glandular hairs of leaves and stems and sticks to the coats of browsing animals from which it is collected and made into cakes. The resin is also collected by boiling the leaves and stems in vats and has the scent of ambergris.
LADY'S MANTLE 5		Max Hoffman said it "would restore feminine beauty to its youthful freshness". An infusion, rubbed on the breasts, restores their firmness.	Make an infusion of the whole plant (excluding the roots) in mid-summer.
LAVENDER 88		It makes scented toilet waters, soaps, hair-creams. Promotes new hair if massaged into the scalp. The dried flowers scent clothes.	The flowers are cut when fully open during July and August.
LEMON 45		The juice of the fruits is used in hair rinses and as an astringent, to tighten the skin and remove wrinkles.	The fruit is gathered almost the whole year, the flowers and fruit appearing together on the trees.
LEMON GUM TREE 62		A lemon-scented oil, obtained from the leaves is used in soaps.	The fresh leaves and twigs are gathered all year and yield a lemon-scented essential oil on distillation. The leaves can be dried and distilled in the same way.
LESSER CELANDINE 139		An infusion of the plant applied to the skin will close up the pores and soon remove wrinkles.	Gather the whole plant early in summer (it dies down quickly well before the end of summer) at soil level.
LILAC 158		It grows wild in Persia and SW China. It is included (with rose and gardenia) in Hermes' wonderful Calèche perfume. The scent of lilac is now obtained from turpentine as terpineol.	The flowers are gathered early in summer and the scent, extracted by enfleurage, is drawn off the pomade by rectified spirit.
LILY OF THE VALLEY 48		The distilled water is astringent and applied to the face closes the pores and removes wrinkles. Its scent is present in Lanvin's Arpège perfume.	The flowers are gathered early in summer and used fresh. The essential oil is obtained by enfleurage.
LIME TREE 163		The flowers make an effective complexion lotion.	The flowers, which are gathered early in summer are used at once or they will ferment.

Plant	Part used	Components and effects	Harvesting and further processing
MADONNA LILY 91		The juice extracted from the bulbs makes an effective anti-wrinkle pomade.	The flowers are gathered June-July, their perfume being obtained by enfleurage. The bulb is lifted in autumn.
MARIGOLD 28		Marigold water is soothing to the eyes. The flowers dye hair yellow and provide a face cream which leaves the skin smooth and silky.	It blooms almost all year except in the coldest weather.
MARSHMALLOW 8		Makes a soothing skin ointment and the water from the boiled roots soothes inflamed eyes.	The roots are lifted in early summer and after cleaning and washing, are boiled with lard or olive oil.
MASTIC 123		A fragrant "gum" of Arabia, burnt as incense and used to strengthen the teeth and gums.	The resinous gum obtained by making incisions in the bark is collected in summer and made into cakes.
MEADOWSWEET 65		The distilled water from the leaves and flowers will relieve tired eyes and is a useful astringent.	The leaves are gathered in summer.
MELILOT 100		From the fresh plant a toilet water is made and an infusion relieves the eyes of soreness and gives them a sparkle.	The fresh plant is gathered in summer.
MIGNONETTE 140		Miel de Mignonette (with honey) makes a soothing non-greasy body lotion. The tiny flowers yield little essential oil, only 0·002% yet its scent is so powerful that it is used in perfumery at a strength of only 1 part in 500 of alcohol.	The flowers are gathered in mid-summer, the fragrance being extracted by enfleurage.
MULLEIN 169		In Titian's day, women of Italy would dye their hair golden by an infusion of the flowers. It is an excellent hair restorer.	The flowers are borne in dense inflorescences in July-August when they are gathered.
MYRRH 22		The fragrant gum is used by eastern women as a body perfume. It is a fixative for perfumes. It is used in the finest soaps and shampoos.	The resinous gum which exudes from the shrub all the year, is collected on the beards and coats of browing animals from which it is removed and made into cakes.
NEROLI 44		The distillation of the flowers is used in the perfume Neroli and to make eau de Cologne.	The flowers, leaves and twigs, and also the fruits yield a fragrant essential oil. The plants bloom almost the whole year, the fruits appearing with the flowers.
NUTMEG 107		It yields an oil which blends with sandalwood and lavender to make soaps; the powder of the ground nut is an ingredient of sachets or scented bags to put amongst clothes.	The trees yield 3 crops a year, the fruits consisting of a fleshy outer covering, the mace, which is removed and dried, whilst the seed or nutmeg which it encloses, takes 6 weeks to dry.
NUTMEG PLANT 113		A decoction of the seeds rubbed on the breasts will bring about their firmness.	The seed capsules are removed late in summer and dried on trays in an airy room.
OAK 138		From the galls made by the gall mite, a dye is extracted to colour the hair black.	The galls, often present on the leaves, are removed in summer and boiled.
OAT 21		Cooked or uncooked oats make a face pack (mask) which clears the skin of impurities and leaves it soft and smooth.	The corn is cut when ripe in late summer and ground into oatmeal which can be stored and used all year.
OLIVE 114		The oil from the fruit is used in skin creams and hair dressing for its nourishing powers.	The ripe fruits are harvested late in summer and placed in hessian sacks for crushing in tubs of water, the green oil rising to the surface for collection.

Plant	Part used	Components and effects	Harvesting and further processing
MARJORAM 115		The dried and powdered leaves were included in many scented powders for they give a "lasting" perfume.	The whole plant (not the roots) is gathered in mid-summer and distilled. An infusion of fresh "tops" added to a beer shampoo increases its effectiveness.
ORRIS 81		The powdered root of the Florence iris is violet scented. It is used in most talcum powders and is an ingredient of Frangipani powder.	The roots of 3–4 year old plants are lifted in autumn, the essential oil being obtained by distillation after the roots have been dried and kept for 2 years, during which time they increase in fragrance.
OIL PALM 59		It produces the palm-oil of commerce which has a violet-like perfume and is used in soaps.	The large fruits, like coconuts, yield upon compression, a greenish oil.
PANDANG 116		A primitive water plant of islands of the Indian Ocean, it is the favourite perfume of Hindu women.	The flowers are gathered for almost the entire year, their essential oil being obtained by distillation.
PATCHOULI 126		Found wild in Bengal, the odour of its leaves is the most powerful of all plants. It was used to impregnate Indian shawls exported to Europe.	The leaves are gathered late in summer and by steam distillation yield a yellowish-green essential oil. The leaves are also dried in the shade and ground to a powder.
PEACH 135		The fruit, put through a blender, makes an excellent face mask for a dry skin.	The large fruits are gathered when ripe in late summer.
PELLITORY-OF-THE-WALL 117		A decoction of the leaves with oil of rosemary, soothes sore hands and face.	Gather the leaves in summer and use fresh.
PEPPERMINT 102		The oil extract is used for fragrance in soaps. A handful in a warm bath will relax and tone the body.	The stems are cut when in bloom and distilled to yield the essential oil.
PINE 122		From the wood and leaves pine oil is obtained to use in bath oils and to impart a refreshing scent to soaps.	The cones and leaf shoots are gathered from the forest floor. Pine oil is obtained by distillation of the wood under steam pressure.
POTATO 153		Peel and wash a freshly dug potato and slice. Rub the pieces on the face, leave for 30 minutes and wash off. It leaves the skin beautifully soft.	The tubers are lifted late in summer and in autumn, before the frosts, and are stored in a frost-free place to use all winter.
PRIMROSE 133		An ointment made from the flowers and lard will soothe chapped hands and face. The juice from the stems removes spots and pimples.	Gather the leaves in spring when young and squeeze out the juice in a blender or mortar. An infusion of the flowers in spring makes an astringent lotion.
PRIVET 90		An infusion of flowers heals a sore skin after sunburn.	Remove the flowers during June and July and infuse in boiling water.
QUINCE 137		The mucilage from the seeds makes an effective cream mascara and is used as a base for cold creams.	The fruits are gathered in late summer when ripe and are cut open to remove the seeds. Soak in water for 15 minutes to form the mucilage.
RAMPION 29		Distilled water of the leaves applied at bedtime "maketh the face most resplendent".	The flowers and leaves are gathered June and July.
RED CLOVER 164		An infusion of the flowers will soothe a chapped face.	The plant is gathered when in full bloom for the high honey content of its flowers.
RED ELM 166		Makes an excellent shaving soap – soothes the skin.	The trees are stripped of the inner bark or bast which is dried and powdered. It is highly mucilaginous.

Plant	Part used	Components and effects	Harvesting and further processing
RED ROSE 143		In the Ashmolean Museum, Oxford, is a recipe for making a perfume and the dried petals are used in all pot-pourris. They make a pleasant toilet water.	Petals are gathered in summer when the flowers are at their best. They can be dried on trays in an airy room when the petals will retain their perfume.
RHATANY 84		The hard woody roots make an excellent dentifrice powder. They whiten the teeth and strengthen the gums.	The shrubs are dug up in late summer and the cylindrical roots cut away and dried in the sun.
ROSEMARY 144		It figures in the finest French eau de Cologne with bergamot and grape spirit. It makes a tonic bath and it is the best of all hair tonics. For dry hair, wash it in rosemary oil.	The "tops" of the shoots are gathered between March-August when in bloom and distilled to produce oil of rosemary. The "tops" placed in a muslin bag will scent a warm bath.
ROSE-ROOT 151		The "poor man's" rose water is made from its roots to sprinkle over clothes.	The roots are dug up in summer and dried in the sun or in a warm, airy room.
SAFFRON 51		It is used to dye the hair golden colour and to make a perfumed body ointment. Crocinum was the most popular perfume of ancient Athens.	The flowers are collected August-September and the stigmas removed. They are dried in a low oven between layers of paper and compressed into cakes.
SAGE 145		An infusion of the leaves colours the hair black and with olive oil, is an effective dressing which imparts a gloss to the hair.	The "tops" are gathered in summer when in flower. The leaves are also dried in a low oven and stored in boxes to use for the same purpose in winter.
SANDALWOOD 149		The essential oil assimilates perfectly with otto of roses. It is also used in "heavy" eastern perfumes. It yields the famous Indian perfume, Abir. It is used as the base of all the "green and woody" perfumes.	The wood of this parasitic tree is cut up into chips which, upon distillation, yield a fragrant oil.
SANICLE 148		An infusion of the plant is a blood purifyer, ridding the skin of blemishes, as it will if applied externally.	It is collected when in bloom in June and July.
SASSAFRAS 150		Native of E Canada and USA the oil extracted from the fragrant wood and bark is used in perfumery.	The shrubs are dug up at all times of the year, the roots being cut up and the oil extracted by steam distillation. The finest oil is obtained from the fruits, gathered in autumn and distilled.
SCARLET PIMPERNEL 10		An infusion of the plant and its juice makes a complexion lotion to relieve sunburn and clear the skin of blemishes.	The entire plant is gathered in summer.
SCENTED-LEAF GERANIUM 118		In the leaves, geraniol and phenylethylalcohol, the chief constituents of attar of roses, are present. It is used for adulterating attar of roses.	The leaves are gathered all the year and distilled when fresh.
SEA-KELP 68		The mucilage with olive oil, imparts a gloss when used as a hair dressing and, also with olive oil, is used as a revitalising skin cream.	The seaweed is collected all the year, dried and burnt, the red ash containing a high percentage of mucilage.
SESAME 152		The oil from the seeds is used in suntan oils, protecting the skin from injurious rays and in face creams.	The fruit is gathered after the monsoon season, the egg-shaped seeds are pressed and they release a pale yellow oil.
SOLOMON's SEAL 129		A toilet water is made from the flowers which "leaves the face fresh, fair and lovely".	The flowers are gathered May-July and distilled.
SOUTHERNWOOD 15		An infusion massaged into the head will prevent hair falling out. For dry hair use southernwood and olive oil.	The leaves are gathered in summer.

Plant	Part used	Components and effects	Harvesting and further processing
SOWTHISTLE 155		The milky juice in a little water is a rejuvenating skin cleanser.	The milky juice is obtained from the stems cut in summer.
STAR ANISE 79		A plant of S United States and China, from the fruit an oil is obtained and is used for fragrance in soaps and hair oils.	The fruits are gathered in September and October and dried, the seeds being distilled for their essential oil.
STINGING NETTLE 167		The leaves purify the blood and improve the complexion. A pint of hot water on a basin of nettle leaves makes a valuable hair rinse.	The whole plant is cut in summer just above soil level (using gloves to handle it).
STRAWBERRY 67		The fruit and its juice is an effective face pack and removes tartar from the teeth, leaving them whiter.	The fruits are gathered June-October and put through a blender.
SUNFLOWER 74		The oil from the seed makes a nourishing face cream.	From the seeds, removed from the dead flowers late in summer and distilled, a pale yellow oil is obtained.
SWEET FLAG 2		Calamine lotion is a product of the rhizome; when dried and ground it makes a scented talcum powder. It is an ingredient of the famous French perfume, Chypre.	The roots are lifted in autumn and after cleaning are distilled or dried in a low oven and ground.
SWEET GRASS 54		A grass, it grows on hills of W Khandesh and from it an oil (to rub on the body) with a rose-like scent is obtained. It was used in W Europe at an early date.	The grass is cut with a sickle in September when the inflorescence is white and the essential oil is obtained by distillation.
SWEET GUM 93		The satinwood of cabinet makers, it is a N American tree, the West's answer to *L. orientale* of the Near East. Liquid storax gives permanence to odours of flowers extracted by maceration.	The gum resin, known as liquid storax, is collected from incisions made in the bark as the sap rises early in summer.
TANSY 160		The leaves soaked in buttermilk for a week make a soothing complexion milk.	Gather the fresh plant during summer.
THYME 162		With rosemary, is a valuable hair rinse and keeps head free from dandruff.	The plants are cut at soil level during mid-summer when in bloom and are distilled.
TOADFLAX 92		A skin cream is made from the fresh flowers and "tops".	The flowers and "tops" are gathered June-October and boiled with lard or olive oil.
TOMATO 95		Use tomato juice on its own as a toning lotion for a greasy skin or with yoghurt as a face pack. Use with oatmeal to make a paste and leave on the face 30 minutes.	Ripe fruits are picked from July-October from the open, when deep red in colour and are peeled and crushed.
TONQUIN 58		A forest tree of Brazil, its black shining seed is almond-shaped and is used for handkerchief perfumes and in sachet powder to place amongst clothes. It is used in Boquet du Champ.	The single-seeded pods containing a large black bean are gathered almost the whole year, the beans being infused in rectified spirit for a month and the essence drawn off. The beans are also dried and ground.
TORMENTIL 131		The juice from the root, after boiling, makes a soothing face cream and skin lotion.	Lift the plant in late summer.
TUBEROSE 128		Its powerful essence is volatile and needs a fixative to give it permanence.	It is unique in that the flowers are gathered at night when their scent is most powerful and it is extracted by enfleurage.

Plant	Part used	Components and effects	Harvesting and further processing
VANILLA 168		The extract of the pods is used to give "lightness" to flowery perfumes, especially heliotrope and wallflower.	The pods, like runner beans, are gathered in autumn, just on the point of ripening and are tied in bundles for export. The essence is extracted by slicing the beans and placing in large jars containing rectified spirit. After a month, the tincture is drained off and used in floral "bouquets".
VERVAIN 170		It was Louis Pasteur who first drew attention to it being an excellent hair tonic. An infusion of the leaves also gives a sparkle to tired eyes.	The whole plant (not the root) is gathered when in bloom in July and August.
VIOLET 172		Fresh flowers in a cup and a little hot milk poured over, makes a valuable "night cream". Violets are also used in perfumery.	The flowers are gathered in spring and early summer and their perfume extracted by maceration.
WALL RUE 19		An infusion of the fronds will rid the scalp of dandruff and promote the growth of new hair.	The fronds are cut during summer and when infused in hot water are mucilaginous.
WALNUT 83		The oil from the nuts colours hair black and acts as an efficient dressing.	The fruits (drupes) are gathered from the ground as they fall in early autumn. The green husks which enclose the shell containing the nut are removed and when boiled, colour the hair brown. The oil is obtained from the nuts by distillation.
WATERCRESS 110		It clears the blood and skin better than anything and an infusion of the leaves applied to the face, leaves the skin soft and smooth.	The juice of the freshly cut plant which is evergreen in all but the coldest winters, is obtained by simmering.
WATER MELON 43		The fruit, cut into sections (slices), re-moisturises and tightens the skin and refreshes in warm weather.	The fruits ripen in summer when they have grown large. They are cut into slices and placed on the face and neck as moisturisers and refreshers in warm weather.
WAX PALM 49		In the axils of the leaves are scales which produce a wax which has a melting point of 84°C and is used for making scented candles. It is known as Carnauba wax.	The wax falls to the ground as the trees are shaken at regular intervals during the summer season.
WEST INDIAN BAY 120		From fresh leaves an oil is distilled which, when mixed with West Indian rum, produces Bay Rum, best of all hair tonic.	The leaves are collected all year, the oil being extracted by distillation.
WHEAT 165		Wheat germ oil is a nourishing skin tonic.	The corn ripens in late summer and early autumn and is harvested as a hard grain. An oil is extracted from the embryo or germ, which is removed to make white bread.
WHITE BIRCH 23		It yields an aromatic oil known as "Russian leather" for it used to be rubbed on the leather bindings of books to preserve them and its fragrance "caught on". It is used in soaps.	The essential oil is extracted by distillation of the wood and bark, in large vats, in autumn. From the leaves, a lotion is distilled during summer.
WILD LETTUCE 85		The juice from the stems makes an astringent skin lotion.	The stems when cut in summer, release a milky juice.
WINTERGREEN 71		A refreshing handkerchief perfume is extracted from the leaves. Also used for fragrance in soaps.	The plants are cut at soil level late in summer, the leaves and twigs being distilled and the oil collected. It is necessary for the plant to be immersed in cold water for 24 hours before it is distilled for the oil develops by fermentation.
WITCHHAZEL/ WINTERBLOOM 73		Makes an excellent skin-cleansing water.	The twigs and leaves are removed at the end of summer and distilled.

Plant	Part used	Components and effects	Harvesting and further processing
WOOD RUFF 18	🌷	Known as "sweet grass" the dried leaves are used to stuff pillows and fresh leaves make a valuable complexion water.	The entire plant is gathered in summer and used in infusion. The dried and powdered plant is placed in sweet bags for its scent improves with keeping.
WORMWOOD 16	🍃 ✿	An excellent remedy for falling hair, used with rosemary to rub into the scalp.	The leaves are gathered in summer and used in infusions. The leaves can be dried in an airy room for winter use.
YELLOW ARCHANGEL 86	🍃 ✿	The leaves macerated in lard and applied to the face will rid it of spots.	The flowers (borne in May and June) and the leaves are macerated in lard or olive oil.
YELLOW LOOSESTRIFE 96	🍃 ✿	An infusion of the flowers and "tops" will relieve soreness of the eyes and acts as an efficient astringent for the skin.	The flowers and leaves are gathered in July and August.
YLANG-YLANG 30	✿	It is blended with otto of Allspice to make the famous Macassar hair oil. It grows wild in the Philippine Islands.	The flowers are gathered throughout summer and their scent obtained by distillation.
ZEDOARY 53	🌿	From the roots, Indian women extract a colouring which imparts a lively tint to their dark complexions.	The roots are lifted in September and October and cleaned and distilled to yield an essential oil. The roots are also dried and ground.

For every aspect of body care

The skin is of two layers, the top layer is the epidermis, the lower, wherein lie the sweat and oil glands, the blood vessels and water cells is the dermis. The dermis contains collagen, which gives the skin its elasticity. Here new cells are continually being formed and make their way up into the epidermis to replace the rough layer of skin which protects the dermis from bacteria and exposure to sunlight. For the skin to be maintained in condition, it must be cleaned constantly so that it will be cleared of the dead cells which cause the pores to become blocked with dirt and sweat. To prevent the pores from becoming blocked, old make-up must be removed each day, preferably at bedtime, so that the skin can breathe during the night and be rejuvenated. If sweat, dirt and excess oils are not regularly removed, the pores will become enlarged and will cease to function properly. The waste material becomes oxidised when exposed to the air, causing it to turn black. Familiar blackheads and greasy looking skin are the result. The skin (like the hair) has a natural acid coating, made up of oil and sweat which protects it from cold and drying winds and from the entry of harmful bacteria, yet it must be constantly removed before it becomes stale and before the pores, through which the skin breathes, become enlarged. Should this happen, the pores will never revert to their original size although astringents will do much to assist with this defect by causing the skin surrounding the pores to swell, thereby partly closing them.

The correct diet and a regular intake of fibrous foods, whereby the bowels are moved regularly and the body rid of toxic materials which would otherwise escape through the pores, is of greater importance than all the beauty aids ever introduced. So too is regular exercise, fresh clean air and deep breathing. Those three verities of good health together with a regular face washing with milk or buttermilk (with rose water or an infusion of herbs collected from the hedgerow added), are the secret of the dairy maid's glowing complexion.

Dry skin will become sore from cold weather or from an excess of sunlight. Dryness also causes wrinkling at an early age, though such skin is usually tight and firm, with no enlarged pores, and so requires no astringents. The aging complexion requires much attention if it is to retain the glow that fresh air and exercise alone could guarantee in youth. Indeed, for all ages, washing the face in warm water and using a honey and almond soap to remove dirt and grease and afterwards rinsing with cold water and the juice of half a lemon, will cleanse and tighten and tone the skin. If done at bedtime, massage into the skin a few drops of almond oil, using a circular movement for the cheeks; a horizontal movement for the forehead. In the morning apply an astringent lotion containing witch hazel and rose water which will close enlarged pores.

As a base for one's make up apply a foundation cream or lotion. This will leave the skin smooth and will make its surface more adherent for face powder. It should be of a soft skin colour, pinky-beige. Calamine lotion,

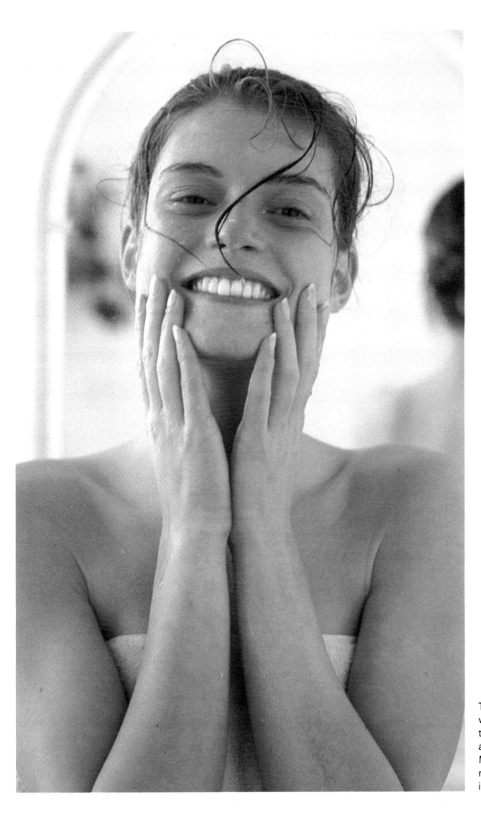

The care of the face begins with washing. A good face soap is the *sine qua non* of all cosmetic and hygienic undertakings. Making your own soap out of nature's garden, is both fun and immensely rewarding.

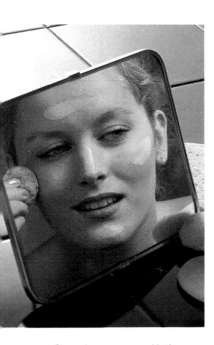

Cleansing creams and lotions are used to remove one's stale make-up and with it dirt and grime which is accumulated during the day and, if not removed at bedtime, will clog the pores, preventing the skin from breathing.

Cold creams and cleansing milks will need beeswax, spermaceti, lanolin, olive and almond oil, borax (as a saponifying agent), and rose water as basic ingredients.

so comforting for sunburn, provides an ideal matt base, at the same time it nourishes the skin.

When using a foundation, apply it gently with a cotton pad. Do not rub it into the pores. It is needed simply as a base, to coat the skin. It is a foundation to work on. Apply it with gentle downward strokes and get it as smooth and even as possible, taking it down under the chin so that there will be no demarcation line between face and neck. Then add the cheek colour, rouge or blush, again applying it as smoothly and inconspicuously as possible. Gently work in the rouge in a circular manner, then apply the powder. This can be made up in several shades but should tone in with the base colour and match the hair and eyes. Powders should give the skin a smooth matt finish and should not soon flake or blow off. Orris, kaolin, rice starch are included amongst the ingredients and are brought to the correct shade required by incorporating one or more of the colour powders obtained from chemists or the manufacturers. Only very small amounts are required to give colour to a powder. Blondes should use a Naturelle shade; brunettes, Rachel.

To make a compact face powder, so that the powders stick together into a cake, a small amount of tragacanth or gum arabic is included when the powder is made up, no more than 1% of the total ingredients. Water is also added to form a stiff paste which is then dried and compressed into a cake. It is applied to the face after wetting and quickly dries on.

To keep the brows with a neat and tidy outline, it may be necessary to remove any hairs out of line with tweezers before make-up begins.

Bathe with eyebright solution to give them a sparkle. Use an eye pencil to pick out the lids and apply a moisturising eye shadow undercoat to the lids before applying the eye shadow.

Apply a cream or liquid mascara with a special brush in an upwards direction with the eyes open, keeping it clear of the eyes. This will make the lashes look thicker and blacker than they are.

Apply a 10 minute face mask to remove dirt and dead cells. Wash off and apply moisturiser to make the skin softer, then an underbase to correct flaws. There should be no line between face and neck. Then a foundation or make up base and smooth on with gentle downward strokes. Apply colour to match the complexion as a powder with a matt finish. Use a little rouge if necessary.

Treat in the same way as the cheeks, applying a make up base with special care about the nose to get it even, and do not work into the skin. Do not apply cheek colour to the nose other than powder thinly applied.

Outline the lips with a lipstick pencil and fill in with a lipstick of a colour to tone with the complexion. Coat with a beeswax and petroleum jelly to prevent the colour coming off too easily.

Remove stale polish once weekly with acetone to which a few drops of olive oil have been added. Soak nails in warm water and push back cuticles with a stick padded with cotton wool at the end. Coat with white iodine or apply a base first and then fresh colour varnish.

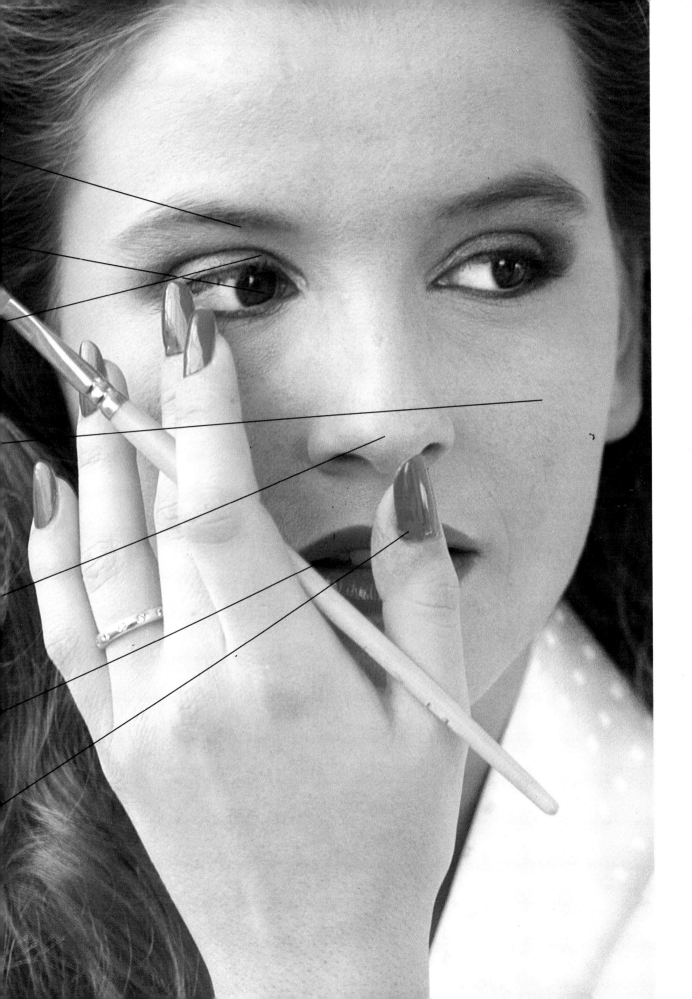

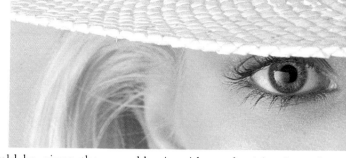

CARE OF THE EYES

Perhaps the facial feature most difficult to make up is the eye. From the time of the ancient Egyptians, eyes have featured most prominently in the world of feminine beauty. The first and most important rule of making up eyes is seeing to their clarity, for no amount of make-up will conceal tiredness and strain.

Greater care should be given the eyes than any other part of the body. An excess of sunlight can do them irreparable harm, so always wear good quality sun-glasses where the eyes are exposed to bright light. This will also prevent the screwing up of the eyes causing "crows-feet" at the sides.

The eyes should be regularly exercised as any other part of the body and this is best done upon rising. The face should be placed in a wash-basin of cold water with the hair held back and the eyes opened and exercised

and boric acid powder (also from the chemist). Place a handful of red rose petals into a jug and just cover them with boiling water. Cover the jug with a piece of plastic to keep in the steam and leave for at least 10 hours. If made in the early morning, it can be used at night. Strain and add the rose water to a $\frac{1}{2}$ teaspoonful of borasic acid dissolved in a small cupful of warm water. Fill the eye bath and bathe the eyes by pressing it around each eye in turn and opening them for about 30 seconds.

Beauty shops in recent years have

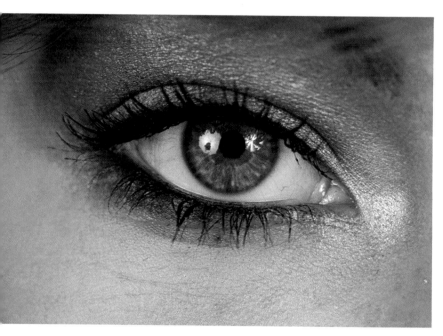

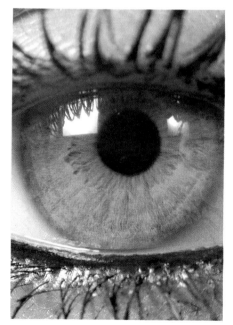

Rest and protection from pollution are paramount in caring for the eyes. Wearing sunglasses is advised against the damaging effects of the sun's brightness. A bath of boric acid and elder flower water is an excellent way to soothe tired and sore eyes, while a few drops of eyebright will give them a natural sparkle.

under water for a few seconds. This will refreshen them and clear them of "sleep". It also gives them a sparkle.

When the eyes are tired or sore from exposure to cold winds or the sun, or to long hours watching television or doing close work, bathe them (using an eye bath from the chemist) with a solution of rose water

enjoyed a greater demand for eyebright than for any other cosmetic, for its lotion really does accentuate the beauty of the eyes, not only relieving tiredness but giving the eyes a brilliance which no other preparation can do. It acts immediately on the mucous lining of the eyes. Running eyes, due to a head

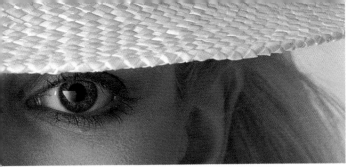

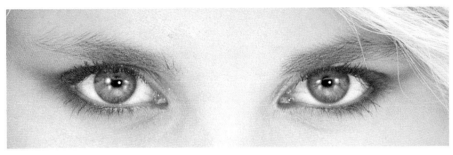

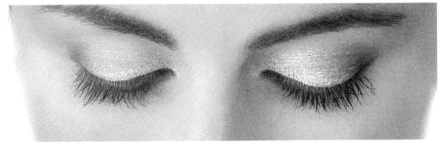

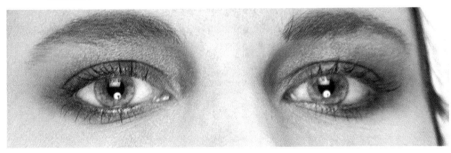

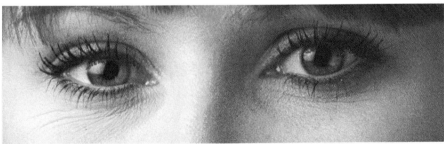

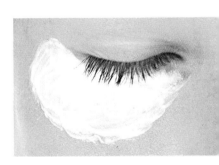

cold or hay-fever, may be stopped at once by bathing them with a handful of the herb infused in ½ litre of milk or water which has been allowed to cool. Use lint or an eye bath to do so. The eyes should be bathed in the lotion before making up when going out for the evening. Before bathing the eyes, use the melon or cucumber treatment as a skin freshener and relax on the bed for 20 minutes with the eyes closed. The sparkle of this will impart the eyes which will be noticed by everyone and will last all evening. The eyes are the most difficult part of the face to make up, but the most rewarding.

Eye make-up is largely a matter of individual preference and colouring, as well as of the fashions of the time. Mascara, applied to the eyelashes to make them look longer and thicker, can be made from a combination of lampblack, gum tragacanth, water and alcohol.

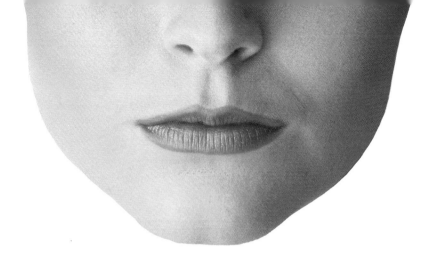

Thy lips are like a thread of scarlet,
and thy speech is comely:
thy temples are like a piece of pomegranate
within thy locks.

Song of Solomon 4.3

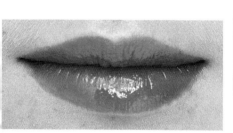 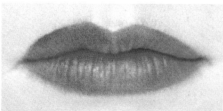 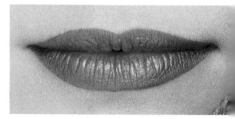

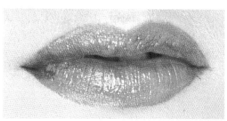 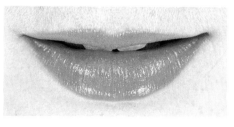

The lips must certainly be the most alluring and sensual of the facial features. For this reason Arab men insist that "their" women go around veiled, covering their lips. Women in most other cultures are still allowed to show theirs off, and even to paint them sometimes to make themselves even more attractive to the opposite sex.

To delineate the lids, an eye pencil is used. Make sure it is soft and smooth and does not "pull" the lids. Eye shadow, green or blue, is applied moist from a cake. The eye lashes are made to look darker and thicker than they normally are, by using mascara in cake or liquid form. Mascaras are usually black, lampblack being used for liquid mascaras, with gum tragacanth, water and alcohol. For a cream mascara, quince seed mucilage is used, together with an equal amount of gum arabic, lampblack and a small quantity of sugar syrup.

Finally, colouring the lips will complete the make up. A lipstick must be smooth and lasting, perfectly harmless and have reasonable plasticity. It should be applied with care; to take in the exact outline of the lips; it must not be applied too thickly or it will spoil the entire make up. One can make lipstick at home from beeswax, white petroleum jelly and spermaceti. Heat the mixture well and add red, pink, coral or orange dye solvents (obtained from various manufacturing chemists) to match one's natural colouring.

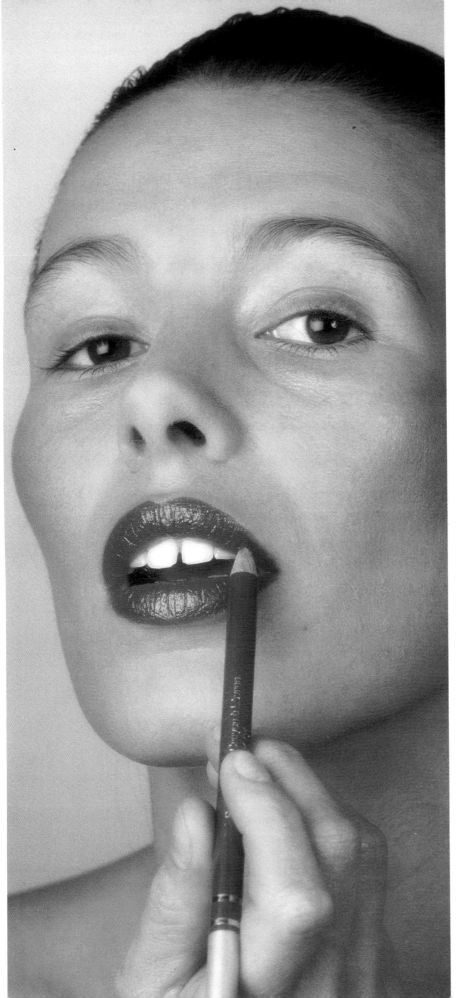

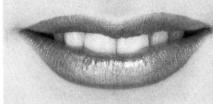

As with the eyes, making up the
lips is, to a large extent, a matter
of personal colouring and taste,
as well as of prevailing fashion.
Whereas in the late sixties and
early seventies no one would go
around in bright red lipstick, in
the late seventies and our
present decade no one would
be seen publicly sporting the
white and fluorescent pearl
shades that were so popular
twenty years ago.

Lipstick can easily be made at
home by combining beeswax,
white petroleum jelly and
spermaceti. Add colouring
(available from various
chemical manufacturers of
dyes) when you heat the
mixture up.

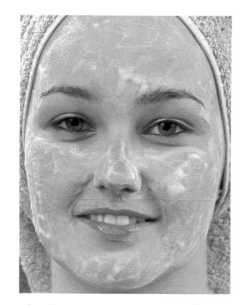

For enlarged pores, mix half a cupful of uncooked oatmeal with 8 ozs (250 g) of yogurt. This should be made up in the morning and refrigerated for 10 hours. Place the face over a bowl filled with boiling water and a handful of rosemary, with a towel over the head to keep in the steam. This will cause sweating and will open the pores still further, clearing them of oil and dirt and also blackheads and blemishes. Then rub the face and neck, lying on the bed with a towel beneath the head and leave for about an hour, then rinse.

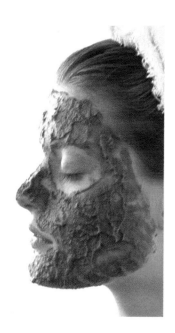

To rejuvenate the face and impart a general sense of wellbeing to tired facial muscles, apply regularly a face pack or mask.

If make up is to be removed during the day, possibly before remaking up for the evening, use a rose water lotion which will also act as an astringent. Leave on for a few minutes, then wash with an almond oil soap. If the skin is dry, add a teaspoonful of glycerine to the rose water and shake well; or instead, add the same amount of olive oil. Or simply smear the face with egg white, saving the yolk as a base for vinegar and olive oil to make a 'mayonnaise' skin cream. Leave on the egg white for 20–30 minutes until the skin has tightened and the pores closed. Wash off in warm water, to which lemon juice has been added and the skin will be tight and firm and beautifully clean and white, the pores closed and any blackheads removed. Better still for a completely rejuvenating facial, relax on the bed during this time, with a towel under the head and the eyes closed.

Follow with a skin freshener. For a greasy skin, pour $\frac{1}{2}$ litre of boiling water over a handful of chamomile flowers and one of rosemary "tops" placed in a jug. Or add a teaspoonful of witch hazel and one of honey. Leave for an hour, then strain and refrigerate. Apply to the skin with cotton wool pads.

For a dry skin, mix a tablespoonful of coconut or almond oil with a teaspoonful of powdered sea kelp and massage into the skin for about 5 minutes. Leave on for 3 minutes, then wash off. Or put half a cucumber through a juicer, add 4 ozs of rose water and $\frac{1}{2}$ oz tincture of benzoin. Refrigerate for an hour, then apply to the face and neck.

A "freshener" contains no alcohol, but a "toner" does and it will tighten the pores after cleansing the skin. Use cucumber juice and white wine for blondes; red wine for brunettes and red heads; or the juice of scented leaf geraniums makes an excellent skin toner.

Follow with a moisturising lotion. This is necessary to replace moisture in the skin cells to keep the skin soft and smooth. Exposure to sunlight and cold wind causes moisture to evaporate more quickly than it is produced and if not constantly replaced, a dry skin and wrinkles will result. A non-greasy moisturiser should be used for greasy skins.

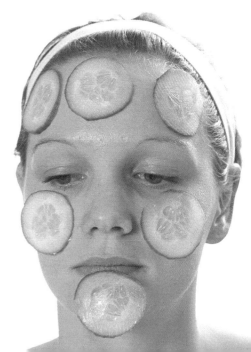

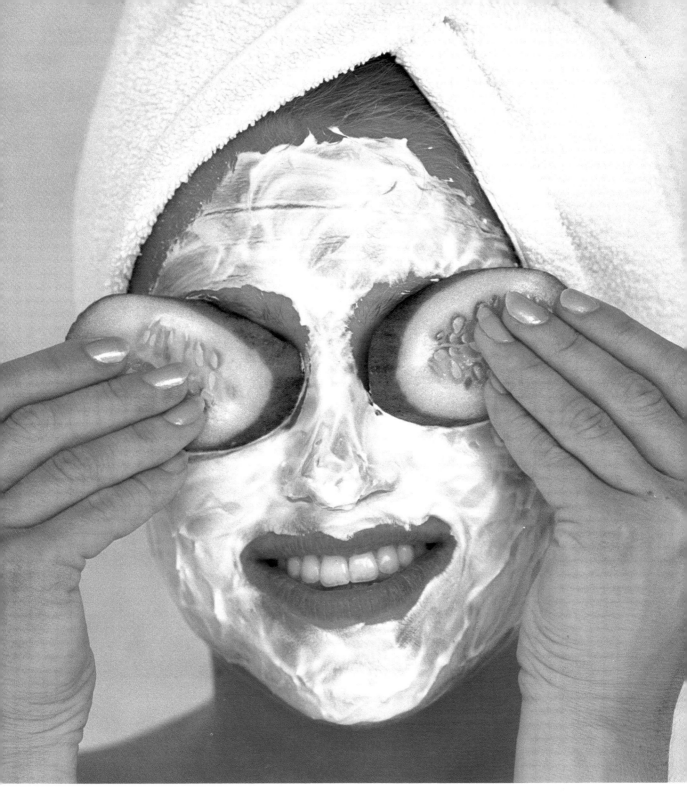

Apply to the face and neck before making up.

For normal skins, make up a moisturiser of egg yolk which supplies the skin with protein; a tablespoonful of almond oil which softens the skin; and a teaspoonful of honey which is nature's best moisturiser. Mix well together and apply with a cotton pad, working it gently into the face and neck. Leave for 30 minutes, then rinse off in warm and then in cold water.

Those living in a dry or cold climate will find a lemon gel face mask an excellent moisturiser. Add

Placed at strategic points on the face, cucumber slices will act as an astringent and tighten pores, and placed on the eyes, they will protect and freshen at the same time.

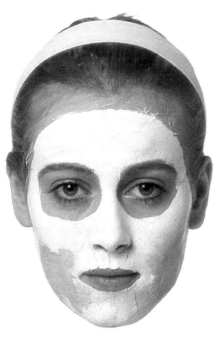

A face pack is especially beneficial for those with an oily or greasy skin. Among the most effective materials to use for a pack are honey, fuller's earth, ripe fruits such as melon, apricot, peach, banana and strawberry, tomato and cucumber.

For a night cleanser for a dry skin which will not only clean but will whiten the skin, add a tablespoonful of lemon juice (the juice of half a lemon) to 4 ozs (125 g) of yogurt and work into the skin with cotton wool. Yogurt is rich in vitamin A and so nourishes the skin over night. If the skin is extremely greasy, use a cupful of buttermilk to which is added a teaspoonful of honey.

hot water to a packet of gelatine and the juice of half a lemon. Refrigerate for 1–2 hours then apply to the face and neck. Leave on for 20 minutes before washing off.

Give your face a treat perhaps once every month with a mask or face pack which will rid the skin of impurities and at the same time replenish the natural oil and moisture lost in so many ways. Allow 2 hours for the preparation and for the uninterrupted time the mask will be on the face.

For a dry skin, reduce an avocado or an apricot and a ripe banana to pulp and afterwards, mix with sufficient milk or cream to work it into a thick paste. For a greasy skin, use 4 ozs of fresh or defrosted freezer-stored strawberries, or several ripe tomatoes, or half a cucumber which has been pulped. Mix with a little milk or yogurt to bring to a paste. Then steam the face over a bowl of hot water poured over a handful of rosemary for 10 minutes to open the pores. Lie down with a towel beneath the head and shoulders and with the mask ingredients ready in a basin, apply them with the fingers to all the exposed parts of the head and neck, after covering the hair with a shower cap. Include the forehead almost up to the hairline in the mask, together with the nose, cheeks, chin and neck, but keep away from the eyes. Relax completely and leave on for at least an hour; two hours is better. Then wash off in warm water containing the juice of half a lemon and rinse in cold. Afterwards, apply an astringent to close the pores.

An egg and honey mask is effective for greasy skins. Separate the whites of two eggs, beat until stiff, then mix

in a teaspoonful of honey and a few grains of alum. Leave on the face for 30 minutes, rinse off and apply an astringent to close the pores.

An alternative for a greasy skin is to make up what is known as a "mud" pack. This has Fuller's earth as a base, an oolite deposit which since earliest times has been used by fullers, men employed to clean the natural oils from sheep's wool. To make a 'mud' pack, add a tablespoonful of Fuller's earth to 4 ozs of yogurt and mix well, adding a teaspoonful of honey and a pinch of bicarbonate of soda. It is applied after steaming the face to rid it of impurities and to open the pores and should be left on for an hour before washing off. For a dry skin, mix a tablespoonful of salad mayonnaise (or make up your own with egg yolk, vinegar and olive oil) with one of yogurt. Add a teaspoonful of Fuller's earth and one of sea kelp powder, mixing in well. Leave on for about 1 hour and rinse off, afterwards using an astringent to close the pores.

In the New World, a face mask would be made of brewer's yeast (2 teaspoonsful) with a tablespoonful of witch hazel and a few drops of water to make into a smooth paste. Leave on for an hour and wash off with cold water into which a teaspoonful of witch hazel has been added. Or use lemon juice instead. A yeast and witch hazel pack, with half a teaspoonful of boric acid powder added is recommended for clearing the skin of blackheads and blemishes. In place of witch hazel, cabbage water can be used with brewer's yeast or oatmeal, together with the boric acid. Leave on the face for an hour and wash off

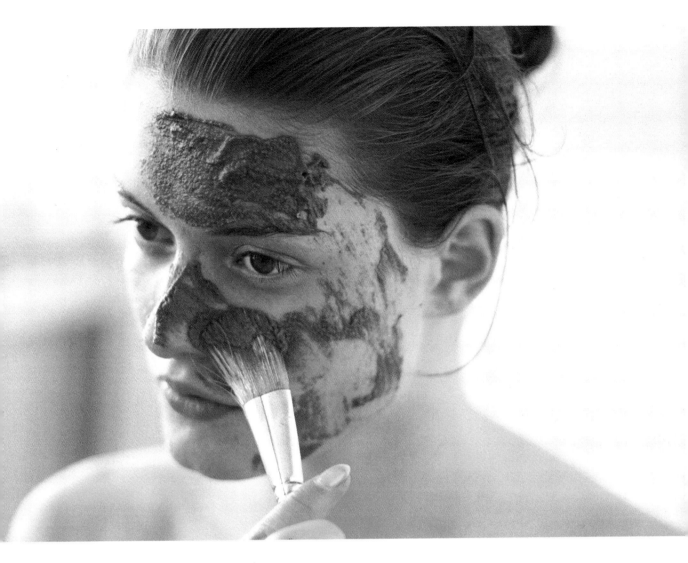

with cold water in which a teaspoonful of witch hazel or lemon juice has been added.

If a face pack is used in the evening, it should be followed by a night cream which will add further nourishment to the skin. John Gerard, writing in 1596 tells of a "Pomatum", made from apples which is specially useful for a dry skin. It is made by coring and peeling several apples, placing them in a pan over a low flame and covering them with lard. Leave to simmer for an hour, stirring occasionally, then turn off the heat and stir in a cupful of rose water and a few drops of tincture of benzoin, turn into pots or jars and allow to cool. It will keep fresh for several months.

The regular use of face packs, moisturisers and creams will keep the skin clean and replenished with the necessary moisture and oils.

If freckles prove troublesome and a few are usually more attractive than not, they may be made to look less conspicuous by applying to them an old remedy made up of glycerine, boric acid and lemon juice. Dissolve a teaspoonful of boric acid in a cupful of hot water. Add a teaspoonful of lemon juice; half a cupful of rose or elder flower water and 1 oz of glycerine and dab onto the freckles with a pad. This should be done at bedtime but if in the daytime, leave on for as long as possible and repeat frequently. The same concoction may be used to impart whiteness to the neck and shoulders.

A pomade to remove wrinkles will include beeswax, honey, the juice of the Madonna lily bulb and rose water.

The best of all astringents, witch hazel, is best used with cucumber or marigold juice and with a teaspoonful of honey. Or use chamomile lotion with a teaspoonful of cider vinegar and one of honey.

Lemon and lime juice from one whole fruit, in 8 oz (250 g) of water will be an effective astringent for a normal skin (do not omit a tablespoonful of tincture of benzoin as a preservative). They will keep fresh in the refrigerator for several weeks.

HAIR –
ONE'S CROWNING GLORY

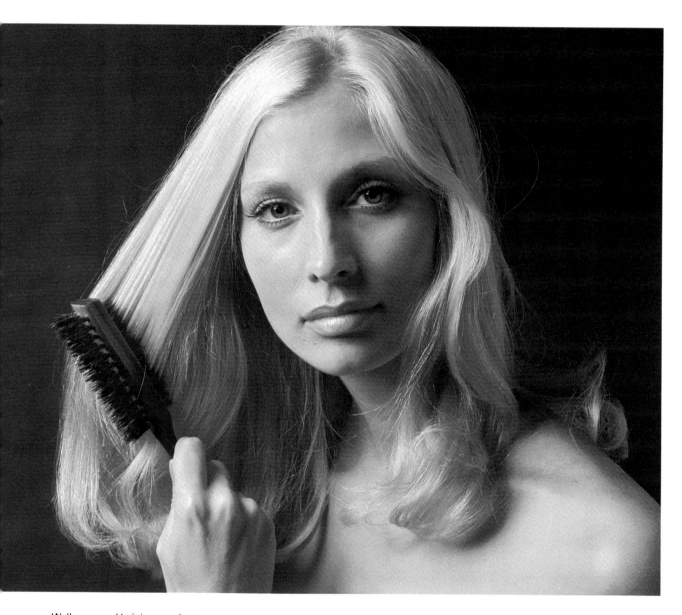

Well-groomed hair is more than simply a matter of regular visits to the hair-dresser. Although hair itself is organically dead material, hair follicles are not. The ancient wisdom of daily brushing is therefore not without credibility.

It is said that a good head of hair is the crowning glory of every man and woman. That men's hair is now being styled as artistically as women's, and that the barber enjoys a status as a hair stylist comparable to that of the hairdresser, is ample evidence of the importance of hair for both sexes.

The hair needs a regular intake of protein-packed foods to maintain it in good condition. Each hair is composed of an outer layer, the cuticle which is made up of the protein, keratin which protects it from bacteria and holds moisture in the hair. An inner layer, the cortex, is where the hair colouring (the pigment) is produced and this surrounds the innermost layer, the medulla. The hair grows from a follicle on the scalp,

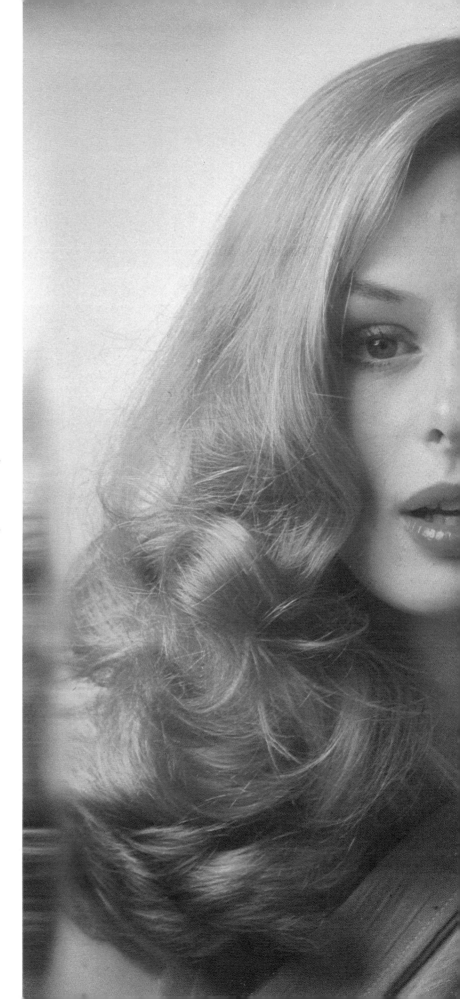

Daily strokes of the brush stimulate the follicles to produce more hair and more oil. Although naturally beautiful hair is given to relatively few, beautiful hair attained through natural means is available to almost every woman.

which is continually nourished by blood and oxygen. Each follicle produces only a single strand of hair and the head of a blonde person may contain up to 150,000 strands; a brunette, perhaps 100,000 and a redhead even fewer.

One's health is reflected by one's hair. A healthy person usually has a head of thick hair which is glossy and appears well groomed. The hair of a person in poor health often looks dull and raggedy, the hair strands breaking easily when brushed. For healthy growth, hair depends on a protein diet, and protein should also be included in shampoos. Fats or body oils provide the gloss. A regular intake of vitamins of the B group and of E and C will feed the hair with its additional needs, and daily grooming will provide it with the care it should have if it is to remain in condition throughout a long life.

Regular brushing night and morning is the first and most important consideration. Always use a bristle brush, made up of natural bristles rather than one made from man-made materials. Brush vigorously to stimulate the scalp, to bring more blood to the follicles and to encourage new hair growth. Brushing will remove old unwanted hair and new hair will take its place. Brushing clears the scalp of dandruff, caused by the flaking of the skin cells due to the drying of oil and moisture from the pores. The too frequent use of alkaline shampoos causes dandruff and falling hair: it dries up the natural oils. As with all other parts of the body, the hair should give an acid reaction, like the skin which is covered in an acid layer, for the

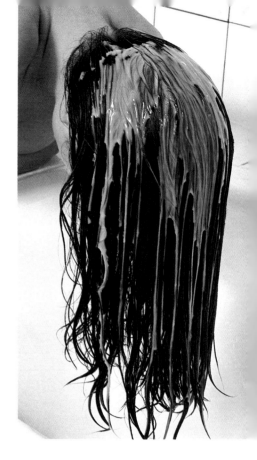

cuticle which protects the hair is composed of overlapping scales, like tiles on a roof. These are raised when in contact with alkalines and so permit bacteria to enter and moisture to escape. This is also the reason why chemical dyes which are alkaline, are bad for the hair. They cause the cuticle layer to swell and in this way allow the colour molecules to reach the cortex. Aniline dyes penetrate to the cortex and fix the colour for considerably longer than natural dyes, but in so doing they weaken the hair. On the other hand vegetable dyes which are slightly acid, coat the hair without penetrating, for they actually tighten the cortex and though are much less permanent, in no way harm the hair.

Much the same may be said of shampoos. To make a shampoo slightly acid, add a teaspoonful of citric acid crystals to it before using, then gently massage it into the hair and leave for 5 minutes. Wash off in warm water and give a final rinsing in almost cold water. Dry gently with a warm towel or preferably with an electric dryer, lifting the hair with a brush whilst holding the dryer with the other hand so that the hair may dry as quickly as possible. If a second person is available, he or she will do it so much better.

An acid shampoo causes the scales of the cuticle to contract, in the same way that astringents cause a tightening of the skin pores, keeping in the natural oils and moisture and preventing bacteria from entering. It should be said that bleaching, colouring, straightening, and waving, using alkaline chemicals are all harmful to the hair, depriving it of natural oils

and moisture. Indeed, most home colouring kits issue a warning that one may be allergic to their contents, and a patch test should always be done on the skin in some unnoticeable place, before using on the hair for they may cause reddening (soreness) of the skin on the scalp and forehead, and at the side of the face and eyes.

The condition of the hair, whether it be dry or greasy will depend to a great extent on one's food intake but either condition can be corrected. Dry hair should be given the warm oil treatment. At bedtime, massage warm olive oil into the hair and scalp. Wrap a warm towel around the head and leave on all night. Wash the hair in the morning with an acid-based shampoo. Dry hair comes from moisture escaping too quickly and more oil can improve this condition. Another corrective method is to follow an acid shampoo with a balsam conditioner which coats the hair, preventing loss of moisture. Another treatment is to warm a tablespoonful

To protect adequately the inner cortex of hair, a slightly acid shampoo is recommended. This is true in general, but for specific hair conditions specific shampoos are needed. Different herbs are ideally suited for different hair problems.

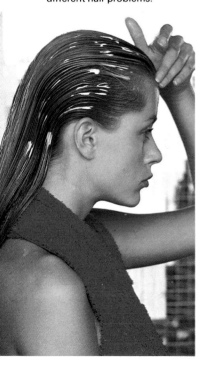

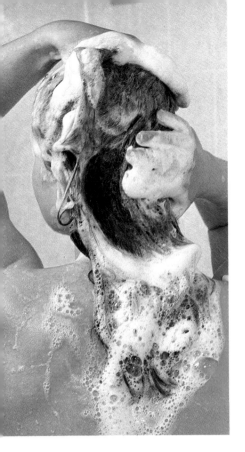

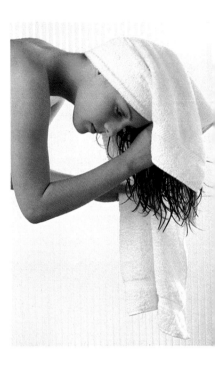

of wheat germ oil with the same quantity of olive, coconut or any vegetable oil and massage the solution into the scalp. Wrap a warm towel around the head and leave for 30 minutes. Then rinse, with the juice of a lemon in a basin of warm water. Massaging the hair has a similar effect to brushing; it draws the blood to the roots and so promotes hair growth.

Greasy hair can be corrected by brushing vigorously with a brush covered with muslin so that bristles penetrate. The grease will collect on the muslin which can then be disposed of. Follow with a lemon juice rinse or use a teaspoonful of citric acid crystals dissolved in a jug of warm water and rinse off in almost cold water.

For a monthly hair tonic, beat up an egg with a cup of milk and dissolve in it a teaspoonful of citric acid crystals or squeeze in the juice of half a fresh lemon. Add a tablespoonful of wheat germ and one of olive or coconut oil and massage into the hair. Cover with a warm towel and leave

for 60 minutes. Then rinse with lemon juice and warm water. Or use 4 oz yogurt beaten up with an egg, into which a teaspoonful of sea kelp powder and one of finely grated lemon rind is added. Mix thoroughly and work into the hair. Leave on for 40 minutes, covering the hair with a shower cap. Then shampoo and rinse.

Rosemary has long been used by countrymen and women as a treatment for falling hair and as an excellent hair tonic. Put a handful fresh or dry in a jug, with a teaspoonful of borax and one of crushed camphor obtained from the chemist. Pour on a $\frac{1}{2}$ litre of boiling water, stir and leave for several hours. Then strain and use, massaging it well into the scalp. The hair should be treated once each week and if it becomes too dry, treat it with an occasional massage of coconut oil.

There are a number of other plants which can be used in place of rosemary for a hair tonic. Chamomile is equally effective: infuse a handful of flowers in a $\frac{1}{2}$ litre of boiling water; when cool, massage into the scalp. Drinking a daily wineglassful of the same infusion is also a soothing boon to tired nerves. A few drops of the essential oil of wormwood, chamomile and rosemary mixed together and massaged into the scalp will be an excellent hair tonic and prevent the hair falling.

Southernwood is also effective in preventing falling hair: infuse a handful of "tops" in $\frac{1}{2}$ litre of boiling water; when cool, massage it into the scalp once weekly.

Another effective method to stimulate the hair glands and bring

Rosemary, depicted below, is nature's cure for dandruff. It is often included in commercially prepared herbal shampoos for this reason.

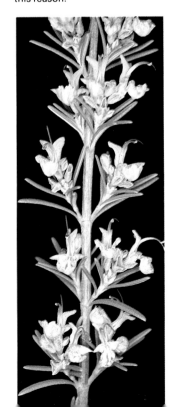

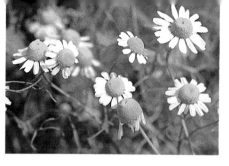

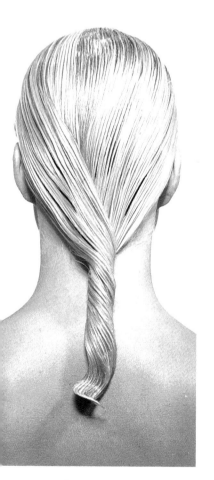

If it is true that blondes have more fun, it is also true that they have more hair (150,000 strands, as opposed to the 100,000 strands of the brunette). Chamomile (above) is an especially effective conditioner and tonic for sun-damaged and dry hair – the particular plague of the fair-haired.

about the growth of new hair is to apply cloths wrung out of hot southernwood and rosemary water to the head for 30 minutes. In S Europe, where the plant abounds, people rub the hair with olive oil and the ash of burnt southernwood stems. This perhaps accounts for their renowned thick black locks.

As a hair restorer and tonic, West Indian bay rum is supreme. Six ounces of bay rum, mixed with one ounce of spirit of rosemary and 3 drachms of tincture of cantharides and used on the hair once weekly, will encourage new hair growth for men and women. Bay rum has been included in gentlemen's hair dressings for more than two hundred years.

Peoples of northern latitudes extolled the virtues of the box tree as a hair restorative. The preacher John Wesley in his Primitive Physic, said that "for baldness, wash the head with a decoction of boxwood" and both the wood and leaves, after simmering for an hour in a saucepan of water, were used for a rinse after shampooing. Modern chemists know that all parts of the box contain the drug 'buxine' in liberal amounts, and this acts as a tonic on the nerves of the head, stimulating hair growth. Those whose hair colour comes somewhere between a blonde and a brunette, will find that box will impart a rich chestnut shade to the hair and leave it with a lovely sheen.

Mullein too, a handsome plant of colder climes, has always been regarded as an effective hair restorer. An infusion of the flowers also strengthens weak hair whilst it gives blonde hair a rich golden sheen. So

too, will lemon juice and water which is the best of all preparations to use on blonde hair.

Rosemary is also to be recommended for clearing the head of dandruff. Mix a few drops of oil of rosemary with 2 tablespoonsful of olive oil and rub well into the scalp at bedtime. Cover with a warm towel to sleep in, or wear a shower cap and rinse with lemon juice and water upon rising.

To give the hair a special gloss for evening occasions, wash it in a large cupful of cider vinegar in a litre of warm water. Wrap a towel round the head and leave for an hour before rinsing.

An infusion of marjoram and sage is a valuable hair tonic. To darken hair, an infusion of sage is both safe and reliable. It is more effective used dry and should be used with tea leaves left in the pot. Place the tea leaves with a handful of sage in a jug and add $\frac{1}{2}$ litre of boiling water. After an hour, strain and apply to the hair after shampooing. The most effective of all hair darkeners is walnut oil or lotion, but it must be used with care. Apply it with cotton wool, being sure to wear rubber gloves and to protect the face for it will stain the hands and forehead also. But of all vegetable dyes, henna has been that most widely acclaimed since earliest times, since it was used by Assyrian men to dye their long hair and beards, and the women of Egypt to impart its reddish colouring to the cheeks. Henna coats the hair, and unlike aniline dyes does not reach the cortex. However, it must not be used for permanently waved hair as it will interfere with the waving bonds. Although aniline dyes do not do this,

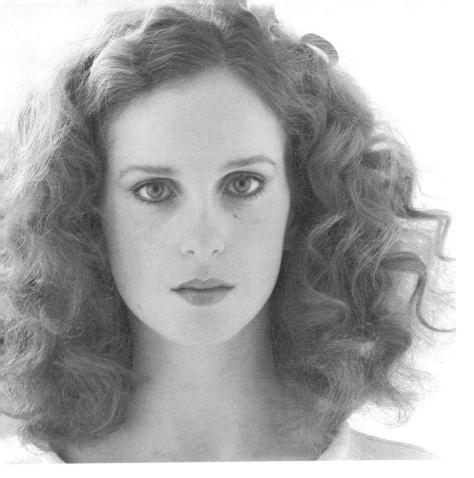

To the many who are not born naturally red-haired, the colour is still attainable from nature. Henna (below) has been used by women for millennia to render their hair various shades of red, from copper to orange red.

being alkaline, they weaken the hair. Permanent waving and the use of aniline dyes have ruined more heads of hair than anything else. Henna imparts a high gloss to hair, and there are hennas of various colours, known as compound hennas. When using henna at home, to impart an auburn shade to the hair, add to the henna paste a cupful of strong tea; a darker shade, mix in a cupful of strong coffee. Henna is a conditioner as well as a dye and when required for this purpose, use a neutral henna. To impart an extra gloss to the hair mix an egg into the paste.

To give the hair a monthly tonic, separate the white from the yolks of 2 eggs and beat until stiff. Mix into a balsam shampoo and leave on the head for 10 minutes. Rinse and then massage the egg yolks into the hair. Leave for a further 10 minutes, wash and dry. Cover the hair line with vaseline (petroleum jelly) and mix the neutral henna into a paste (it should not be too sloppy). Brush the henna into the hair from the roots to the ends, doing it in sections until the whole head has been treated. Cover with a piece of thin plastic tied round at the front and leave for at least 1 hour. Then rinse in a bowl of warm water containing the juice of a lemon and dry.

Do not use henna on hair which has been treated with metallic dyes which impart a metallic coating of copper, silver, or gold to the hair.

Those who set their own hair in its natural waves can prepare a setting lotion by obtaining a packet of gelatine from the supermarket and slowly melting it over a low flame in a pan with a cupful of water. Then add a small teaspoonful of lemon juice and one of eau de Cologne and it will be ready to use.

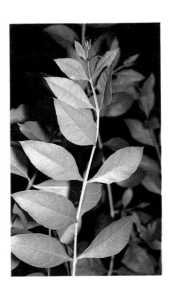

Henna, available in neutral shades, is an excellent hair conditioner.

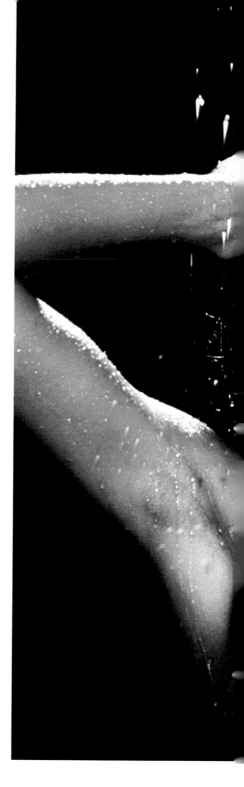

There is no better way to relax the whole body and even to remove the strains of modern stressful life than to lie supine in a warm bath. Although less relaxing, a shower is also a refreshing stimulant to the skin pores, and is perhaps more hygienic than a bath.

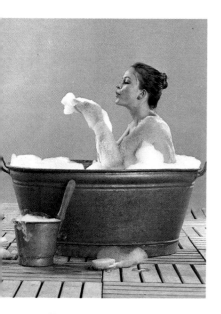

The danger of too frequent bathing – the drying up of the skin's natural oils – is easily compensated by the inclusion of bath oils in the water.

Next to Godliness is said to be cleanliness. A daily bath or shower will not only clear the skin of stale perspiration that blocks the pores and causes blackheads and blemishes, but the friction of towel on the skin gives it a healthy glow. As with all things, moderation should be used in selecting the temperature of the bath (or shower) water; have it comfortably warm rather than hot. A bath is preferable to a shower on several days a week for only in a bath can the body be given a thorough soaking and impurities be dissolved from the pores, whilst bath oils replace the body's natural oils needed to keep the skin soft and supple and free from any scaling. A warm bath relaxes the muscles and, if taken at bedtime, usually encourages sound sleep.

The flowers and leaves of a number of plants relax and tone the skin when placed in a bath. Roman soldiers after a long march would relax in baths containing dry bay leaves or rosemary. Those of north Europe would use fresh or dry balm leaves, pine leaves, pennyroyal or water mint, each of which gives the water a refreshing smell. The flowers of chamomile or elder have the same effect. Fragrant agrimony and bergamot can also be used.

To include the plants in the bath water, place them in a muslin bag. Tie the bag closed with string, and put it in the bath as the water is run in.

For centuries a milk bath has always been considered the height of luxury; since Nero's wife, Poppaea bathed in donkey's milk and rose water.

To make a cleansing and toning milk bath at home: dissolve 2 large cupfuls of dried milk in 2 litres of warm water; add 2 cupfuls of chamomile tea previously prepared from the flowers (fresh or dry) and stir in 2 large spoonfuls of honey until dissolved; pour into a bath of warm water and soak the body thoroughly for 10 minutes before using soap. A

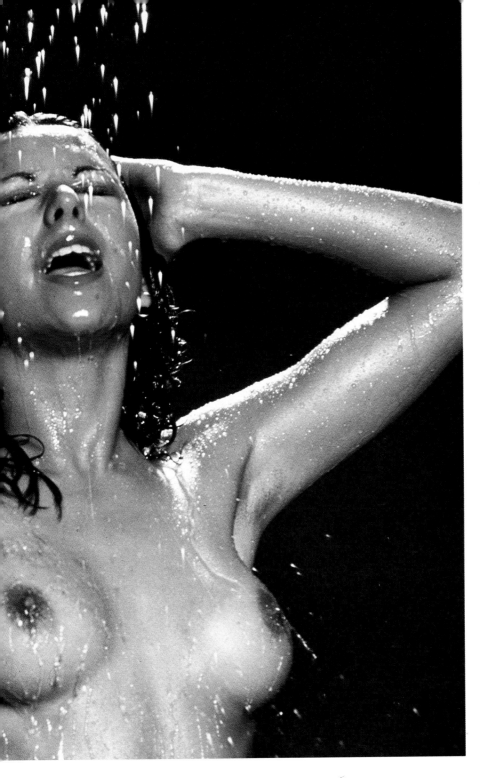

Different herbs provide different comforts in the bath water, lavender and balm being especially effective as a calmative and rosemary and pine as a stimulant.

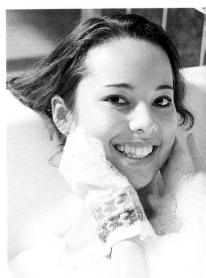

Extract of chamomile is the all-time favourite bath additive, being suited both to the fresh skin of an infant and the tired flesh of the mature adult. Donkey's milk, when available, is also a welcome addition to any bath.

bath oil for dry skin can be made from several ingredients including corn or olive oil and either apricot or cucumber juice, with yogurt, milk and eggs. (See Recipes.) It is especially effective for those living in a warm climate.

For an "after-bath" or "after-shower" spray for normal skins, mix 4 oz of rosemary or red rose water with 4 oz of fresh milk and refrigerate for an hour before using. Place in a sprayer and apply the full force to the body. For greasy skin, use 2 tablespoons of milk, the same of witch hazel and lemon juice, and 8 oz of chamomile tea with 3 oz rosemary or red rose water. Refrigerate before

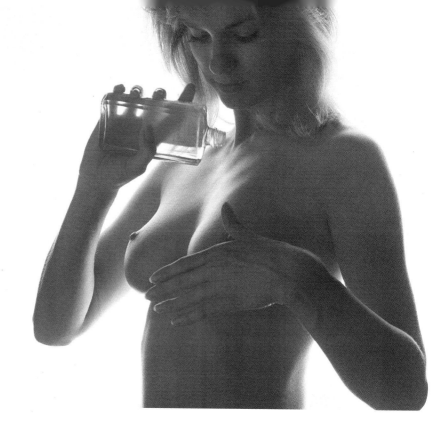

The practice of anointing the body with oil is especially recommended for sun-dried skins. Breasts which have been exposed to the sun are even more in need of oil than other parts of the body, since the skin of the breasts is more sensitive than that of other areas.

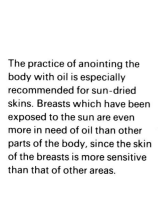

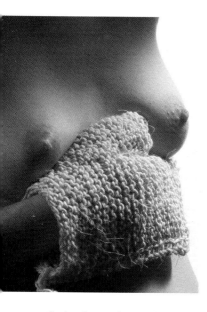

Curiously, certain practices that one would associate with the more perverse elements of medieval penitance – such as self-flagellation with birch branches and rubbing the body with hemp – are making a comeback in the world of twentieth century body care. Rubbing the body with a hemp mitt stimulates the pores and makes the skin feel good.

using. Allow to dry on before dressing.

If the skin tends to be dry and there is a shower room in the home, smear corn or olive oil over the body, beginning at the neck and working down to the legs and feet. Then turn on the shower to "hot" but do not stand under it. Draw the curtains to create a Turkish bath atmosphere. Turn off the shower and stand in the steam for several minutes. Then stand out again and repeat the process. Stand under a warm shower and use a good quality toilet soap to wash off the oil, which will by then have soaked into the skin.

The shower cubicle can also be used to refreshen the body after taking a shower. Before going in, fill a litre size plastic spray bottle with not quite a litre of soda water into which the juice of a grapefruit or lemon has been placed. After drying, stand back into the cubicle, draw the curtains and spray the body from neck to legs. Stand for several minutes to allow the moisture to drain off and the rest to dry on before dressing or better still, relax on the

bed for half an hour with the face covered in pieces of cucumber held in place with a cold flannel.

Skin has a natural acid coating made up from sweat and oils which work to the surface through the pores, protecting it from harmful bacteria and keeping out the cold. Alkalines (also present in hair dyes of chemical composition) will destroy this acidity layer and as soaps are alkaline, only those of the highest quality and enriched with natural oils should be used.

MAKING YOUR OWN SOAP

To make a toilet soap of pleasing perfume, enriched with olive, palm or almond oil, place several bars of ordinary yellow or green curd soap, cut into thin wafers, in an iron pan over a low flame. Add water and put the lid on. Melt the soap in the steam created in the pan, adding more soap every half-hour until the whole is of a uniform soft consistency. You can then stir in any one of the vegetable oils and extinguish the flame. As the mixture begins to cool, add perfume, but not if you have used palm oil. Pour into a frame made with hard wood sides and a base. The sides should have slots to take thin strips of wood which will divide the box into sections and the soap into bars when it has set. This will take 2 or 3 days or longer. The partitions are then re-moved and the bars cut into sections each about $1\frac{1}{2}$ inches or 4 cm thick, the bars being about 3 inches or 7 cm in length and 2 inches (5 cm) wide. Trim the sharp edges off the tablets and stand each on its side to complete the setting or hardening which may take 6 months. The longer soap is kept, the harder it becomes and the more economic it is. Such a soap will have low alkalinity and contain the oils for a natural skin food. Where palm oil is used, the pale green colouring can be accentuated by the addition of a small amount of chlorophyll.

Soaps can be perfumed with vari-ous flower and leaf scents. The fra-grance of orange blossom is obtained by using otto of neroli to curd soap and the smell of sandalwood is ob-tained from otto of sandalwood and a small amount of otto of bergamot. The refreshing scent of Brown Wind-sor soap is obtained from ottos of caraway, cloves, thyme and lavender and the brown colour from burnt sugar or caramel. Medicated soaps are made by adding the various medi-caments to curd soap. Sulphur soap is that most widely used; it cleanses the skin of blemishes. Flowers of sulphur are added, and mixed in thoroughly whilst the soap is soft and still warm.

The soap bars are made up as described.

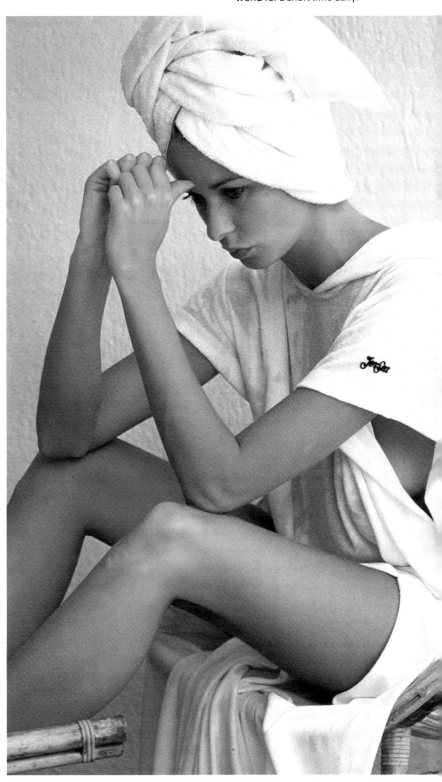

CARE OF THE FEET AND LEGS

In medieval times, people used Soapwort or Bouncing Bet, a perennial weed found by ponds and streams, which creeps over the waste ground rooting at the nodes. Its leaves and stems when crushed yield the principle saponin, which creates a rich lather when mixed with water. Indeed, the word "soap" comes from the plant's botanical name, *Saponaria*, from the Greek, *sapon*. Pliny often mentioned in his writings that soap making was discovered by the Gauls who made it from tallow and ashes.

The primary soaps are divided into hard and soft. Hard soaps contain soda as the base; soft soaps have a potash base and are made from lard. The finest soaps are only slightly alkaline (nearly neutral) and are known as curd soaps, these being hard soaps made from pure soda and tallow. Oil soaps are made from olive or palm oil and pure soda and contain very little water in combination. Here, the odour and colour of the palm oil is unchanged, the odoriferous principle resembling that of orris.

Taking each part of the body in turn, we begin with the most important: the feet which control one's gait and posture. One quarter of the bones in the body are present in the feet. After bathing, dry the feet thoroughly, especially between the toes for dampness left for any length of time will encourage "athlete's foot". This is due to a fungus which attacks the skin between the toes causing cracking and flaking and considerable soreness.

Excess moisture, caused by the feet sweating in warm weather may also cause "athlete's foot", to soak up this moisture, it is advisable to use plenty of talcum powder on the feet after bathing and before putting on shoes. Use the powder again at bedtime, especially between the toes. A home-made powder is made from orris root and wheat or rice starch, together with a small quantity of powdered cloves or sandalwood. It is also applied with a puff to all those parts of the body where perspiration proves troublesome.

Those who are on their feet for

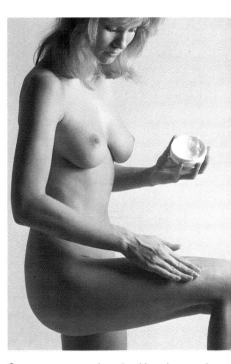

Creams to massage into the skin to improve its elasticity include olive, almond and sesame oil and for baths, to relax tired and aching limbs, there is bergamot, the mints, rosemary and extract of horse chestnuts.

long periods each day should pay particular attention to the feet. The ancient Greeks believed them to be the most important part of the body and would spend long hours caring for them. To harden the skin, to prevent calluses from forming on the bottoms of the feet, rub the soles upon rising each day with lemon juice in a small amount of water. Once each week, soak the feet in a warm footbath in which are placed herbs such as rosemary, catmint or wild thyme, and afterward massage them with olive oil. Do this at bedtime and put on a pair of old socks kept for the purpose and sleep in them. The oil will soak into the feet overnight and leave them soft and supple by morning.

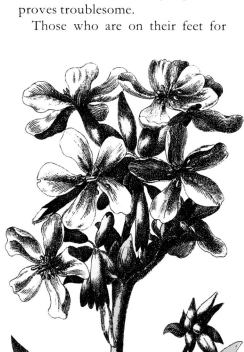

See that the toe nails are trimmed once each week, first soaking them in warm water for 20 minutes to soften them. Once a week massage warm olive oil into and around the nails and sleep in socks. If painting the nails, first apply a base (as with finger nails) to protect them from absorbing colour to which some people are allergic.

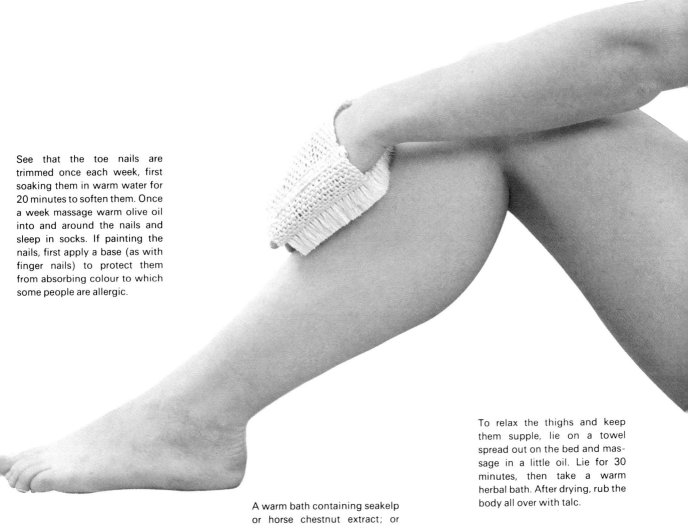

A warm bath containing seakelp or horse chestnut extract; or herbs such as rosemary, balm or bay will relax the muscles of the legs and thighs. After drying, gently massage them with a little olive oil or almond oil and sleep in old stockings.

To relax the thighs and keep them supple, lie on a towel spread out on the bed and massage in a little oil. Lie for 30 minutes, then take a warm herbal bath. After drying, rub the body all over with talc.

Soak for 15 minutes daily in a bath or bowl or warm water and treat with olive oil massaging it well in as for the nails. After washing the feet, dry well between the toes and apply talc to take up any surplus moisture. To prevent callouses forming beneath the feet, rub the soles daily with lemon juice or witch hazel.

CARE OF THE HANDS AND NAILS

The feet can be cared for by a daily soaking in a bath, and by the application of various dusting powders, particularly at night. A simple massage of oil will do wonders for tired overworked feet.

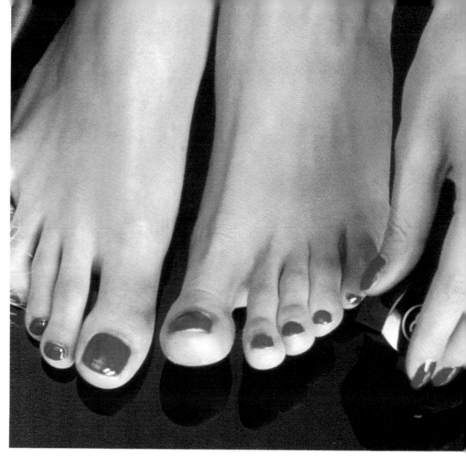

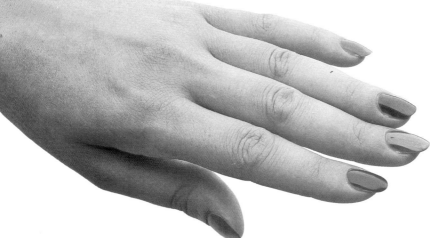

The care of the hands is as important as the feet, and well groomed hands are as noticeable as a well groomed head of hair. As hands are constantly in use, they become stained and the nails discoloured if not given constant attention. If the hands and nails become discoloured, rub half a lemon over them and afterwards, rinse them in white wine vinegar made slightly warm. Then place the hands in warm water and using a soft soap and nail brush, scrub them hard, especially the nails. After drying, soak the nails for 5 minutes in warm olive or almond oil, then massage the oil into the hands, paying particular attention to the fingers and backs which in cold weather and from the use of detergents for washing clothes and crockery become chapped. A teaspoonful of honey mixed with the oil will improve the treatment. Then wrap the hands in a warm towel for 5 minutes, remove and again massage in the oil. Then put on a pair of cotton gloves kept for the purposes and sleep in them. By morning the hands will be soft and beautifully white and any soreness will have healed completely. This care should be given the hands once every week, before going to bed. It will take about 15 minutes and will keep the hands and nails attractively white and smooth.

Another way to care for the hands is to massage a mixture of a tablespoonful of almond oil and a cupful

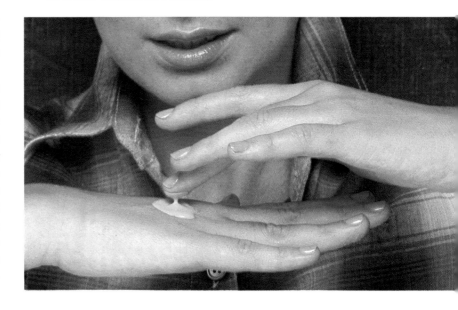

To strengthen the nails, soak them daily for 5 minutes in warm almond (or olive) oil. For discoloured nails, clean them with lemon juice and scrub them in white wine vinegar.

of buttermilk into the hands at bedtime. Wear cotton gloves and sleep in them and wash the hands in warm water upon rising.

Similar to the hair and skin, nails are made up of keratin. Alkaline detergents and poor quality soaps weaken the nails and cause them to split so it is advisable to wear rubber gloves when using detergents or indeed, when doing any work which will stain the hands. The best of all nail "varnishes" is white iodine from sea kelp which strengthens and protects them. Acetone which is used to remove coloured nail varnish is dry-

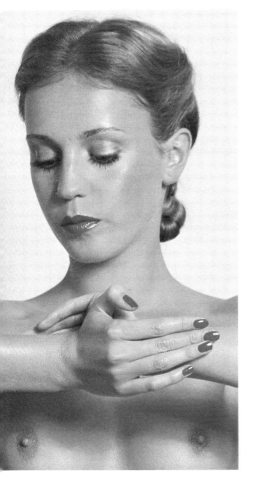

ing and harsh, so after using (which should be only once weekly), soak the nails in olive oil for a few minutes before washing the hands.

Nails need protein to keep them strong and this must be provided in the diet. They should also be kept as dry as possible, water harms nails, and they should be manicured every few days to keep them at the right length and to press back the cuticles. This is done with a small stick with a wad of cotton at the end, after first softening the cuticles in warm water. The nails should always be dry before manicuring. Use a pair of sharp scissors for trimming them and an emery (sand paper) file rather than a metal one. Always file the nail in the same direction. Manicuring is best done before bedtime and the nails and hands then treated with olive oil.

TO SOFTEN HARD OR CHAPPED HANDS

Mix a teaspoonful of honey with two of almond (or olive) oil and massage into the hands after washing them in warm soapy water and drying. Put on a pair of old cotton gloves, kept for the purpose, and sleep in them. Wash the hands in warm soapy water in the morning and they will be soft and white. Repeat a second night if necessary.

Hand creams, needed to replace loss of moisture and oil from the hands through having them too long in water, will contain carrageen moss which provides mucilage, as does sodium alginate which may be used as an alternative.

OTHER PARTS OF THE BODY

Oils to massage into the skin to improve its elasticity include olive, almond and sesame. For an after-bath oil, almond, olive and sunflower oils can be used and for home-made toilet soaps, stearic acid and coconut oil provide abundant lather as well as nourishing properties for the skin.

To firm the breasts after child feeding or illness, mix collagen with a teaspoonful of tincture of arnica (from the chemist or by treating the roots of the flowers with spirits of wine) and massage gently into the breasts using a circular movement. This should be done daily for a month or so.

Everyone wants to have a beautiful suntan, and indeed the sun is essential for the maintenance of a healthy body. Care should always be taken to avoid the sun when it is strongest and to protect the skin against too strong a dosage of the sun's brightest rays. Nature's best suntan oil is a combination of almond, sesame, olive and coconut oils.

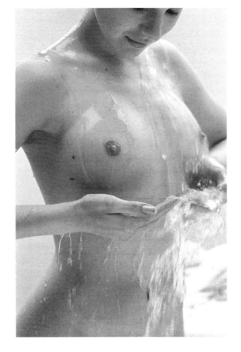

Firm breasts are as important to a woman as a good head of hair. Gentle exercising as described will be an advantage. To firm them after feeding babies, countrywomen would use Lady's Mantle, a prostrate perennial of grassy mountainous slopes of colder climes. Women would make an infusion of the flowers and soak cloths in it while still warm, and place them on the breasts while lying down for half an hour daily. The writer, Max Hoffman, who knew of its virtues in this respect, said the plant "had the power of restoring feminine beauty however faded, to its early freshness".

Women of the Mediterranean countries would use the seeds of *Nigella sativa* instead to make an infusion to apply in the same way. They would also rub the powder of the ground seeds on their breasts at night. Extract of arnica may also be used to tighten the breasts.

Care of the neck is important in preserving one's youth, for nothing shows the advancing years more than wrinkles and bagginess of the skin beneath the jaws and around the neck. Gentle exercises such as the following should be done night and morning throughout one's life: move the head to the right and to the left then, move the head in as wide a circle as possible, first clockwise, then counter-clockwise, several times each way but not so often as to cause dizziness. At bedtime, massage in a nourishing skin food. Begin just beneath the ear with a downwards movement then round and upwards and the same for each side of the neck. Make up a skin food or ask the chemist to do it for you to this recipe: $1\frac{1}{2}$ ozs of almond oil; $\frac{1}{2}$ oz lanolin; $\frac{1}{2}$ oz spermaceti; $\frac{1}{2}$ oz witch hazel, benzoin, and a few drops of tincture of benzoin (to prevent its turning rancid). To make the neck and shoulders soft and white, use this mixture as a rub; 12 ozs elderflower water, $\frac{1}{2}$ oz glycerine and 3 drams powdered borax. This will display the shoulders to advantage when revealed by an off-the-shoulder evening frock. Or alternatively, use 4 ozs almond oil with 8 ozs rose water, not forgetting to add the benzoin. Or use juice with almond oil and a few drops of benzoin to massage into the neck, bosom and shoulders.

Greatest of all revitalisers is the sun, worshipped by the Egyptians as the greatest of all the deities for its healing powers. All growth relies on the sun without which the earth would be in perpetual darkness. Its short ultra-violet rays bring about the formation of vitamin D, the enemy of rickets and malformation of the bones; its long rays acting on the nervous system, being relaxing, comforting and toning. It is stimulating to the blood vessels, improving the circulation and causing a sense of well-being. But the sun's rays are powerful, hot enough to fry an egg on a pavement and too long exposure will do the same to the skin, burning the epidermis and the rays may even reach down to the dermis beneath, causing blistering and burning large areas of skin. If exposing the body to the sun at the beginning of summer, do so only for 10–15 minutes on the first day and increase this by a few minutes daily. Make sure to cover the eyes with a thick cloth to protect them. To protect the skin, massage into the body each day before sun bathing begins, an efficient sun-tan oil or lotion. This will give a healthy tan to the skin and prevent any soreness. The best of all sun-tan oils is sesame oil, but if it is not available, use one of the lotions containing para-aminobenzoic acid which will allow certain ultra-violet rays to penetrate the skin but will prevent any burning. Never sleep in the sun but move the body about frequently so that any one part does not become too exposed. After sun-bathing, massage the oil into the body rather than wash it off, for it will feed the skin.

Instant relief can be given to those parts which have become over-exposed to the sun by the application of calamine lotion, which can be obtained from a chemist and which also makes an excellent base for face powders. Or use the juice of half a cucumber put through a juicer with a small cupful of milk and pat it onto the sore area with lint or cotton wool. If no cucumber is available, use vinegar and water (half and half).

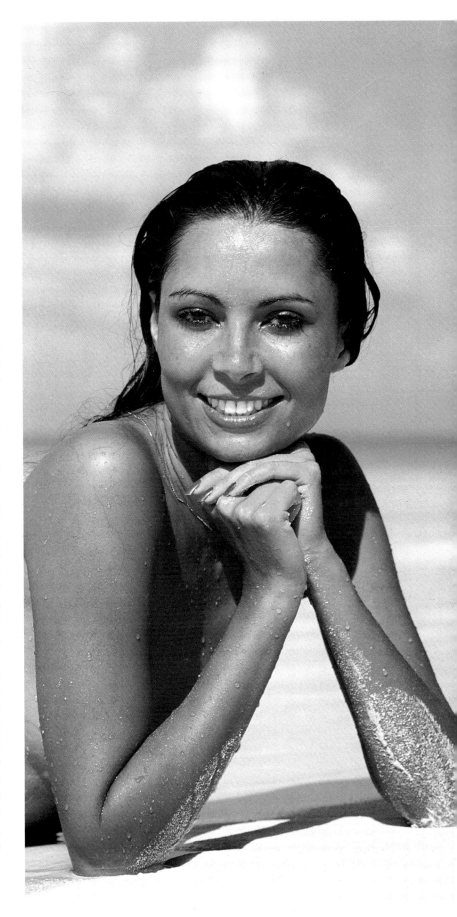

Cosmetics and perfumes of the east

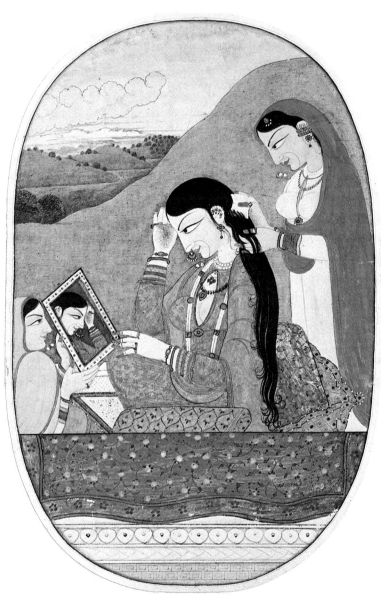

Oriental women spend several hours daily on the care of their jet black hair which they keep in condition with oil in which gall nuts have been heated and to which is added a mixture of herbs, cloves, gum arabic, henna leaves and flowers of the pomegranate.

After the fall of the Roman Empire, after centuries of unrivalled splendour and good living, these fineries spread eastwards, first to Constantinople where on the byzantine domes, the Crescent replaced the Holy Cross, the followers of Mohammed taking with them a love and a knowledge of the aromatic gums of Arabia where the prophet was born and where he died. By the tenth century, Muslim suzerainty stretched from Araby to the Indus, encompassing the whole of Alexander's Macedonian empire where the conqueror obtained his love of fragrant substances.

It was an Arabian doctor, Avicenna, practising in the tenth century, who was first to obtain a volatile oil from flowers, the attar, by distillation, for until then, the only known perfumes were sweet gums and resins, exudations obtained from the stems of plants. Avicenna is believed to have used the rose of a hundred'petals, R. centifolia, in his experiments and he has described the methods he used to obtain the attar, confirmed by other writers of the time.

To the peoples of the East, the rose was the favourite of all flowers for it gave of its perfume in many ways. The petals of the red rose, R. rubra or R. gallica increase in perfume when dry and the longer they are kept the stronger it becomes. From the flowers of the Damask rose, attar and sweet scented water is obtained.

The Turkish people took their love of bathing from the Romans, introducing the idea of steam-heated baths. The sweating caused by the heat opened the pores and rid the skin of impurities. The body was then washed with the fragrant soaps and massaged with scented oils. "... by thy scent my soul is ravished", wrote the Persian poet Sadi, author of *Gulistan*, a poem about a garden of roses which is the most exquisite of all Persian writings.

Oriental women in their anxiousness to please their menfolk, attend to their toilet as their most urgent occupation. "Nowhere are the women more beautiful, nowhere are they better skilled or more practised in the art of arresting or repairing the ravages of time", wrote the Italian, Sonnini, in his *Travels*.

Robert Browning, in *Paracelsus*, tells of the lavish use of fragrant flowers and resins by Hindu women to dress their

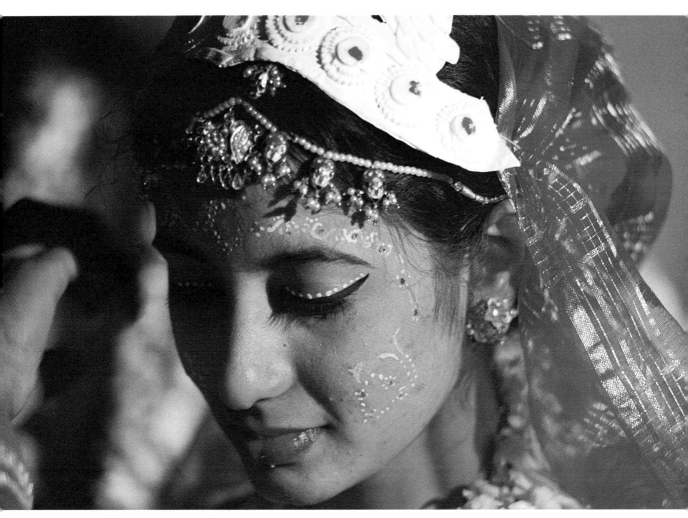

A Hindu bride made up for the wedding ceremony. A complexion powder known as batikha to whiten the face and body is widely used in the East.

hair:

Heap cassis, sandal-buds and stripes
  of labdanum, and aloe-balls,
Smear'd with dull nard, an Indian
  wipes
From out her hair.

In Eastern countries where water is scarce, people make use of spices and resins to burn as incense, to fumigate clothes and bedding and to purify the body.

At Hindu marriages, the bride receives from her husband, a toilet or beauty box containing a glass bottle filled with otto of roses, one of rose water, a spice box, a hair comb, a box of powder called soorma to darken the eye lids and another containing kohl to darken the eyelashes, also a box holding betel nuts to chew in order to sweeten the breath. Kama, the god of love of Indian myth-

ology is always depicted with his Cupid's bow and five arrows, each of which is tipped with the blossom of a scented flower. Each arrow can pierce the heart through the five senses. One of the most

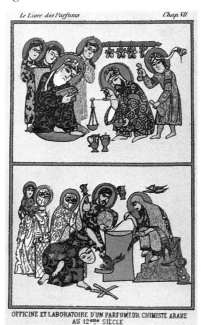

An Arab perfumer selling his wares. It was an Arabian doctor, Avicenna, practicing in the 10th century, who first obtained a volatile oil from flowers by distillation. Until then the only known perfumes were sweet gums and resins, exudations obtained from the stem of plants.

It is common practice in the Indonesian islands, as well as in the Philippines and in many islands of the Pacific, to anoint one's head with fragrant oil and to adorn it with wreaths of scented flowers which form a natural enfleurage in the oil of the hair, giving it a perpetual fragrance. Below, a Balinese dancer. Slender hands and long fingernails (here artificially elongated) are an essential feature to the beauty of classical Indonesian dancers (opposite).

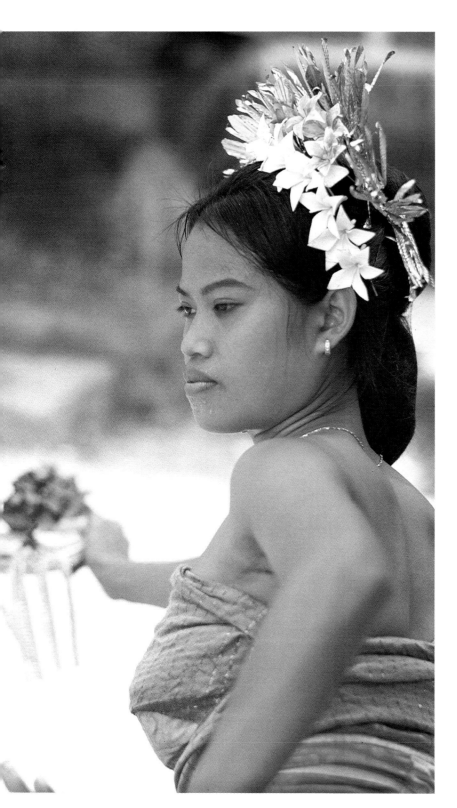

popular of all Hindu perfumes is jasmine sambac. It is produced at Ghazepore, situated on the left bank of the Ganges above the Holy City of Benares, where all Hindu hope to visit to ensure their salvation in the life hereafter.

The sambac jasmine was mentioned in the earliest known treatise on flowering plants written by Chi Han in the third century AD. It was cultivated for its perfume from Peking to Canton, the unopened buds of the flowers being taken to the cities each day to decorate the hair of Chinese girls. The buds were also placed in tea giving China tea its unique quality.

The jasmine gardens in Kwantung Province extend for miles along the banks of the Pearl River. In *An account of the Interesting Objects in Kwantung Province*, by Li T'so Yuan (1777) there is a charming description of jasmine buds used to decorate the hair: after the fragrant buds are placed in the hair at eventide, they begin to open, becoming brighter under moonlight and more fragrant with human warmth, their scent lingering until dawn.

Carl Thunberg, the Swedish naturalist and explorer, gives a similar picture of Batavian women. They anoint their hair with fragrant oil, then tie it into a large knot on top of the head and adorn it with wreaths of scented *Nyctanthes tuberosa*, a small tree native of the Indonesian islands which bears white star-like flowers with the scent, according to Thunberg, of orange blossoms. "The whole house", he wrote "is filled with the scent, enhancing if possible, the society of the fair sex".

The women of Thailand also adorn their heads with fragrant flowers which form a natural enfleurage in the oil of the hair and give it a perpetual fragrance. The Tagal women of the Philippine Islands also pay particular attention to their long jet black hair, treating it daily

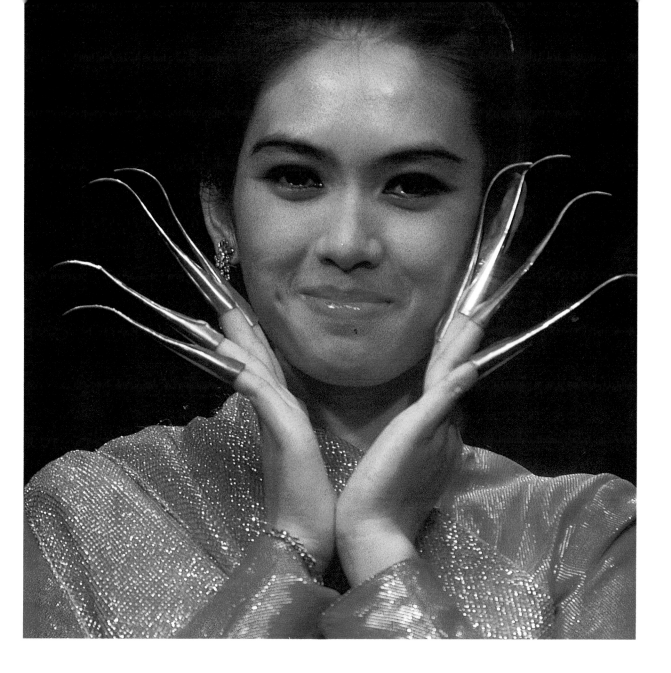

with coconut oil. The oil of coconut, in great demand in Western hair dressings, is used also by the women of Tahiti: it is usually scented with oil of sandalwood. Tahitian women massage their bodies with an oil they call monoi which keeps the skin soft and smooth as well as sweet-smelling in the tropical heat.

Indian women use a preparation known as Urgujja to massage into the body. It is composed chiefly of otto of rose and essence of jasmine. Indian women also make a body oil from "gingelly" seeds. The oil in the seeds becomes impregnated with the perfume of jasmine or the flowers of *Cananga odorata* with

which they are placed in boxes for several days before the flowers are renewed. This process continues for 3–4 weeks.

The most popular dusting powder amongst Eastern women is Abeer. Its chief ingredients – sandlewood, aloes, rose petals, zedoary and a few grains of civet – are pounded in a mortar until they become a fine powder. Zedoary is the tuberous root of *Curcuma zedoaria*, a plant of the ginger family, native of China and Bengal. An extract of the roots, amongst the most important articles of perfumery and cosmetics in the East, is used by Indian women to enliven the colouring of their normally dark complexions.

With flowery headgear and face paint, an African school girl (overleaf) is going to the school opening. The need artificially to beautify face and body, using make up to frighten off enemies and illnesses or to attract the opposite sex, is a constant of human culture since time immemorial.

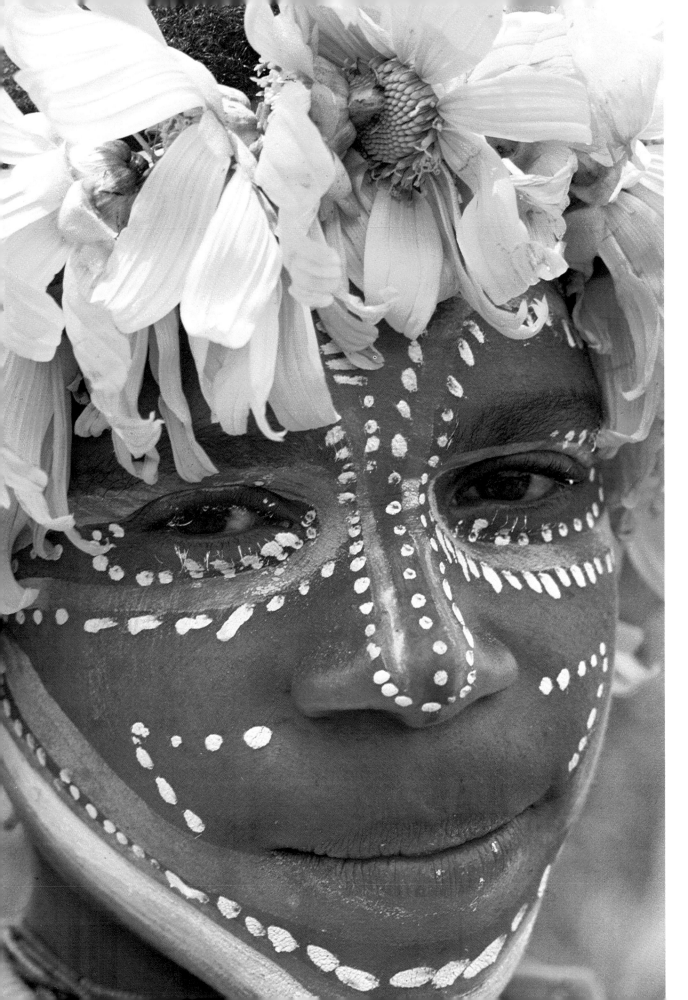

The home cosmetician

REFERENCE SECTION III
In this section the most common cosmetic preparations are listed for the various parts of the body. The reader will find at a glance the beauty aid he is looking for under the appropriate heading. The recipes include instructions on how to prepare specific herbal products along with notes about related applications.

There are cosmetics for all purposes: to improve the quality of the skin, nourishing it and clearing it of spots and blemishes; for the eyes, to remove tiredness and to give the eyes a sparkle; for the hair, to impart a healthy gloss, for its colouring and to prevent it from falling out, whilst correcting any dryness or excess greasiness. And there are prepara-

banned substances. Certain other substances are permitted in limited amounts only and these must be listed on the product. This directive came into force 1 January 1980. The Food and Drug Administration (FDA) of the U.S.A. requires by law that all ingredients used in cosmetics and hair dyes be labelled, so that users with skin allergies to any of them could take notice of the contents.

A number of ingredients contained in hair dyes have been proved to be cancer-causing when fed to animals and these may be dangerous to humans when penetrating the scalp, and a number of toxic chemicals used in cosmetics may irritate the skin. These are used mostly as preservatives and are now being replaced by others which are less dangerous. The American FDA now prohibits the use of nine chemicals once used in hair dyes. Natural hair dyes take time to improve the colour but also condition the hair. Cosmetics without chemical preservatives will not have as long a life but will be safe to use, whilst the use of natural oils in creams and body oils will not deprive the skin of fat-soluble vitamins as does mineral oil.

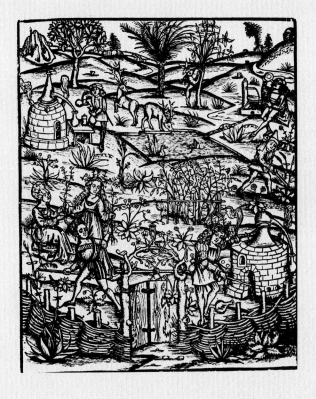

Above, a woodcut from the *Liber de Arte Distillandi* (Book of the Art of Distillation) by Brunschwyg Hieronymus, which appeared around 1500 in Strasburg.

tions for maintaining all parts of the body in condition and to give it a sense of well being.

The recipes given contain only natural ingredients. Toxic chemicals included in cosmetic preparations which were dangerous for users, compelled the European Economic Community to issue a directive making it an offence to make or sell cosmetics containing any of these 350

Astringent lotions

Plant	Preparation	Notes
157 Benzoin	The gum resin of styrax benzoin provides benzoic acid, which prevents fats from turning rancid and gives permanency to perfumes. A few drops of tincture of benzoin, added to equal parts of witch hazel and rose water and applied to the face and neck, tightens the skin and closes enlarged pores.	It should be kept under refrigeration and used once weekly.
23 Birch	An effective astringent complexion lotion is made from the leaves by infusing a handful in a pint (0·5 litre) of boiling water and straining when cold.	
90 Common Privet	Place two handsful of flowers in a saucepan and add a pint (0·5 litre) of water. Heat for several minutes over a low flame. Cool and strain and add 2 tablespoonsful (1 fluid ounce) of witch hazel or rose water. Bottle and cork tightly and keep under refrigeration.	
36 Cornflower	Infuse a handful of the flowers in a half-pint (0·25 litre) of boiling water and allow to cool. With the addition of a teaspoonful of witch hazel, this infusion makes an effective astringent lotion.	
112 Ground Ivy	Make an infusion of the whole plant (roots excluded) by adding a large handful to a pint (0·5 litre) of boiling water; strain and cool. This proves an effective astringent and will clear the skin of spots and pimples.	Take a wineglassful daily of the infusion for the same effect and to tone the system.
77 Hop	Obtain a perfumed water from the newly opened flowers by placing them in a still or kettle. The distillation is an effective astringent lotion.	Can be used to provide a pungent and pleasant-smelling handkerchief perfume.
139 Lesser Celandine	Take a large handful of the plant and infuse in a pint (0·5 litre) of boiling water for 15 minutes. When cool, add a teaspoonful of lemon juice and apply to the face with lint pads. It will tighten the skin, remove wrinkles, and close large pores.	
139 Lesser Celandine	An ointment made by heating a large handful of the plant, with flowers of elder and houseleek and the leaves of the common plantain in 1 lb (0·5 kilo) of pure lard, will rid the skin of pimples and sores. After heating for 20 minutes, strain and allow to cool off before pouring into screw-top jars.	
48 Lilly of the Valley	The distilled water obtained by heating 1 lb (0·5 kilo) of flowers in a kettle of water and collecting the steam in a jar (see Red Rose) makes an effective astringent lotion and leaves the skin white and soft.	
163 Lime	Add the juice of a lime (or lemon) to 2 large cupsful (8 fluid ounces) of water and to it add 1 tablespoonful (½ fluid ounce) of simple tincture of benzoin as a preservative.	This simple solution is best suited to dry and normal skins; for an oily skin, witch hazel is preferable.
65 Meadowsweet	Place a handful of flowers in a bowl and pour over them a half-pint (0·25 litre) of boiling water. When cool, strain, and add a teaspoonful of witch hazel for an effective astringent lotion.	A similar infusion of the flowers will bring comfort to tired eyes and give them a sparkle.
44 Neroli	The finest neroli otto is obtained from orange flowers, by distillation and by maceration and is known as "neroli pétale". "Neroli bigarade" is obtained from flowers of the Seville or bitter orange. The essence or esprit is obtained by "washing" 2 oz (60 g) of pomade with 4 pints (2 litre) of rectified spirit. Mixed with elder flower or rose water, it is an effective astringent, closing large pores almost at once.	

Plant	Preparation	Notes

| 143 | Red Rose | Gather 1 lb (0·5 kg) of scented red or deep pink rose petals and put in a large kettle half filled with water and over a low flame. Attach a length of rubber tube to the spout, leading to a large glas jar; before reaching the jar, the tube should pass through a bowl of cold (preferably iced) water to cool the steam, so have the tube of sufficient length. Pure rose water of rich perfume will continue to drip into the jar until all the water in the kettle has evaporated. Pour into smaller bottles and cork or screw down. Apply to the face and neck to tighten the skin and remove (and prevent) wrinkles. "Mock orange" blossom (*philadelphus*) is also unharmed by heat and can be used instead of roses.
Always use scented red or deep pink rose petals so that the rose water will be of a pleasing pink colour. If pale pink or white roses are used, the colour will be a "dirty" shade of grey or pale brown.
An even simpler method of making rose water, but one which will not be as concentrated, is to place 1 lb (0·5 kg) of rose petals in a saucepan and cover with a half-litre of water. Put on the lid to prevent the steam escaping and simmer over a low flame for 30 minutes. Allow to cool, keeping the lid on, then strain into a glass jar with a screw-top. Store in a refrigerator.
To make an astringent: Stir into a tablespoonful ($\frac{1}{2}$ fluid ounce) of glycerine placed in a bowl, a small cupful (4 fluid ounces) of alcohol, then twice the volume of witch hazel and three times that of rose water. Pour into bottles, cork tightly and keep under refrigeration. | |

| 151 | Rose-root | Though not nearly as powerful in its scent and astringent qualities, rose-root water is a useful substitute for that made from the petals. The roots are lifted in autumn (when plants are divided) and pieces of the succulent roots are removed, cut up, and washed clean, whilst they are replanted. Place 1 lb (0·5 kg) of root in a saucepan with a lid and add 1 pint (0·5 kg) of water. Simmer over a low flame for 1 hour (with the lid on), then strain into bottles when cool and keep under refrigeration. | |

| 37 | Sweet Fern | Make an infusion of a handful of the fresh leaves in a half-pint of boiling water or hot (but not boiling) milk; apply to the face, after the removal of make-up, and let it dry; will remove blackheads and pimples and close up large pores. | |

| 93 | Sweet Gum | The resin which exudes from the bark is used to give permanence to flower odours. A fluid drachm mixed with a cupful (4 fluid ounces) of rose water and a tablespoonful ($\frac{1}{2}$ fluid ounce) of witch hazel will prove to be an efficient astringent lotion, tightening the skin and closing large pores. | |

| 92 | Toadflax | The distilled water is an efficient astringent, closing large pores and removing wrinkles. The addition of a teaspoonful of lemon juice or witch hazel to every $\frac{1}{2}$ pint (0·25 litre) of water will give greater efficiency. | |

| 83 | Walnut | An infusion of a handful of the leaves in a $\frac{1}{2}$ pint (0·25 litre) of boiling water, will be an effective astringent when applied to the complexion. | A wineglassful taken daily will rid the skin of blemishes. |

| 73 | Witch Hazel | To a teacupful (4 fluid ounces) of rose water made by distillation, add 2 tablespoonsful (1 fluid ounce) of witch hazel, obtainable from a chemist or druggist and 1 table-spoonful ($\frac{1}{2}$ fluid ounce) tincture of benzoin. Apply to the face and neck at night. Rosemary water can be used as an alternative to rose water. | For a neutral skin. |
| | | Mix 4 tablespoonsful (2 fluid ounces) of calomine lotion; 4 of witch hazel and 2 tablespoonsful (1 fluid ounce) of pepper-mint essence with a teaspoonful of cider vinegar. Add 1 | For an oily (greasy) skin. |

[handwritten at bottom: Calomine lotion : cooling, pink covering creme f. sunburn + measles]

Plant	Preparation	Notes
Witch Hazel (continued)	tablespoonful ($\frac{1}{2}$ fluid ounce) tincture of benzoin as a preservative. Apply to the face and neck with cotton wool pads after steaming open the pores and leave on.	
16 Wormwood	Place a handful of rosemary tops and one of wormwood in a large screw-top glass jar and over them add 2 pints (1 litre) of malt vinegar. Leave in a sunny window for a week, then add 1 oz (30 g) powdered camphor, leave for 24 hours, strain and bottle. In place of rosemary and wormwood, red rose petals and sweet marjoram can be used. Treat in the same way. Use undiluted on the face, neck and forehead to tighten the skin or add a little of the malt vinegar to a half basin of ice cold water. This is an effective cooler on a hot day and will clear the skin of perspiration and close the pores.	

Complexion lotions

Plant	Preparation	Notes
12 Angelica	Dig up the root of a two-year old plant. Clean and slice it before placing in a pan with a $\frac{1}{2}$ pint (0·25 litre) of water. Add a tablespoonful of honey and simmer for 20 minutes; the liquid will be honey-coloured and aromatic. Cool and strain into a bottle and use as a complexion lotion. Keep in the refrigerator.	
171 Brooklime	Make an infusion of a handful of the hollow stems and leaves in a pint (0·5 litre) of boiling water; let cool. Apply to the face with lint pads to remove spots and blackheads to leave the skin soft and clean.	A wineglassful of the infusion taken daily will clear the blood and give the same results. It is also a good idea to include the plant in salads in place of watercress.
61 Centaury	Take a handful of the whole herb, fresh or dry, and add to a pint (0·5 litre) of boiling water; allow to stand until cold. Applied to the face, the infusion will take away blemishes and leave the skin soft and smooth.	It is also a blood purifier and tonic, is equally effective when taken internally. Drink a wineglassful daily.
156 Chickweed	A handful of the fresh herb, with 1 oz (30 g) of ground ivy or wood sage infused in a pint (0·5 litre) of boiling water will, if applied to the face and neck when cool, take away spots and pimples and firm the flesh.	It is a blood purifyer, used fresh in salads or cooked like spinach.
145 Clary	A handful of fresh tops in a pint (0·5 litre) of boiling water will, after straining and cooling, make a soothing complexion lotion. If $\frac{1}{2}$ oz (15 g) of the seed is steeped in cold water for 24 hours and one drop of the mucilage is placed on a pimple or infected blackhead, it will draw it and quickly heal the skin.	
70 Cleavers	To make a lotion to remove freckles and ease sunburn, place a handful of the fresh herb in a saucepan and cover with a half-pint (0·25) litre) of water. Simmer for 20 minutes, strain, and apply to the face either warm or after having been refrigerated for 30 minutes.	A wineglassful taken hot or cold will clear the skin of impurities and leave it soft and smooth.
159 Costmary	Place a handful of leaves in a bowl of buttermilk for 24 hours and strain. This will make a soothing lotion especially effective for a dry or sunburnt skin.	
17 Cuckoo-pint	Dig the tubers in autumn; slice and boil them for 10 minutes in a pint (0·5 litre) of water to remove some of the starch and toxic properties. Drain off the liquid, then add a half-pint of milk to the tubers and simmer slowly for 20 minutes. Strain into bottles when cool and apply to the complexion; it will rid the face of pimples and leave the skin soft and white.	

Plant	Preparation	Notes
142 Damask Rose	Add a cupful (4 fluid ounces) of rose water to one of creamy milk and mix with the milky juice of $\frac{1}{2}$ lb (0·25 kg) of almonds put through a blender. Apply to the face and neck with lint pads. Leave on for an hour before washing off.	
161 Dandelion	To $\frac{1}{2}$ lb (0·25 kg) of fresh roots and the same amount of horseradish, add a pint (0·5 litre) of water or milk and simmer for 10 minutes. Strain and bottle and apply as a complexion lotion at bedtime. Let dry on.	
60 Horsetail	Cut the flowerless stems in pieces late in summer and place in a large saucepan. To make an infusion, cover with 2 pints (1 litre) of water, add a tablespoonful of honey and simmer for 20 minutes with a lid on. Strain, and when cold, add a tablespoonful ($\frac{1}{2}$ fluid ounce) of witch hazel and refrigerate. Apply to the face and neck to tighten the skin, close the pores, and leave your face free from blemishes. Horsetail water obtained by distilling the leafy stems is even more effective and will remove almost at once, any soreness caused by an infected blackhead. For which purpose, a small bottle of it should always be at hand. Distil the leafy stems using a kettle and tube and collecting in a glass jar.	
163 Lime Tree	The flowers are not readily accessible, but if they can be gathered in early summer, a handful infused in a half-pint (0·25 litre) of boiling water, will, after being strained and allowed to cool, make an effective complexion lotion. For greater efficiency, add equal parts of rose water and use after refrigeration.	
29 Rampion	To a large handful of flowers and leaves (the "tops"), add a pint (0·5 litre) of boiling water and leave for 15 minutes. Strain and add a teaspoonful of lemon juice and bottle. Apply to the face at bedtime after removing make-up and leave to dry on. It will leave the complexion smooth and white by morning.	
164 Red Clover	The high honey content makes an infusion of the flowers especially healing for skin made sore by wind or sun. Place a handful of flowers in a bowl and pour over them a pint (0·5 litre) of boiling water. Let stand for 10 minutes, strain and apply to the face with lint pads and leave to dry on.	
40 Succory	Make an infusion of a handful of the blue flowers in $\frac{1}{2}$ pint (0–25 litre) of boiling water and allow to cool. After straining, work in a teaspoonful of honey. The lotion will leave the skin soft and white.	
73 Witch Hazel	Dissolve $\frac{1}{2}$ oz (15 g) of borax in a pint (0·5 litre) of water over a low flame. Let cool, then stir in a cupful (4 fluid ounces) of alcohol and a half-cupful (2 fluid ounces) of witch hazel. Pour into bottles and cork tightly. Keep under refrigeration.	
72 Wood Avens	Make an infusion of 2 oz (60 g) of the fresh or dry root with the same amount of angelica root in boiling water. Strain and cool, and apply to the face with lint pads to take away any soreness caused by sunburn and to leave the skin soft and smooth. It will also take away freckles if applied persistently.	
18 Woodruff	A large handful of the fresh plants placed in a saucepan with $\frac{1}{2}$ pint (0·25 litre) of water and a teaspoonful of honey and simmered for 10 minutes. Strain and cool; add an equal amount of rose-water. Bottle and keep under refrigeration and use as complexion lotion, especially at bedtime after removing make-up. It will leave the skin smooth and white and remove blemishes and wrinkles.	The dried and powdered leaves are placed with lavender and marjoram in sweet bags to put amongst clothes.

Complexion milk

	Plant	Preparation
161	Dandelion	For a complexion milk: Place $\frac{1}{2}$ oz (15 g) each of beeswax and white soap shavings with a tablespoonful ($\frac{1}{2}$ fluid ounce) of green oil in a pan and partly immerse in a bowl of boiling water to melt. Blanch 4 oz (120 g) of sweet almonds and then pound them in a mortar, at the time slowly adding 1 pint (0·5 litre) of rose water. Then stir in a fluid ounce of the juice of dandelion root until well mixed in to make a thick white emulsion. It is now slowly added to the saponaceous mixture, mixing in all the time by beating it. Then slowly add 2 cupsful (8 fluid ounces) of rose essence, mixing thoroughly. Leave for 24 hours to settle, then strain into bottles, leaving behind the precipitate.
147	Elder	Blanch 4 oz (120 g) sweet almonds and remove the skins. Place in a mortar and pound, using a pint (0·5 litre) of elder flower (or rose) water to create a thin emulsion. Put through a muslin sieve, allowing it plenty of time to run through. In a separate pan over a very low flame, place a cupful (4 fluid ounces) of elder flower (or rose) water and into it shave a small tablet of white soap, stirring until it melts. Then slowly add $\frac{1}{2}$ oz (15 g) each spermaceti and white beeswax this allows time for their partial saponification by the soap. Place the mixture in the mortar and allow the almond emulsion to trickle into it very slowly, blending it carefully. With equal care, work in $\frac{1}{2}$ pint (0·25 litre) of alcohol, strain and bottle.
39	Feverfew	Place a handful of leaves and flowers in a pan and cover with a $\frac{1}{2}$ pint (0·25 litre) of milk. Simmer for 20 minutes, let cool, and strain into bottles. It will nourish a dry skin and remove blackheads and pimples.
69	Fumitory	An infusion of the whole plant (excluding the roots) in a $\frac{1}{2}$ pint (0·25 litre) of either hot water or milk, will, after straining, make a soothing complexion lotion, removing freckles caused by long exposure to the sun and any dryness of the skin.
129	Solomon's Seal	For every fluid ounce of the distilled water obtained from the flowers, mix a cupful (4 fluid ounces) of milk of sweet almonds obtained by putting 1 lb (0·5 kg) of almonds through a blender. It will make an admirable complexion milk, removing spots and pimples and leaving the skin soft and white. It will also take away any soreness of the skin caused by long exposure to the sun or drying winds.
110	Watercress	Bruise a handful of the stems and leaves in a saucepan and add a half-pint (0·25 litre) of water or milk. Simmer over a low flame for 10 minutes to release the juices and put in a teaspoonful of honey. When dissolved, strain into bottles. Apply to the face and neck, after removing make-up, at bedtime and let dry on. It will remove blemishes and leave the complexion soft and white.
85	Wild Lettuce	Dissolve the juice of the whole plant in a $\frac{1}{2}$ pint (0·25 litre) of hot water in a saucepan; let cool. The water should be thick and milky. Apply to the face and to any part made sore by sun or drying winds, to leave the skin soft and smooth and to take away soreness.

Cleansing lotions/cold creams

	Plant	Preparation
9	Almond	Heat in a saucepan over a very low flame 4 oz (120 g) of white beeswax, remove from the heat and stir in 1 pint (0·5 litre) of almond oil. Slightly warm a large cupful of rose water and stir

Handwritten notes:
8 :
15g wax, 75ml oil, 1½ tbsp
7/8 tsp borax

90g sweet almond oil, 15g white wax, 30g Lanolin,
30g Rosewater, 10 drops Jasmin oil, 10 drops Rose Geranium
or other scented oils.

Plant	Preparation	Notes
Almond (continued)	in a teaspoonful of borax, then add it slowly to the wax and oil, mixing it well in before it becomes cold. Add a few drops of oil of rose to perfume it, mixing it well in, then pour into porcelain jars with screw tops.	
9 Almond	Mix together a small cupful (4 fluid ounces) of sweet almond oil and one of bitter almond oil and place in a pan over a low flame. Stir in 1 oz (30 g) of flaked honeydew soap until it has melted. As it cools, pour into a screw-top jar and store in the refrigerator.	
9 Almond	Beat up the yolks of 4 eggs with $\frac{1}{2}$ lb (0·25 kg) of honey, then mix in a cupful (4 fluid ounces) of sweet almond oil. Blend in 4 oz (120 g) of blanched and ground almonds to make it into a thick paste or emulusion. Massage into the skin and leave on for 30 minutes. Wash off with lukewarm water.	
13 Chamomile	To a small handful of chamomile flowers (fresh or dry) and one of rosemary tops placed in a basin, add a pint (0.5 litre) of boiling water and leave until cold. Strain and place in the refrigerator for several hours, then dip in cloths, wring out excess moisture and apply to the face for 5 to 10 minutes, going over the procedure several times.	For an oily skin.
13 Chamomile	A simple but effective skin lotion is made by placing 2 handsful of chamomile flowers (fresh or dry) in a saucepan and adding a pint (0·5 litre) of water. Simmer over a low flame for 5 to 10 minutes, strain and let cool. Add a teaspoonful of witch hazel or lemon juice for every pint (0·5 litre) of liquid. Bottle and refrigerate.	
13 Chamomile	Make up a pint (0·5 litre) of chamomile "tea" from a handful of flowers. Strain when cool and mix in 2 tablespoonsful (1 fluid ounce) of creamy milk and 1 tablespoonful each of lemon juice and witch hazel. Refrigerate for an hour and apply to the face and neck with lint pads.	
47 Coconut	The oil is extracted from the shell of coconuts and is included in most face creams as it nourishes the skin. To make a cream, take 1 oz (30 g) white beeswax and warm it; mix in 4 fluid ounces of coconut (or sunflower) oil. Then slowly blend in a cupful of water into which a teaspoonful of borax has been dissolved. To blend water with oil calls for some practice. As it cools, add a few drops of rose oil to perfume it and pour into screw-top jars. It will be a cream of pleasing consistency.	
159 Costmary	Place a handful of leaves in a pan and cover with a cupful (4 fluid ounces) of olive oil. Simmer for 20 minutes over a low flame then strain and work in half an ounce (25 g) of white beeswax and the same of spermaceti to make a thick cream. Before it cools, pour into screw-top jars.	
132 Cowslip	Make an infusion of a handful of flowers and their stalks in a pint (0·5 litre) of boiling water; allow to cool. For greater effectiveness, add a tablespoonful of witch hazel after straining. The solution will cleanse the skin of perspiration and dirt.	
52 Cucumber	Place 1 oz (30 g) each of white beeswax and spermaceti in a glazed bowl in a sink part-filled with boiling water. After they have melted, stir in 1 pint (0·5 litre) of olive oil. Remove the bowl from the water and stir in the juice of 2 cucumbers put through a blender, agitating the mixture the whole time as the juice is poured slowly in and whilst the contents of the bowl are still warm. Before it sets, pour into small glazed screw-top jars; it should set to a creamy consistency and be a pale green colour.	

Plant	Preparation	Notes
46 Horseradish	Lift and clean the roots, then slice them into a saucepan and to every 1 lb (0·5 litre) of milk and simmer for an hour over a low flame. Strain and bottle and apply as a lotion to the face and forehead. Keep any surplus in the refrigerator.	To clear the skin of blackheads and pimples.
21 Oats	Stir into a large carton of buttermilk or yogurt, half a cupful (about 2 oz or 60 g) of finely ground oatmeal and place in the refrigerator for several hours. Lie down and apply the contents thickly to the face and forehead. Leave on for 30 minutes and rinse off in lukewarm water containing a little lemon juice.	To reduce large pores and clear the skin of impurities.
144 Rosemary	Melt together 1 oz (30 g) each beeswax and spermaceti and 2 oz (60 g) camphor ice in a large pan partly immersed in boiling water. Stir in a cupful (4 fluid ounces) of almond oil, then remove the pan and slowly work in a ½ pint (0·25 litre) of rose water, stirring all the time. When thoroughly mixed to a creamy consistency, add a teaspoonful (1 fluid drachm) otto of rosemary and pour into screw-top jars.	
155 Sowthistle	Cut the stems into small pieces and place in a saucepan with a ½ pint (0·25 litre) of water and simmer for 15 minutes. Strain off the milky juice and mix with an equal quantity of fresh milk. Apply to the face and forehead at bedtime, after removing make-up, and let dry on. It will remove the greasy film, together with blackheads and pimples.	
128 Tuberose	Place 1 oz (30 g) each of beeswax and spermaceti in a pan which is partly immersed in a bowl of boiling water. When melted, stir in a cupful (4 fluid ounces) of almond oil and one of tuberose water, obtained by distillation. Add this slowly and stir continuously to keep the cream agitated. Stop stirring occasionally to scrape the cream from the sides and mix it well in. It will help the water to mix if it is first slightly warmed. Now add a few drops of essence of tuberose and pour into glazed screw-top jars, whilst still warm. It will set to a stiff creamy consistency.	

Moisturisers

Plant	Preparation	Notes
119 Avocado	Put an avocado through the blender and mix a teaspoonful of honey to it; add the same of lemon juice and sufficient yogurt to make it into a stiff cream. Refrigerate for 30 minutes, then massage into the face and neck until the cream has disappeared and leave on over-night.	
45 Lemon	First steam open the pores or place a hot towel over the face for several minutes, then apply a lemon gel mask. Reduce a packet of lemon gelatine in a basin to a paste by adding a cupful of hot water. Add the juice of a lemon and place in the refrigerator for 20 minutes to firm up. Apply to the face and forehead. Leave on for 20 minutes and wash off in luke-warm water.	To use in a dry, warm climate.
43 Water Melon	There is no better method of refreshing the body in hot weather and giving the complexion a "fresh" appearance than to cut a water melon into slices and to place them over the face and neck whilst lying down for 30 minutes in a darkened room. It will be still more effective if the juice of half a lemon (or a lime) is squeezed onto it and it has been refrigerated for 20 minutes. It will reduce the body temperature, tighten the skin and remoisturise it.	If lemon juice is used, cover the eyes with a damp cloth to protect them. this will, in any case, relieve tired eyes.

Plant	Preparation	Notes

Night creams

9 Almond	Melt 1 oz (30 g) of white wax with 2 fluid ounces of almond oil over a very low flame and stir in a small cupful (2 fluid ounces) of rose water. Pour into small screw-top jars and leave to set. It will be about 24 hours before the cream is ready to use.	If you wish face creams to last for any length of time, add a few drops of alcoholic tincture of benzoin before filling the pots.
98 Apple	Put 1 lb (0·5 kg) of peeled and cored apples through the blender and add the juice and pulp to 1 lb (0·5 kg) of lard warmed in a pan over a low flame. Simmer and stir until well mixed, remove from the flame and add several drops of benzoin and a cupful (4 fluid ounces) of rose water, stirring all the time. Strain into screw-top jars and use as a night cream, massaging it well into the face and neck.	Massage the cream into the breasts to make them soft and plump.
119 Avocado	Put an avocado through a blender (after removing the stone) and mix the juice into a cupful (4 fluid ounces) of warm almond oil, stirring until it is thoroughly mixed. Add a small quantity of white beeswax to make it set and whilst still warm, pour into a screw-top pot. Massage a little into the face and neck at bedtime, until it is absorbed.	
124 Common Plantain	Gather a handful of plantain leaves together with a handful of southernwood, black currant and angelica leaves and one of elder flowers and place in a saucepan with a cupful (4 fluid ounces) of almond or olive oil. Simmer for 30 minutes and strain off the oil. Rewarm the oil and add 1 oz (30 g) white beeswax or lard before removing to cool. Pour into screw-top jars before the mixture sets. It will make a nourishing night cream.	
124 Common Plantain	Fill a saucepan with the leaves and add the juice of a lemon and 1 pint (0·5 litre) of water. Simmer for 20 minutes, strain and when cool, add a fluid ounce of witch hazel. Bottle and keep under refrigeration.	
6 Garlic	Break up a bulb into several cloves and place in a saucepan with 1 lb (0·5 kg) of lard and heat gently for 30 minutes. Leave for several hours after turning off the heat, then add ½ oz (15 g) beeswax and slowly reheat. Remove the garlic cloves and pour into screw-top jars to solidify. Use as a night cream.	
92 Toadflax	Gather the tops of the flowers, which are rich in honey, when the plants are in bloom. Boil (simmer) the tops in ½ pound (0·25 kg) of purified lard or a cupful (4 fluid ounces) of olive oil into which ½ oz (15 g) beeswax has been placed to make the mixture set better. As it cools, add a few drops of rose oil and strain into screw-top jars. Work into the skin after removing make-up at bedtime.	

Skin tonics

45 Grapefruit	Remove the skin (rind) from a grapefruit and cut into small pieces. Put through the blender, then mix with a small carton of yogurt to make a paste. Refrigerate for an hour, then smear over the face and neck. Leave on for 30 minutes until you feel your pores tightening. Wash off in lukewarm water and the face will be completely refreshed.	
153 Potato	There is nothing better than a raw potato to make the skin taut. Peel and wash and cut into thick slices. After cleaning the face and neck, open the pores by wrapping a hot towel round the face neck, or put your face over a bowl of hot water with a towel over, to keep the steam from escaping. After 5 minutes, rub the pieces of potato over the face and neck and leave the juices 15 minutes to dry on. Then moisturise and make up.	The potato pieces will be more effective and more refreshing if refrigerated for 10 minutes before using.

Plant	Preparation	Notes
74 Sunflower	Melt an eggcupful of lanolin in a pan over a low flame and stir in a cupful (4 fluid ounces) of sunflower seed oil. Remove from the heat and stir in a teaspoonful of wheat germ oil and a half cupful (about 2 fluid ounces) of witch hazel. Bottle and refrigerate and massage a little into the face and neck at bedtime.	
165 Wheat	The embryo or germ, removed in the refining of flour, yields wheat germ oil, which is one of the finest of skin tonics. Obtainable from chemists or drug stores, 1 fluid drachm (a teaspoonful) when mixed with 4 fluid drachms (a table-spoonful) of witch hazel will make an admirable skin lotion which is astringent and will replace the skin's natural oils. Apply to the face and neck at bedtime.	

Soothing skin preparations

Plant	Preparation	Notes
99 Cajuput	To rub on the skin after exposure to the sun or a drying wind, use 1 part cajuput oil, obtained by distillation of the leaves and twigs, to 2 parts olive or almond oil. If cajuput oil is in short supply, use half and half (equal parts) with oil of rosemary.	
90 Common Privet	Gather a shoe-boxful of flowers and place them in a shallow bowl in a sunny window. Cover with a pint (0·5 litre) of olive oil and leave for a week in the sun. Strain into bottles and gently massage into the skin at bedtime. By morning your skin will be soft and smooth and will have lost any soreness.	
52 Cucumber	Take a piece of cucumber, 1 in (2·5 cm) thick, remove the skin and place the piece in a bowl. Cover with lemon or lime juice and let stand for 1 hour. Then gently rub the cucumber over the face, taking care not to allow it to come into contact with the eyes. Leave on for 30 minutes then wash off in warm water. This treatment will leave the skin tight and beautifully soft and smooth.	
52 Cucumber	Slice a cucumber and put through the blender. Mix the juice or pulp with a small teaspoonful of honey and one of witch hazel and apply to the skin with lint pads. Leave on for 20 minutes and rinse off.	
52 Cucumber	Slice and put a small cucumber through the blender and mix with an equal amount of yogurt or cream. Refrigerate for an hour, then massage into the face and neck until it is absorbed and leave on over-night.	
52 Cucumber	First treat 2 lbs (1 kg) of pure lard with a little gum benzoin (see Tonquin), then place in a large glazed bowl with $\frac{1}{2}$ lb (0·5 kg) spermaceti. Melt by placing the bowl in a wash-basin partly filled with boiling water. Keep the spermaceti and lard constantly in motion and when melted pour into a mortar or bowl and work in the juice of 2 cucumbers which have been put through a blender. Whilst still warm, pour into screw-top jars until set into a smooth pomade. Then it is ready for use.	
138 Oak	Heat for 10 minutes 1 oz (30 g) of dried and powdered galls with 4 oz (120 g) of purified lard containing a few drops of tincture of benzoin (benzoated) to prevent its turning rancid, or use a cupful (4 fluid ounces) of olive oil. Strain and pour into screw-top jars. Apply to the skin made sore by blackheads.	If olive oil is used, add a few drops of oil of clove and use as a hair dressing instead of walnut oil.
133 Primrose	Gather a large handful of fresh flowers, with their stalks and pound them into 1 lb (0·5 kg) of fresh lard. Leave for 2 days, heat gently and strain. When cool, repeat the process, leave for 2 more days, then strain the lard into screw-top jars and let set.	

Plant		Preparation	Notes
148	Sanicle	A large handful of the plant, at its most effective when just coming into bloom in mid-summer, immersed in a pint (0·5 litre) of boiling water, with a teaspoonful of honey added, will, after straining, make an ideal astringent lotion and will soothe skin made sore by sun or drying wind.	The plant can be gathered and dried at this time and stored in a shoe-box for similar use in winter.
152	Sesame	Mix together 20 parts sesame oil with 10 parts each olive and almond oil, adding one at a time and stirring thoroughly until blended, then work in a small measure of a sun-screening agent.	If warming is required to mix the ingredients, do not add the sun-screening agent until the mixture is almost cool.
160	Tansy	Place a handful of tansy leaves in a pan and pour over them a large cupful of half milk, half water. Put on the lid and simmer for 15 minutes over a low flame. Allow to cool, then strain and apply to the skin with a lint pad and let dry on. Another method is to soak a handful of tansy leaves in a large cupful of buttermilk for several days, then strain and apply to the skin, leaving it to dry on. The juice from a handful of leaves put through a blender and mixed with a small cupful of orange juice and a teaspoonful of honey is a tonic drink and is a good treatment to clear the skin of impurities.	
131	Tormentil	It is the root that has healing and tonic properties. Wash and clear pieces of root and place in a saucepan together with a $\frac{1}{2}$ lb (0·25 kg) of lard for every 1 lb (0·5 kg) of root; or use a cupful (4 fluid ounces) of olive oil to the same amount of root, together with $\frac{1}{2}$ oz (15 g) of beeswax for it to set better. Simmer for 21 minutes over a low flame and strain into screw-top jars to set. The juice of the fresh root (after washing and cleaning) is also a good treatment for warts. Apply to the wart for several days and it will disappear and heal the skin around it. A decoction of the root will clear the skin of blemishes and leave it soft and smooth.	

Nourishing creams

Plant		Preparation	Notes
9	Almond	To a jar of almond cream, mix in a teaspoonful of honey and 1 oz (30 g) of crushed sweet almonds (meal), which can be obtained by putting a handful of whole almonds through a blender or buying already pulverised from a supermarket. This will add roughage to the cream mix which is gently massaged into the skin for several minutes, left on for 10 minutes, and washed off in lukewarm water. It will take away any greasiness and leave the skin soft and smooth.	To remove the "dead" layer of surface skin from the face and to nourish the skin.
9	Almond	Mix 2 tablespoonsful (1 fluid ounce) of almond meal (ground almonds) with a small carton of yogurt (rich in vitamin A) or sour cream. Apply to the face and neck and leave on for an hour. Rinse off in lukewarm water.	For a dry or blemished skin.
52	Cucumber	Put a sliced cucumber through a blender and to every 4 tablespoonsful (2 fluid ounces) of juice, add 1 tablespoonful ($\frac{1}{4}$ fluid ounce) tincture of benzoin and a pint (0·5 litre) of distilled water. Place in the refrigerator for several hours before applying to the face and neck. Leave on for 20 minutes and wash off. It will leave the skin soft and smooth.	
28	Marigold	Gather 1 lb (0·5 kg) of the newly opened flowers and place in a large glass jar with a screw-top and cover with spirits of wine. Leave in the sun for a week, shaking continually. Then strain off the essence. Heat a pound (0·5 kg) of pure lard and when melted, stir in the essence. Add a teaspoonful of tincture of benzoin to preserve it, and as it cools, pour into screw-top jars and use as a night cream. It will leave the skin soft and smooth and remove any soreness.	_Skin cleaner: Add 3 tbsp of marigold petals to 1 pint of boiling water simmer for 5 min, cool, strain and bottle, use as a moisturiser, softener and tonic._

Plant	Preparation	Notes

| 21 | Oats | Mix together the beaten yolks of 2 eggs; a tablespoon of honey; a cupful lanolin; and the same of crushed (ground) almonds or of oatmeal. Stir in the juice of half a lemon and a few drops of tincture of benzoin if to be kept for any length of time (although it is best made and used fresh). Massage into the face, neck and forehead with a circular movement and leave on for 15 minutes. Then wash off in lukewarm water. |

| 114 | Olive | Mix 2 tablespoonsful (1 fluid ounce) of olive oil with the yolks of 2 eggs, stirring in until the yolks are fully absorbed. Apply to the face with a pad, leave on for 30 minutes, then wash off in warm water containing a little lemon juice. |

| 166 | Red Elm | Take 2 oz (60 g) of marshmallow leaves and boil in 2 pints (1 litre) of water for 20 minutes. Then strain or remove the marshmallow leaves.
Melt together 1 lb (0·5 kg) of refined lard and 3 oz (90 g) beeswax in a saucepan over a low flame, then stir in slowly the extract of red elm and marshmallow until completely mixed in and pour into screw-top jars before the mixture becomes cold and sets. Red elm has the power of preventing cream from becoming rancid. Use a little to massage into the face and neck at bedtime. |

| 86 | Yellow Archangel | Heat one pound (0·5 kg) of fresh leaves and a cupful (4 fluid ounces) of olive oil in a pan over a low flame with 1 oz (30 g) of beeswax. Remove from the flame and let the leaves remain to macerate for an hour or so, then remove them and replace with others. Put back the pan and reheat the contents, simmering for 10 minutes, then strain into jars to set. |

To remove wrinkles

| 56 | Carrot | Take a large garden carrot or several wild carrots and put through the blender. Add a teaspoonful of olive or almond oil and mix well in. Place in the refrigerator for 1 to 2 hours, then apply around the eyes and cheeks. Leave on for 30 minutes and relax on the bed with the eyes closed. Then wipe off with warm water. |

| 132 | Cowslip | Place 1 lb (0·5 kg) of lard in a large saucepan and heat slightly over a low flame until it melts. Add ½ lb (0·25 kg) of cowslip flowers and macerate for 48 hours. Reheat and strain, adding more flowers to the warm lard. Leave for another 48 hours, reheat and strain into screw-top jars. Massage a little into the face, especially around the eyes, and neck at bedtime. |

| 91 | Madonna Lily | Use the juice of 2 bulbs put through a blender after removing the outer scales and place in a small pan. Add 2 tablespoonsful of honey and 2 oz (60 g) white beeswax and mix together over a low flame, adding half a small cupful of rose water or marigold water. Pour into screw-top jars and when cold and set firm, massage a little into the neck and at the side of the eyes at night. |

| 167 | Stinging Nettle | Infuse ½ lb (0·25 kg) of stinging nettle "tops" in ½ pint (0·25 litre) of boiling water for 20 minutes. Strain and when cool add a tablespoonful of witch hazel and apply to the face and neck with a lint pad. Let dry on. |

| 96 | Yellow Loosestrife | Make an infusion of the flowers and leaves in ½ pint of boiling water and leave for 15 minutes. Strain and apply to the face and neck to remove blemishes and wrinkles. |

Plant	Preparation	Notes

Face masks and face packs

9 Almond

Put ½ lb (0·25 kg) of sweet almonds through a blender to make almond meal or use ground almonds from the supermarket. Mix with a little milk or water to make a smooth paste and smear over the face and neck. Leave on for 30 minutes then wash off in lukewarm water and massage a little almond oil into the skin. It will remove spots and leave the skin soft and smooth.

105 Banana

Beat up 2 egg yolks and an eggcupful of almond or olive oil until thoroughly mixed. Then beat in a ripe (but not over-ripe) banana. Smear over the face and neck. Leave on for 30 minutes and rinse off in lukewarm water containing a little lemon juice.

47 Coconut

Mix together in a basin a teaspoonful of sea-kelp powder (dried and ground) and 2 tablespoonsful (1 fluid ounce) of coconut oil. Massage into the face, neck and forehead for several minutes, leave on for 30 minutes and rinse off in lukewarm water into which a few drops of lemon juice have been added. it will remove blemishes and leave the skin soft and smooth.

135 Peach

Mash 2 tablespoonsful of powdered milk with a teaspoonful of honey and a ripe peach or apricot. Smear on the face and neck and leave on for an hour before washing off in warm water containing a little lemon juice. *or cider apple vinegar.*

you may replace the honey by lemon juice and the peach/apricot by strawberry, if not allergic to it.

102 Peppermint

Mix to a paste 4 oz (120 g) brewer's yeast and a tablespoonful (½ fluid ounce) of witch hazel. Add a few drops of peppermint essence to improve its astringent qualities. Apply to the face and forehead, and lie down with the eyes closed. Leave on for 30 minutes. Then wash off in lukewarm water containing a little lemon juice, and apply a moisturising lotion.

102 Peppermint

Mix a tablespoonful of fuller's earth with a 4 oz carton of yogurt. Add a teaspoonful of honey; 2 or 3 drops of peppermint essence (obtainable from a chemist or druggist) and a pinch of bicarbonate of soda. Apply to the face and neck with lint, and leave on for 30 minutes. Rinse off in warm water. It will remove all greasiness from the skin.

166 Red Elm

Mix a teaspoonful of the powdered bark of red elm with enough hot water to form a creamy consistency. When cool, apply to the face. Leave on for 20 minutes and wash off in warm water containing a teaspoonful of lemon juice. The mask will rid the skin of blemishes and leave it smooth and clean. It is soothing and healing.

68 Sea Kelp

Make up some salad mayonnaise and mix together a teaspoonful of fuller's earth (obtainable from chemists) and one of sea kelp powder. First cover the face with a thin layer of egg yolk, then apply the mud pack. Leave on for 30 minutes, then rinse off.

Mayonnaise, massaged into the skin, provides all that is necessary to maintain it in a soft healthy condition, for egg yolk provides protein; olive oil improves skin texture; and malt vinegar gives the acid mantle which the skin needs.

67 Strawberry

Mash 4 oz (120 g) of freshly gathered stawberries with 2 tablespoonsful of powdered milk and one of lemon juice. Smear over the face and neck and leave on for an hour. Wash off in warm water containing the juice of half a lemon or a little cider apple vinegar.

From the wild fruits, chemists prepare a tincture that is highly effective for sore skin.

Plant		Preparation	Notes
95	Tomato	Use the juice of 2 or 3 ripe tomatoes put through a sieve and mix with a small carton of natural yogurt. Then stir the mixture into a basin of oatmeal which has been boiled with a little water for 20 minutes to make a smooth paste and allow to cool. Lie down and apply thickly to the face (shielding the eyes with pads) and leave on for 30 minutes. Relax with the eyes closed. Rinse off in cold water. It will leave the skin soft and clear of blackheads and pimples and will take away the greasy film.	
73	Witch Hazel	Mix together 2 heaped teaspoonsful (1 oz or 30 g) of brewer's yeast and sufficient witch hazel to make a smooth paste. Refrigerate for 20 minutes, then smear over the face and neck. Leave on for 30 minutes and wash off in lukewarm water.	

Eye lotions

Plant		Preparation	Notes
4	Agrimony	Make an infusion of a handful of fresh "tops" in a pint (0·5 litre) of boiling water; let cool. Strain the mixture and use it to bathe the eyes. Agrimony is second only to eyebright in its ability to make the eyes sparkle.	A wineglassful of the same infusion sweetened with a little honey will, if taken daily, purify the blood and clear the skin of spots and pimples.
13	Chamomile	Infuse a handful of flowers (the central boss contains the valuable qualities) in 1 pint (0·5 litre) of boiling water and leave until cool, then pour into an ice cube container and place in the refrigerator for several hours until the cubes are iced through. Remove a cube when required and rub it around the eyes and over the closed lids for several minutes. The eyes will be completely refreshed and the "tired look" will disappear. The eyes are now ready to be made up.	
146	Clary	Place a handful of leaves or tops in a saucepan, cover with a cupful (4 fluid ounces) of milk or water and simmer over a low flame for 10 minutes. Strain and when lukewarm, bathe the eyes with lint or use an eye bath.	One drop of the complexion lotion (q.v.) in the eye will remove the most stubborn intrusion and heal any soreness.
124	Common Plantain	The juice of the leaf or flower stems of the common plantain, diluted with a little water (preferably distilled) and dropped into the eyes will clear them of inflammation and leave them bright and clear.	
36	Cornflower	Infuse a handful of flowers in $\frac{1}{2}$ pint (0·25 litre) of boiling water and allow to cool. The lotion will ease the eyes of soreness and give them a sparkle.	
147	Elder	Elder flower water sold by beauticians is obtained by distillation of the flowers in a still; at home it is done with a kettle and tube. A simple substitute is made by pouring 1 pint (0·5 litre) of boiling water onto 2 large handfuls of elder flowers placed in a bowl. Allow to soak for 12 hours, strain and bottle. Keep under refrigeration. Use to bathe the eyes at bedtime.	
64	Eyebright	To a large handful of the herb (excluding the roots) placed in a basin, add 1 pint (0·5 litre) of boiling water and allow to stand until almost cool; then strain. Bathe the eyes with lint pads or an eye bath.	The water dissolved in gelatine makes a soothing gel to apply at night.
66	Fennel	Place 1 oz (30 g) of seed in a pan, cover with a pint (0·5 litre) of water and simmer for 20 minutes over a low flame. Strain and cool; pour into bottles. In an eye bath or applied to the eyes with lint, this infusion will take away inflammation and give the eyes a sparkle.	

Plant		Preparation	Notes
28	Marigold	There is nothing better for sore or inflamed eyes than to bathe them in marigold water. Place a large handful of flowers in a saucepan and add ½ pint (0·25 litre) water. Simmer for 20 minutes, strain and use whilst slightly warm.	
100	Melilot	Make an infusion of a large handful of the plant in ½ pint (0·25 litre) of boiling water; strain and allow to cool. This proves a good remedy to eyes.	
137	Quince	The mucilage eases sore or tired eyes, leaving them clear and sparkling. Place a teaspoonful of seeds in a jam jar and add ½ pint (0·25 litre) of water. Stand in a large saucepan containing hot water and simmer for several hours, until the water in the jar has become milky with the mucilage. Strain into another jar. For the eyes, use a teaspoonful (1 fluid drachm) mixed with a tablespoonful (½ fluid ounce) of rose water and apply with lint pads or with an eye bath. This mixture should be applied at bedtime: by morning the eyes will take on a new brightness and will be free of any soreness.	
40	Succory	Make an infusion of a handful of the blue flowers in ½ pint (0·25 litre) of water; allow to cool. The infusion will remove tiredness and inflammation from tired eyes or eyes that have been exposed to strong sunlight.	
92	Toadflax	An infusion of the "tops" in boiling water, after straining and allowing to cool, can be used in an eye bath to ease tired eyes and give them a sparkle.	
170	Vervain	Make an infusion of a large handful of the plant in a pint (0·5 litre) of boiling water and let stand for 20 minutes before straining. When cool it will soothe inflamed eyes and give them a sparkle.	Taken warm at bedtime with a teaspoonful of honey, it will promote sound sleep, the best of all beauty aids.
96	Yellow Loosestrife	Make an infusion of the flowers and leaves in ½ pint of boiling water and leave for 15 minutes. Strain and apply to the eyes with lint pads at bedtime to remove soreness and to give them a sparkle. Dilute the application with an equal amount of water.	

Dentifrices and mouth wash

Sage leaves + sea salt

Plant		Preparation	Notes
136	Blackthorn	The juice, when thick, has the same uses as gum acacia. Rubbed onto the gums it strengthens them, preventing the teeth from becoming loose and causing them to take on a glistening whiteness. An infusion of the leaves in boiling water, which has been allowed to cool, has similar if less effective qualities. Use it as a mouth wash.	
36	Cornflower	A handful of the flowers infused in ½ pint (0·25 litre) of boiling water and allowed to cool, makes an admirable mouth wash.	
22	Myrrh	Place 1 oz (30 g) each of honey; gum myrrh and red sanders wood (or cedarwood) in a large glass jar and cover with 2 pints (1 litre) of spirits of wine. Leave for 14 days to macerate, then strain into bottles and use a few drops in warm water as a mouth wash. It will also improve the whiteness of the teeth.	A few drops of tincture of myrrh adds staying power to perfumes.
81	Orris (Iris)	To 1 lb (0·5 kg) of precipitated chalk, mix 1 oz (30 g) powdered rice starch and 1 oz (30 g) powdered orris root (which is more than a year old so that it is richly scented).	
84	Rhatany	Dry and pulverise the reddish-brown roots and mix with an equal amount of orris root, together with a little powdered charcoal; or use gum myrrh and prepared chalk. Rubbed onto the teeth, the powder will remove tartar and leave the teeth white and shining.	

[Handwritten note beside Marigold: Or 1 oz of Fennel seeds in 1/2 pint of water, used in the same way will take away inflammation and give the eye a sparkle] X

[Handwritten note beside Cornflower: + the same infusion will ease the eyes of soreness and give them a sparkle] X

Plant	Preparation	Notes

| 67 Strawberry | Strawberry juice is an excellent dentifrice. Put several large fruits through a blender and brush onto the teeth. Leave on for a few minutes. Dissolve a teaspoonful of bicarbonate of soda in a cup of warm water and use as a mouth wash. Then dust the brush with the bicarbonate and brush onto the teeth. Rinse the mouth with a cupful of warm water containing a few drops of tincture of myrrh. Though the process takes only a few minutes, it will remove tartar and stains and leave the teeth white and glistening, the breath sweet and the gums free of any soreness. | |

Hand creams

| 9 Almond | Mix a teaspoonful of honey with two of almond (or olive) oil and massage into the hands after washing them in warm soapy water and drying. Put on a pair of old cotton gloves, kept for the purpose, and sleep in them. Wash the hands in warm soapy water in the morning and they will be soft and white. Repeat for a second night if necessary.
To strengthen the nails, soak them daily for 5 minutes in warm almond (or olive) oil.
For discoloured nails, clean them with lemon juice and scrub them in white wine vinegar. | Remember that acetone used to remove nail varnish is drying, so add a few drops of almond (or olive) oil to it when it is used and do so only once each week. |

| 38 Carrageen Moss | Place 1 lb (0·5 kg) of the seaweed carrageen, or Irish moss, in a saucepan, add 2 pints (1 litre) of rose water and a cupful (4 fluid ounces) of glycerine. Let soak for 18 hours, then heat to 140°F (60°C) for 2 minutes and let stand for 48 hours. Remove the moss and add a small cupful of alcohol and a few drops of oil of rose, then bottle and cork. | |

| 38 Carrageen Moss | Gather and wash clean of sand, 1 lb (0·5 kg) of the seaweed fronds and soak for 48 hours in a saucepan containing a cupful of glycerine. Warm slightly for a few minutes and allow to cool, removing the fronds before it is completely cooled. Pour into a jar or bowl until it is set into a stiff cream. Applied to the hands (and face) it will remove any soreness, but as it is slightly sticky, it is advisable to sleep in old gloves kept for the purpose. | |

| 78 Common St. John's Wort | Warm a cupful (4 fluid ounces) of olive oil in a pan. Then add 2 large handsful of common St. John's Wort flowers to the warm oil and half a pint of white wine. Leave for 24 hours, stirring often. Warm slightly and strain. Replace over a low flame and melt in ½oz (15 g) white beeswax and pour into screw-top jars. | |

| 147 Elder | Obtain a pot of petroleum jelly and heat it until it liquifies. Pour into a saucepan and add to it several handsful of fresh elder flowers. Leave for about 40 minutes, gently reheating as it cools. Put through a sieve whilst still warm and pour the liquid into screw-top jars to solidify. Rub on the hands at bedtime and sleep in an old pair of cotton gloves. | |

| 8 Marshmallow | Infuse 1 lb (0·5 kg) of freshly dug and cleaned root and ½ lb (0·25 kg) each of flax seed and fenugreek in 4 pints (2 litre) of water for about a week. Press out the mucilage through muslin and gently heat. Add 2 pints (1 litre) of olive oil and boil until the water has evaporated. Add 2 tablespoonsful (1 fluid ounce) of turpentine and 1 lb (0·5 kg) white beeswax, stirring until the preparation has achieved the consistency of an ointment. Allow to cool and pour (before it becomes cold) into glazed screw-top jars. | |

Plant	Preparation	Notes
168 Vanilla	Place 2 oz vanilla pods (sliced) with 8 oz (240 g) of pure lard, 4 oz (120 g) each of spermaceti and gum benzoin and 2 large cupsful (12 fluid ounces) of almond oil in a porcelain bowl, part submerged in a large saucepan of water heated to 175°F (80°C) for several hours. Let cool, but whilst still warm, strain into porcelain screw-top jars.	If vanilla pods (beans) are not available, add a teaspoonful of vanilla essence to the mix as it cools.

To soothe tired feet

Plant	Preparation	Notes
60 Horsetail	Gather a large handful of stems, chop them up and place in a large jug. Pour over a litre of boiling water and let stand for 10 minutes. Strain into a foot bath or large bowl and add more hot water. Sit with the feet in the water for 10 minutes, dry them and rub them with witch hazel or surgical spirit and let dry on. This could be done once a week in summer. If horsetail is not available, marshmallow or stinging nettle can be used instead.	
14 Arnica	A few drops of tincture of arnica, obtained by treating the freshly dug roots of the flowers with spirits of wine, in a footbath of warm water, will remove soreness or tenderness from the feet. Rub them afterward with surgical spirit and let dry on.	Do not take arnica internally and do not use externally if the skin shows sensitiveness to it.

Breast lotions

Plant	Preparation	Notes
14 Arnica	To firm the breasts after child feeding or illness, mix callagen with a teaspoonful of tincture of arnica (from the chemist or by treating the roots or the flowers with spirits of wine) and massage gently into the breasts using a circular movement. this should be daily for a month or so.	
5 Lady's Mantle	To firm breasts which sag from child-bearing or old age, make an infusion of the fresh plant (1 lb or 0·5 kg) in 2 pints (1 litre) of boiling water and after 5 minutes strain and place in it cloths for covering the breasts. Wring out surplus moisture and leave on for 10 minutes. A daily repetition for several weeks will restore a youthful firmness to the breasts.	The same infusion with a teaspoonful of lemon juice will be an effective astringent lotion, and it is styptic, stemming the flow of blood from cuts (whilst shaving) or sores and healing the skin.
113 Nutmeg Plant	An infusion of the seeds of Nigella sativa (1 oz or 30 g to 4 pints or 2 litre of boiling water) and straining will provide a lotion which since earliest times, Egyptian women have used to firm the breasts. Whilst still warm, wring out cloths or towels and place over the breasts, leaving on for 10 minutes. Repeat until the liquid is used up. or rub the breasts with the lotion at bedtime and let dry on.	

Hair rinses

Plant	Preparation	Notes
98 Apple	Mix a large cupful (8 fluid ounces) of cider apple vinegar in 2 pints (1 litre) of warm water; or put a large cooking apple through the blender and mix the juice with a cupful of malt vinegar; or obtain a pack of pure apple juice from the supermarket and mix a little with some malt vinegar (also obtainable at the supermarket). Partly dry the hair and cover with a shower cap, complete the drying in a warm room. The hair will take on an attractive gloss and golden tint.	
76 Barley	Malt vinegar, obtained by the oxidation of fermented malt wort (can be purchased at a supermarket), when mixed with equal parts of warm water and applied to the face and neck with lint pads, is an excellent astringent and rinse for fair hair. It leaves the hair soft and glossy and brings out the colour. With beer (also from barley malt), it makes an efficient setting lotion.	

Plant		Preparation	Notes
13	Chamomile	Collect and dry the flowers of chamomile in a warm oven, turning them often. When quite dry, take a cupful and reduce to a powder. Add an equal amount (by bulk) of kaolin powder with a little water; mix to a creamy paste. Massage well into the hair and leave on for 30 minutes. Rinse off in lukewarm water containing a little lemon juice.	
13	Chamomile	Over a handful of freshly opened flowers, and 1 of rosemary tops, placed in a saucepan, pour 1 pint (0·5 litre) of boiling water. Allow the infusion to cool before using as a rinse after shampooing. It will give the hair a lustrelike sheen and enhance its golden colour.	
154	Golden Rod	A handful of fresh flowers infused in 1 pint (0·5 litre) of boiling water and used as a rinse, will impart a golden sheen to fair hair and improve its texture.	
144	Rosemary	Place 2 oz (60 g) of fresh rosemary leaves or tops in 2 pints (1 litre) of water and simmer slowly for 10 to 15 minutes. Then massage into the scalp each day, morning and night. Spirits of rosemary are even more effective. They are obtained by treating oil of rosemary with spirits of wine, which can be purchased at a chemist or drug store. To make oil of rosemary, treat 1 lb (0·5 kg) of fresh tops, preferably in early summer when in bloom, with 2 litres of proof spirit. Allow to stand for a week, then collect the oil by simple distillation.	
144	Rosemary	Place a large handful of "tops" in a saucepan with 2 pints (1 litre) of water, clean rain water if possible. Simmer for 20 minutes over a low flame, strain and let cool. After shampooing the hair, finish with the rosemary rinse. It will add a lustre and bring out the colour.	
170	Vervain	Make an infusion of a large handful of the plant in 1 pint (0·5 litre) of boiling water. Let it stand for 20 minutes before straining. Massage this infusion into the scalp to stimulate hair growth. Used as a rinse, it will impart a brightness to fair hair.	

Shampoos

Plant		Preparation	Notes
87	Bay	Gather a few bay leaves and dry them. Crush them with a rolling pin and mix with them a handful of dried chamomile flowers and one of rosemary. Place in a large jug and pour over a litre of boiling water. Strain after 2–3 minutes and mix in a teaspoonful of soft or liquid soap and apply to the hair massaging it well in. Use a herbal rinse after shampooing or a little lemon juice or cider apple vinegar in warm water.	
55	Hound's Tongue	Gather a handful of leaves and dry them and with them mix a handful of dried chamomile flowers. Place in a large jug and pour onto them a litre of boiling water. Leave for several minutes and strain. Stir in a teaspoonful of liquid soap and shampoo the hair. Rinse with a herbal preparation.	Shampooing is drying to the hair and before each shampoo, it is advisable to rub olive oil or coconut oil into the scalp and to leave on for 20–30 minuts. It is nourishing to the hair roots.
115	Marjoram	Remove the stems when in bloom in mid-summer and use fresh, with an equal amount of rosemary or dry in an airy room to use in winter. To use fresh, place a small handful of each in a large jug and pour over 1 litre of boiling water. Let stand for several minutes, strain and add a small cupful of beer, working it well into the hair. Use a herbal rinse afterwards.	
88	Lavender	The essential oil is obtained by distillation of the flower spikes (see red rose) and it is the tiny green bracts enclosing the flowers (4 lbs or 2 kg will yield 1 fluid ounce) which yields the oil. A little on the finger tips massaged nightly into the scalp for several weeks will cause new hair growth to appear.	

Plant	Preparation	Notes

| 163 Lime | Obtain the juice by putting a lime through a blender (or by the prepared juice from a drug store or supermarket) and mix with a teaspoonful of glycerine. Massage thoroughly into the scalp, and cover the head with a shower cap overnight. Rinse in the morning with a little pure lime or lemon juice in 2 pints (1 litre) of warm water or use cider apple vinegar. | |

| 115 Marjoram | A handful of the leaves and flowers, with one of sage or rosemary (or both) infused in 1 pint (0·5 litre) of boiling water and allowed to cool will, if daily massaged into the scalp, prevent loss of hair. It should be done daily (making a fresh infusion) for several weeks. Afterwards, treat the hair with a little olive oil to prevent it becoming too dry. | |

| 115 Marjoram | Distill the shoots of sweet marjoram (which should be cut as they are just coming into flower) by placing them in a still or kettle and collecting the oil in a bowl or glass jar. Rub this tonic into the scalp and hair to promote the growth of new hair and to give the hair a pleasing gloss. The oil, rubbed over the body, with equal parts of olive or almond oil, will keep the skin soft and supple. An infusion, made by boiling the "tops" in water, rubbed into the scalp and hair will keep the hair healthy and glossy. | |

| 149 Sandalwood | Mix a teaspoonful (1 fluid drachm) of sandalwood oil, obtained by distillation of the wood chippings with a large cupful (4 fluid ounces) of coconut oil and massage into the hair. This will promote new hair growth and give the hair a brilliant gloss. | |

Hair dressing preparations

| 120 Bay Rum | Immerse 1 lb (0·5 kg) of bay laurel or West Indian Bay leaves in a jar with 1 pint (0·5 litre) of alcoholic rum. Leave for 10 days and strain, adding to it half the amount of water. Pour into screw-top bottles and keep under refrigeration. Massage it well into the hair and scalp twice weekly. A dark brown fragrant oil is obtained from the distillation of the round pea-sized fruits of *Pimenta acris*. This is mixed with Jamaica rum and water in equal parts and massaged into the hair and scalp. It will promote the growth of hair and add lustre to it. | Europeans will use the leaves of bay laurel and rum. |

| 63 Clove | Heat and mix 1 lb (0·5 kg) benzoated lard with a cupful (4 fluid ounces) of almond oil and 2 tablespoonsful (1 fluid ounce) of palm oil. Strain through muslin and whilst still warm add 2 tablespoonsful of otto of lemon or eau de Cologne and a small teaspoonful ($\frac{1}{2}$ drachm) of otto of cloves. It will make a pleasantly scented cream to use as a hair dressing and give the hair a healthy look. | |

| 104 Gum Benjamin | The oil extracted from the seeds by distillation is odourless, but does not become rancid, and is used in hair dressing, creams and suntan lotions. For a hair dressing, mix 2 tablespoonsful (1 fluid ounce) of oil of ben with 1 litre of cocounut oil and keep in a dark place when not in use. | It is now superseded by styrax benzoin. |

| 20 Gum Tragacanth | First dissolve $\frac{1}{2}$ oz of gum tragacanth in 3 fluid ounces (20 centilitres) of alcohol in a medium size saucepan. Stir in 2 tablespoonsful (1 fluid ounce) of castor oil and half that amount of glycerine, holding the pan over a very low flame and stirring all the time. Slowly add $\frac{1}{2}$ pint (0·25 litre) of water, stirring until all the ingredients are thoroughly mixed. Then cool and pour into a bottle. If desirable, a few drops of fragrant oil can be added before the mixture has cooled. | |

Plant	Preparation	Notes
127 Jacob's Ladder	To keep the hair black and to impart a gloss cut the plant in summer when in bloom and break into small pieces. Place a pan containing $\frac{1}{2}$ pint (0·25 litre) of olive oil and simmer over a low flame for 30 minutes, until the oil has turned jet black. When cool, strain and pour into a bottle and use as a hair dressing.	
45 Lemon	Dissolve a packet of gelatine in a basin, in a cupful of hot water. Add a small teaspoonful (1 fluid drachm) of lemon juice and one of eau de Cologne or oil of rosemary, its chief ingredient, and use as a setting lotion for the hair.	
79 Star Anise	The oil from the seeds contains shikimol, which is identical to saffron, hence its pleasing perfume. The oil is obtained by distillation of the seeds and is mixed with olive or coconut oil at a strength of 1 part in 10. Massaged into the scalp, it will promote the growth of new hair and impart a healthy gloss to it.	
58 Tonquin	Grind $\frac{1}{2}$ lb (0·25 kg) of beans, place in a large bowl and cover with 2 lb (1 kg) of melted fat, or use warm olive or almond oil. If hot lard is first macerated with powdered gum benzoin for several hours, it will partly perfume the fat and at the same time prevent its turning rancid. Macerate the beans for 24 hours, which is best done in a very low oven to keep the fat slightly warm. After 24 hours, strain (whilst warm) through muslin into screw-top jars and allow to set. The oil or grease will then have taken on the fragrance of the tonquin beans and will keep the hair healthy and glossy.	Vanilla beans (pods) can be used in the same way.
30 Ylang-Ylang	The fragrant otto is obtained by maceration and is drawn from the pomade by treating with rectified spirit (see cassie). To give it lasting fragrance, it should be mixed with a few drops of oil of cloves which it resembles in scent. It is included in Macassar hair oil as a substitute for oil of cassie.	

To clear the scalp of dandruff

Plant	Preparation	Notes
111 Catmint	Gather a handful of leaves and "tops" when in bloom, place in a pan and add 1 pint (0·5 litre) of boiling water. Let stand until cool, then massage into the scalp for several minutes and rinse off with warm water containing a little lemon juice.	
144 Rosemary	Into half a small cupful (about 2 fluid ounces) of warm olive or coconut oil, add a few drops of oil of rosemary and massage into the hair and scalp, or use an old but clean brush, kept for the purpose, to brush the oil into the hair. Leave on overnight, covering the hair with a shower cap. In the morning, rinse with warm water and cider apple vinegar or lemon juice.	
162 Thyme	Gather a handful (about 4 oz or 120 g) of "tops", which are most potent when just coming into bloom, and infuse in 1 pint (0·5 litre) of boiling water for 15 minutes. A handful of sage or rosemary could be included for greater efficiency. Strain and massage into the scalp to remove dandruff and use as a rinse to darken the hair and give it healthy gloss.	Oil of thyme is used in medical soaps. After flaking and melting white soap, the oil is added and the liquid soap poured into poached egg dishes to set.
19 Wall Rue	A handful of fronds and one of chamomile flowers infused in 1 pint (0·5 litre) of boiling water for 20 minutes will remove dandruff and prevent falling hair if daily massaged into the scalp. For greater efficiency, add a few drops of oil of rosemary to the lotion. Equally effective is an infusion of a handful of the closely related common maidenhair fronds in the same amount of water. This will make a mucilaginous paste which, massaged into the scalp, acts in the same way.	

Hair conditioners

	Plant	Preparation	Notes
119	Avocado	Put an avocado (rich in vitamin E) through the blender and to the juice or pulp, beat up the yolks of 2 eggs. Massage well into the scalp and hair and leave on for 30 minutes. Rinse thoroughly in lukewarm water containing a little lemon juice or cider apple vinegar.	
68	Sea Kelp	Beat up the yolk of an egg with a 4 oz (120 g) carton of yogurt; mix in a teaspoonful of finely grated lemon rind and a teaspoonful of sea kelp powder. Massage into the hair and scalp, leave for 30 minutes, then shampoo the head and rinse in warm water to which has been added a few drops of lemon juice.	
74	Sunflower	Mix 1 small cupful (2 fluid ounces) of wheat germ oil and the same of sunflower seed oil, warm slightly and massage into the scalp and hair. Cover the head with a shower cap and leave for 30 minutes. Then follow with a citric acid or lemon juice and water rinse (see Wheat).	
165	Wheat	Beat 1 tablespoonful ($\frac{1}{2}$ fluid ounce) of milk into 1 raw egg yolk, then add 1 cupful (4 fluid ounces) of water into which the juice of $\frac{1}{2}$ lemon has been squeezed. Stir in a tablespoonful of glycerine and one of wheat germ oil. Massage into the hair and scalp and leave for 60 minutes. Rinse with 2 pints (1 litre) of water into which a teaspoonful (1 fluid drachm) of citric acid crystals (or cider apple vinegar) has been dissolved.	

Hair colourants

	Plant	Preparation	Notes
27	Box	Place a handful of leaves and "tops" of the shoots with one of sawdust in a saucepan and simmer in an alkaline solution for 30 minutes. Strain and apply to the hair whilst still warm, especially at the roots.	This solution will help promote the growth of hair, for the plant contains buxine which stimulates the nerves of the scalp.
78	Common St. John's Wort	Collect and dry a handful of leaves, grind them to a powder and mix a small cupful with $\frac{1}{2}$ pint (0·25 litre) of hot water to form a paste. Massage well into the hair and leave for 20 to 30 minutes. Rinse in lukewarm water containing a little lemon juice.	
89	Henna	First feed the hair with balsam and protein conditioners before using henna, which is the dried and finely powdered leaves of *Lawsonia inermis*. As a conditioner, use a neutral henna. To dye the hair, there are compound hennas for black, dark brown and red-heads. (Do not use henna on blond or bleached hair, or on grey hair; or on hair previously treated with metallic dyes). Mix the henna into a stiff paste with water and for extra gloss, stir in an egg yolk. Tea will darken red henna, and coffee, black henna. Red wine will give an auburn finish. Cover the hair-line with vaseline, then brush in the henna with a small nail brush, from the roots outwards to the end of the hair strands, going over the head in sections. Wrap the hair in a sheet of plastic (having previously covered the shoulders with a plastic sheet) and put on a shower cap. Leave for at least an hour, preferably two, then rinse off in warm water mixed with a little lemon or lime juice. The hair will take on a brilliant gloss.	
80	Indigo Plant	You can obtain an indigo dye (blue-black) from the dried leaves, by soaking them in water. This dye has been used by Eastern women to colour the hair blue-black for centuries. It is mixed with an equal amount of henna and made into a paste with hot water. Massage it well into the hair, particularly at the roots, leave on for 30 minutes and rinse off in lukewarm water.	

Plant	Preparation	Notes
169 Mullein	Make an infusion of a handful of the flowers in 2 pints (1 litre) of boiling water and allow to stand for 20 minutes before straining. The infusion makes a rinse which imparts a rich golden colour to fair hair.	Mullein water, to which a few drops of oil of rosemary have been added, is an excellent hair restorative if rubbed into the scalp daily.
138 Oak	Galls, which are round excrescences produced on the twigs of oak trees by the larva of the mite, can be used to dye hair black. Infuse a large handful of the freshly gathered galls in 1 pint (0·5 litre) of boiling water and leave for 10 minutes. Strain, and whilst still warm, apply as a hair rinse, working it well into the hair and at the roots.	
97 Purple Loosestrife	Collect and dry the leaves of purple loosestrife, then grind or roll to a powder. Mix 1 oz (30 g) of the leaves with ½ pint (0·25 litre) of hot water to form a thin paste and massage well into the hair combing it out afterwards. Leave on for 20 minutes and rinse in lukewarm water containing a little lemon juice.	
51 Saffron	Immerse a pinch of saffron grains (powder) in 1 pint (0·5 litre) of boiling water and let stand for 10 minutes. The water will take on a bright yellow colour. Use a wash after shampooing and let dry on. Fair hair will acquire a rich golden tint.	
145 Sage	Make an infusion of a handful of "tops" or the dried leaves in 1 pint (0·5 litre) of boiling water and let stand for 10 minutes before straining. Thus treated, sage will darken the hair and give it a lustre if massaged into the scalp and hair after shampooing. Let dry on and afterwards massage in a little coconut oil if the hair is dry.	
83 Walnut	The oil, obtained by distillation of the nuts, is jet black and has been used for centuries to colour men's hair and impart a gloss to it. If the green outer husks are boiled (1 lb or 0·5 kg) in 1 pint (0·5 litre) of water and strained after 15 minutes, the liquid used as a rinse, will colour brown hair a darker shade.	

Shaving creams

Plant	Preparation	Notes
59 Oil Palm	Mix in a pan placed in a larger pan containing hot water, half a small cupful (about 2 fluid ounces) of stearic acid and add a tablespoonful (½ fluid ounce) each of palm and coconut oil. Add 1 teaspoonful (1 drachm) of sodium hydroxide, 1 tablespoonful of glycerine and 1 small cupful (4 fluid ounces) of water, stirring all the time. Then add another ½-cupful of stearic acid. Stir it in well and allow to cool and set. The palm oil will provide its own violet perfume.	
106 Wax Myrtle	The fruits or berries of the bog myrtles are covered in white wax. This wax is removed by boiling and skimming from the water when cool. The fruits are then reheated and more wax skimmed off, the whole process being repeated several times. The wax is made into cakes to solidify and is included in face creams and ointments in place of beeswax.	

After shave lotions

Plant	Preparation	Notes
50 Coriander	Take 2 oz (60 g) of seed which should be a year old for their orange perfume to be pronounced, and place in a pan with a tablespoon of honey and 1 pint (0·5 litre) of water. Simmer over a low flame for 20 minutes and when cool, add a tablespoonful (½ fluid ounce) of witch hazel and strain into bottles. If kept under refrigeration, the lotion will be especially refreshing when used.	
147 Elder	Pour 1 pint (0·5 litre) of boiling water onto 2 large handfuls of elder flowers placed in a bowl. Allow to soak for 12 hours, strain and bottle. Keep under refrigeration.	

Plant	Preparation	Notes

Foundation creams/powders

| 49 | Carnauba Wax | Heat 1 oz (30 g) of wax to 84°C (its melting point) and stir in 1 cupful (4 fluid ounces) of almond oil and 1 oz (30 g) white beeswax. Remove from the heat and add a few drops of rose oil as perfume then, as it cools, pour into screw-top pots. |

| 20 | Gum Tragacanth | Mix together 1 part powdered orris and 1 part kaolin with 4 parts rice starch. Add the required colour and a few drops otto of rose to give it perfume and mix with 1 drachm gum tragacanth to act as a binding agent. |

| 81 | Orris | Mix together 4 oz (120 g) of rice starch and 1 oz (30 g) powdered orris root with 1 oz (30 g) kaolin. Add the prepared colour and a few drops otto of rose. Keep in a closed box. |

| 123 | Pistachio | Pistachio nuts and almonds, after having been put through a milling machine, make a fine-grain complexion powder which is smooth and soft to apply and adheres to the skin without flaking. Mix together ½ lb (0·25 kg) each talc, rice starch and pistachio starch and add a few drops otto of rose and of lavender, mixing well in. Without the addition of colouring matter, the powder will be white and prepared colours are obtainable from chemists (drug stores). Blondes should use a peach or naturelle colouring; brunettes need rachel. Colourants are added after brushing the powders through a fine sieve. |

| 149 | Sandalwood | Mix with 3 lb (1·5 kg) of rice starch, 1 teaspoonful (1 drachm) each of otto of rose and otto of sandalwood. Work ½ drachm of rose-pink colouring from the chemist and keep mixing until the powder is evenly blended throughout. Pour into suitable containers. It will give a matt-like finish. |

Rouge

| 11 | Alkanet | Lift, clean and dry the roots of alkanet in a low oven, or use them fresh. Slice into a basin or bowl and cover with spirits of wine. Leave for 7 days. This will draw out the red colouring matter from the rind. Strain into a saucepan containing ½ lb (0·25 kg) of lard and heat gently, stirring all the time until the red colouring is well mixed in. Let cool, but before it becomes cold, add a few drops of tincture of benzoin as a preservative and pour into pots to set. |

| 33 | Safflower | Immerse a handful of flowers in a pint (0·5 litre) of boiling water to extract the red dye. This is then mixed with finely ground rice powder and kaolin (3 parts rice powder to 1 part kaolin) to make a smooth powder. |

| 33 | Safflower | Mix the red dye (obtainable from chemists or druggists) with equal parts rice powder and kaolin, and stir into twice the amount by weight of lard or petroleum jelly which has been melted over a low flame. The result should be a cream rouge of soft consistency. Pour into screw-top jars. |

Mascara

| 49 | Carnauba Wax | Heat over a low flame and mix together 4 oz (120 g) carnauba wax and the same amount of beeswax. Add 2 oz (60 g) stearic acid and 1 oz (30 g) triethanolamine and 1 oz (30 g) of colouring (lampblack) mixing well. Pour into suitable containers and allow to set firm before using. |

| 20 | Gum Tragacanth | Heat a small amount (1·5 g) of gum tragacanth in ½ pint (0·25 litre) water, stirring until it has melted. Remove from the heat and mix in a tablespoonful (½ fluid ounce) of alcohol and |

Plant	Preparation	Notes
Gum Tragacanth (continued)	a teaspoonful ($\frac{1}{2}$ oz or 15 g) of lampblack. Cool and pour into screw-top jars.	
137 Quince	Make up a sugar syrup by dissolving in a saucepan, a cupful of sugar in a $\frac{3}{4}$ cupful (3 fluid ounces) of water over a low flame. Stir in 1 oz (30 g) of gum arabic until dissolved. In a basin, soak an eggcupful of quince seed in $\frac{3}{4}$ cupful of water for several hours and to it add the gum arabic and liquid sugar, stirring until well mixed. Add a few drops of alcoholic tincture of benzoin as a preservative and keep under refrigeration. Do not forget to add the mascara colouring to your taste, perhaps black, blue or green.	

Lipstick and lip salves

11 Alkanet	Place 2 oz (60 g) each white beeswax and spermaceti in a bowl, partly submerged in a sink of boiling water to melt the wax and add 2 oz (60 g) of washed and chopped alkanet root. Leave for several hours, constantly renewing the hot water. Strain and work in a cupful of almond oil and add a few drops of otto of rose as a perfume. Pour into screw-top jars and let cool.	
24 Annatto	The fleshy orange pulp enclosing the seeds is used in commerce to colour lipsticks, for it blends well with wax and oil. Place 2 oz (60 g) each white beeswax and spermaceti in a bowl, partly submerged in a sink of boiling water to melt them and work in a small quantity of annatto (the dried pulp). Stir in a cupful (4 fluid ounces) of warm almond oil and pour into old lipstick cases to solidify.	
141 Castor Oil Plant	Mix 9 parts lanolin with 1 part castor oil and keep in a dark place. Apply a little after using a lipstick to give additional gloss to the lips. For a lip salve, heat and mix 1 part each white beeswax and spermaceti and 2 parts castor oil, adding a little pink colouring if desired. When blended, pour into screw-top jars.	
114 Olive	To 2 teaspoonsful (1 fluid ounce) of olive oil, add enough beeswax to fill a eggcup, place into a small saucepan. Add a handful of tips of young rosemary shoots and simmer for 30 minutes. Then add a cupful (4 fluid ounces) of rose water for fragrance and whilst still warm, strain into screw-top face cream jars and allow to set. Apply to the lips when sore or as a base before using a lipstick.	

Essences and perfumes

103 Champac	The fragrance of the perfume is obtained by enfleurage as for jasmine and tuberose and extracting the scent from the pomade by rectified spirit. Use 2 pints (1 litre) of spirit to every 2 lb (1 kg) of pomade. Leave for a month, shaking up daily, then strain off the perfume and bottle, adding a few drops of sandalwood oil as a fixative.	
31 Elemi	The white gum resin collected from incisions made in the bark has the lemon scent of verbena after being digested for a month in rectified spirit and frequently shaken up. It is strained and included in "bouquets" and used to perfume toilet soaps.	
26 Frankincense	Place 1 oz (30 g) of the gum in a jar and cover with $\frac{1}{2}$ pint (0·25 litre) of rectified spirit. Leave for a month, shaking daily, then drain off and bottle, adding a few drops to home-made perfumes to give them more permanence. It also gives a balsamic perfume to home-made toilet soaps.	

Plant	Preparation	Notes
75 Heliotrope	The perfume of the flowers is difficult to extract and is usually reproduced synthetically. Place 1 lb (0·5 kg) of benzoated lard in a pan which is partly immersed in a bowl of boiling water. To the melted fat, add a handful of flowers and let them remain for 24 hours, adding more hot water every so often. Then remove the flowers, reheat the fat and water and add fresh flowers. Repeat the process for 5 or 6 days. When cold, the pomade is chopped up and placed in a large glass jar.	
75 Heliotrope	Cover with rectified spirit and leave for a month in a warm room, shaking up daily. Strain through cotton wool. The resulting spirit is an essence or extract of heliotrope and is admirable for mixing in "bouquets" or for use as a handkerchief perfume, whilst the perfumed pomade is suitable for hair dressings.	
82 Jasmine	Flowers of white jasmine are collected when newly opened and are embedded in a tray of fat. To $\frac{3}{4}$ lb (0·36 kg) of animal fat and $\frac{1}{4}$ lb (0·12 kg) of lard, add 2 pints (1 litre) of water into which has been dissolved a teaspoonful of alum. Bring to the boil and when the fats have dissolved, strain and allow to cool. Collect the fat on the surface, remove and reheat. Add a few drops of benzoic acid to prevent the fat turning rancid. Pour the fat into 2 fairly shallow dishes of similar size and allow to set. Place the flowers to a depth of 2 in (5 cm) over the fat of one dish and over them place the inverted second dish with the rims in contact. Leave the dishes undisturbed for 2 days and nights, then remove the flowers and replace with fresh ones. Continue this process every 48 hours for about a month or until the plants have finished flowering, by which time the fat will have fully absorbed the perfume. The fat from both dishes is then scraped into a large glass screw-top jar and the same amount (by bulk) of spirits of wine is added. The jar is placed in a warm dark cupboard for 2 months and is shaken up each day to extract the perfume. The liquid is then strained through muslin and a drop of sandalwood oil added as a fixative, to intensify and preserve the scent. After straining off the otto, the pomade left behind will still contain the perfume. It is re-heated and mixed with an equal amount of olive oil and a little beeswax so that it will set better. Pour into small screw-top jars to set. It will make a deliciously scented body ointment or pomade for the hair.	
109 Jonquil	The method is described under Jasmine, jonquil (narcissus) flowers being used instead.	
42 Labdanum	The gum resin is used as a fixative for perfumes, like myrrh, the "cakes" being treated with spirits of wine and, after several weeks, strained and a few drops added to flower scents to prolong their fragrance, to give them a lasting quality.	
158 Lilac	The fragrance is obtained by enfleurage in grease, and is drawn off the pomade by rectified spirit as for cassie and tuberose. To give it permanence, add $\frac{1}{2}$ oz (0·15 g) of tincture of benzoin or extract of vanilla for every pint (0·5 litre) of essence. Use the essence as a handkerchief perfume; the pomade for hair dressings.	
44 Neroli	Place 1 tablespoonful ($\frac{1}{2}$ fluid ounce) of otto of neroli pétale; the same of otto of rosemary; and double the amount of otto of bergamot orange in a glass container and to them add 10 pints (5 litre) of grape spirit. In place of the otto of orange, equal amounts of otto of orange and lemon peel can be used. The grape spirit gives eau de Cologne its unique fragrance. Allow to stand for several days before bottling and use as an astringent or to rub over the body after bathing in summer when its coolness will be especially refreshing.	

Plant	Preparation	Notes
144 Rosemary	Oil of rosemary (or that of any other herb) is obtained by soaking 1 lb (0·5 kg) of rosemary tips (most potent in summer) in 1 gallon (4 litres) of proof spirit in a screw-top jar. Allow to stand for 10 days, then distill, as described for making rose water.	The oil (a few drops) may be added to a warm bath or used to massage into the scalp. It is an excellent hair restorer.
128 Tuberose	The essence is extracted from the pomade (the fragrance of the flowers being obtained by enfleurage in darkness, an artificial inducement for the flowers to "work" harder in giving their perfume) by placing in a large jar and for every 2 lb (1 kg) of pomatum, adding 2 pints (1 litre) of rectified spirit. Leave for a month, shaking daily, and strain off the essence through cotton wool. To every pint (0·5 litre) add $\frac{1}{2}$ ounce of tincture of benzoin or of extract of vanilla to give permanance.	
168 Vanilla	The pods are sliced and placed in a large glass jar and covered with alcohol to extract the perfume. For every 1 lb (0·5 kg) of pods use 1 pint (0·5 litre) of alcohol and leave for 5 to 6 weeks, shaking daily. The tincture is then strained off and is ready to use in floral "bouquets" in which no single odour predominates.	
172 Violet	The perfume is obtained by maceration. A large handful of flowers is thrown into a porcelain pan in which 2 lb (1 kg) of benzoated lard has been melted over a low flame. The flowers are allowed to remain for 8 hours and are then removed with a strainer, the fat reheated and fresh flowers thrown in. The process is repeated 6 or 7 times until the fat is saturated with the scent of the flowers. When cool, the olive-green essence is obtained by treating the solidified pomade with rectified spirit for a month. After straining, the washed pomatum is reheated to use in hair dressings.	

Toilet waters

Plant	Preparation	Notes
50 Coriander	To 1 lb (0·5 kg) of lemon balm leaves, add 2 oz (60 g) of lemon peel; and 1 oz (30 g) each of nutmeg, cloves, coriander seed and chopped angelica root. Place in a home still or an old kettle with 1 pint (0·5 litre) of orange blossom or elder flower water and 2 pints (1 litre) of alcohol. Slowly distil, if using a kettle, collecting the toilet water, which is passed through a tube beneath cold water, in a large jar.	This celebrated toilet water was made by the nuns of the Carmelite Abbey of St. Just in the 14th century, and was used all over Europe.
88 Lavender	Place the flower spikes, together with some pieces of canella bark, in a simple still or use a kettle filled with water. Put over a low flame and collect the distillation from a tube passed through cold water. The condensation will drip into a glass jar and will continue until the water in the kettle is used. Add the same amount of rose water and it will make a pleasant body lotion.	It is also astringent and is used as a complexion water.
10 Scarlet Pimpernel	Make an infusion of the whole plant (not the roots) with boiling water for 15 minutes. After straining, apply to the face. This infusion will rid the skin of blemishes and soreness caused by exposure to sunlight.	An ointment from the juice is equally effective.

Toilet soaps

Plant	Preparation	Notes
23 Birch	From the distillation of the bark of the Silver Birch, *betula alba*, a dark brown perfumed oil is obtained for use in soaps. To make a brown Windsor soap, use 2 tablespoonsful (1 fluid ounce) of birch oil to every 1 lb (0·5 kg) of white soap, and to make up the soap cakes see Red Rose, using in this case birch oil instead of otto of rose. Birch soap is an effective skin disinfectant and helps get rid of blemishes.	

Plant		Preparation	Notes
57	Carnation	The scented otto is obtained by maceration and is drawn from the pomade by rectified spirit. To give it more permanence, add a few drops of oil of cloves. The otto is added to home-made toilet soaps and is also included in "heavy" or Eastern perfumes.	
54	Citronella	Oil of lemon grass is used to impart a verbena-like perfume to soap (see Red Rose for the method of making it). It can also be used to adulterate rose oil, for it has a high geraniol content and blends as effectively as oil of the rose-scented pelargonium.	
107	Nutmeg	The nuts, after the removal of the arillus or outer covering, are placed in a still (or kettle) filled with water, and the vapour (steam) driven through a rubber tube into a glass container or bowl where the oil separates from the liquid which forms. It is blended with oil of sandalwood or lavender (or both) to impart its fragrance to home-made soaps.	
143	Red Rose	Obtain a small phial of rose oil (or of rosemary or verbena) from the chemist or drug store and add a few drops to a large cupful of water brought to the boil in an enamel pan. Have ready, thinly cut pieces or shavings from a bar of pure white soap and add them to the boiling water. They will quickly dissolve. Then pour into small rounded containers used for poaching eggs (there are usually 4 to a pan) and allow to cool. the mix will set into circular "cakes" and leave no trace of soap other than that which can be removed by warm water when removed from the containers. The cakes are pure and pleasantly scented; the longer they are kept, the harder and more lasting they become. All kinds of perfumes can be used.	
150	Sassafras	From the oil distilled from the ripe fruits under steam pressure, a perfumed toilet soap is made (see Red Rose). The oil is used in perfumery, for its fragrance is lasting and it blends with other less expensive perfumes.	
118	Scented-leaf Geranium	The essential oil, geraniol, which resembles otto of rose, is obtained by distillation of the leaves of any of the rose-scented pelargoniums, using a simple still or a kettle and collecting the oil which rises to the top of the distillate. For making toilet soap, see Red Rose.	
71	Wintergreen	The leaves and stems must be soaked in cold water for 24 hours for the oil to develop by fermentation. Then they are placed in a still and the resulting oil is drawn off. A few drops may be included when making toilet soaps.	

The bath and after

Plant		Preparation	Notes
134	Apricot	Mix together 2 tablespoonsful (1 fluid ounce) of melted butter and two of olive oil. Leave for an hour, then mix in 1 teaspoonful (1 fluid drachm) of cider apple vinegar; 2 tablespoonsful (1 fluid ounce) of witch hazel; the juice of 3 apricots put through a blender together with a small carton of yogurt. Stir in 2 beaten eggs and $\frac{1}{2}$ pint of milk and put through the blender, adding another $\frac{1}{2}$ pint (0·25 litre) of milk after. Place in a plastic bottle and keep in the refrigerator until required. There will be enough for 6 baths, adding about a cupful each time.	
13	Chamomile	Pour 1 litre of boiling water in a saucepan over a large handful of chamomile flowers. Mix in 2 tablespoonsful (1 fluid ounce) of honey and when cool, strain. Make up separately 2 pints (1 litre) of powdered milk, using a cupful of the powder, and mix together. Add it to a bath of comfortably hot water and relax in it for 20 minutes adding more hot water if necessary.	

Plant	Preparation	Notes
3 Horse Chestnut	Boil 1 lb (0·5 kg) of horse chestnuts until the outer skins are soft enough to remove. Then boil the nuts for 30 minutes more in 1 pint (0·5 litre) of water, simmering over a low flame, and strain off the juice. Whilst still warm, add 1 small teaspoonful (1 fluid drachm) of pine oil and 1 of triethanolamine oleate. When cool, bottle and add a little to a warm bath as the water runs in. It will tone the flesh and leave it firm.	
28 Marigold	Boil together 1 lb (0·5 kg) barley meal and 2 lb (1 kg) of bran. Add a large handful of borage leaves; 1 of lemon balm; and 1 of marigold flowers. Simmer together for 30 minutes and add to a warm bath. Soak in it for 30 minutes, adding more warm water as the bath cools. Afterwards, rub down the body briskly with a warm towel.	To cleanse the skin of impurities.
100 Melilot	Place the plant in a muslin bag, together with several bay laurel leaves and a handful of rosemary "tops". This "herb bouquet" will provide a fragrant bath, toning the body.	
59 Oil Palm	Mix together equal amounts of palm oil, almond oil and olive oil (say, a small cupful, or 4 fluid ounces, of each), with $\frac{1}{2}$ cupful (2 fluid ounces) of wheat germ oil and keep in a closed bottle in the dark, using a little to massage into all parts of the body after bathing or swimming. The palm oil will provide a pleasing violet fragrance. If sunbathing afterwards, substitute sesame oil for the almond oil and add a sun screening agent obtainable from a chemist or drug store.	
122 Pine	Mix 1 teaspoonful (1 fluid drachm) of pine oil with 1 tablespoonful ($\frac{1}{2}$ fluid ounce) of nonyl phenol in a jug or basin. Add 1 fluid ounce of triethanolamine alkyl sulphate (from a chemist or drug store) and mix in a pint (0·5 litre) of water in which balm or bergamot have been infused. Pour into the bath as the water runs in.	
15 Southernwood	Simmer in a pan for 10 minutes a handful of leaves (the "tops" of the shoots being most potent) of rosemary, lemon balm, bergamot, hyssop, southernwood and lemon thyme, together with a handful of chamomile flowers. There should be altogether about 1 lb (0·5 kg) of herbs to 2 pints (1 litre) of water. Then strain and when cold, add to the liquid $\frac{1}{5}$ part of brandy or whiskey, which will keep it potent for 2 months. Use a little in a warm bath, for it will tone the flesh, cleanse the skin of impurities and relax the muscles.	
74 Sunflower	Mix together a cupful (4 fluid ounces) of sunflower oil and the same of almond oil with 2 tablespoonsful (1 fluid ounce) of wheatgerm oil and the same of olive oil. Keep in a screw-top bottle and massage a little into the body after drying it.	
110 Watercress	Watercress juice is included in foam bath gels and the water in which the plant has been boiled for 10 minutes when added to a warm bath, will tone up the flesh and bring relief to tired muscles.	

Dusting powders

Plant	Preparation	Notes
25 Boldo	All parts of the plant, the twiggy shoots, the pea-sized fruits, and the leaves are fragrant. After drying in the sun, they turn red and the perfume increases in strength. When dry, they are ground into powder and mixed with equal amounts of orris root and French chalk to make an attractively scented talcum powder.	
32 Canella	The bark has the scent of cinnamon and when dried and pulverised, is mixed with an equal amount of orris root and powdered chalk and put through a sieve. It is then placed in a container which should be kept tightly closed.	

Plant	Preparation	Notes

| 82 | Jasmine | Place a layer of white jasmine flowers in a strong cardboard box (a shoe box is ideal) and cover the flowers with a 1 in (2·5 cm) layer of starch or French chalk. Then add another layer of flowers and more starch and so on until the box is full. After 48 hours, sift the powder through a fine sieve onto a layer of fresh jasmine flowers in another box, adding more flowers and chalk (starch). Throw away the old flowers and leave for another 48 hours and repeat the process. Then sift the scented chalk and mix with it a few grains of civet or ambergris. Put into old talcum powder boxes and apply to the body with a large powder puff. | |

| 81 | Orris | Lift and dry the root of a three-year-old orris (iris) plant, replanting pieces of root with leaves attached to maintain a supply and using the rest of the rhizomes (roots) to make a powder. Scrape or lightly peel the roots and dry in a low oven with the door ajar. When dry, the roots will be hard and woody. The longer they are kept, the more pronounced their perfume. Use a small milling machine to grind to a fine powder, then mix 1 lb (0·5 kg) with 5 lb (2·5 kg) of rich starch and add a few drops of otto of bergamot orange and of cloves, mixing well. It should be kept in a box with a tight fitting lid and should be applied to the body with a large puff. | |

Deodorants, body oils & lotions

| 14 | Arnica | To a cupful (4 fluid ounces) of witch hazel, add 1 tablespoon-ful ($\frac{1}{2}$ fluid ounce) of tincture of arnica (from the chemist or drug store) and 1 teaspoonful (1 fluid drachm) of glycerol. Shake up well and store in a screw-top bottle under refrigeration. | |

| 130 | Balsam Poplar | The buds exude a resin with a balsamic scent which is used as a fixative for perfumes and to make a skin cream or unguent. First place the buds in a large glass jar to treat with spirits of wine to remove the resin. Leave for several days, frequently shaking up. Strain and add to warm lard, to which 1 cupful (4 fluid ounces) of almond or olive oil has been added. Just before it is cool, pour into screw-top jars and massage into the body for sunburn or when exposed to drying winds. | |

| 140 | Mignonette | The fragrance of mignonette, jasmine and white lilac is obtained by enfleurage (see jasmine). Otto of mignonette, one of the most powerfully scented of the whole floral kingdom is obtained by pouring alcohol onto the pomade (1 pint or $\frac{1}{2}$ litre to each pound or 0·5 kg of pomade) leaving for 2 weeks. After filtering, add 2 tablespoonsful (1 fluid ounce) to extract of tolu to give it greater permanence. | |

| 51 | Saffron | Melt over a low flame 1 cupful (4 fluid ounces) of olive oil and one of almond oil and add a pinch of saffron, stirring until the mixture is completely blended and has attained a rich yellow colour. Pour into bottles and use after bathing or swimming, to massage gently into all parts of the body after drying. | |

| 149 | Sandalwood | Mix 1 teaspoonful (1 fluid drachm) of sandalwood oil, obtained by distillation of the wood chippings with a large cupful (4 fluid ounces) of cocounut oil and massage into the body after bathing. | |

| 74 | Sunflower | Partly warm $\frac{1}{2}$ cupful of sunflower or almond oil (about 2 fluid ounces) and massage it into all parts of the body, while sitting on a shower-room stool. Then create steam in the shower cubicle. Turn off the hot water and stand in the steam for 5 minutes before creating more steam and repeat several times. Then wash the body with warm water and almond soap. | |

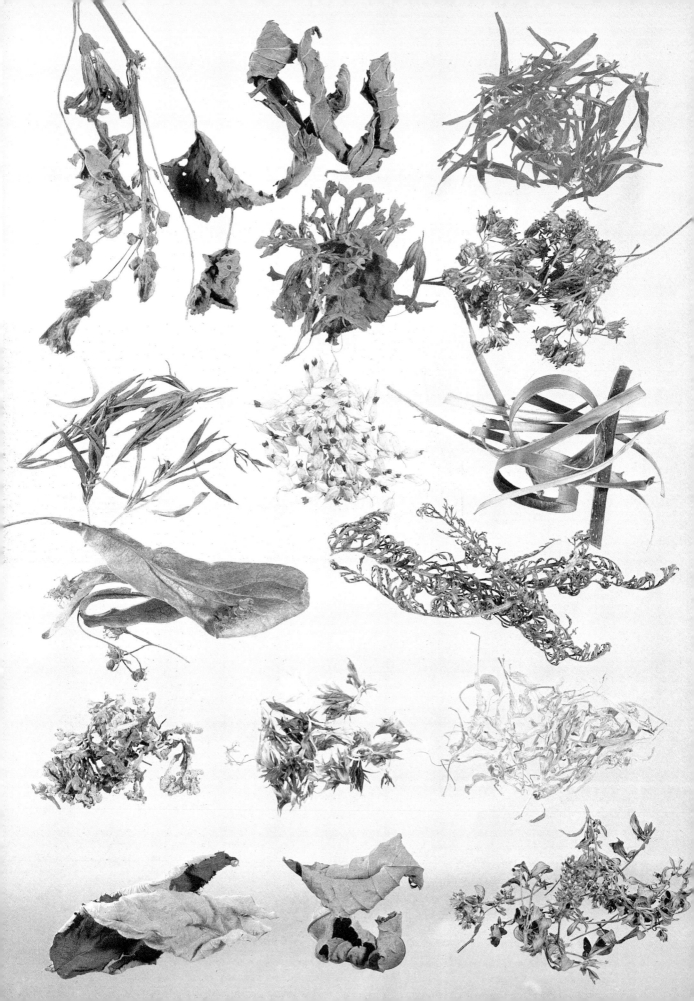

Preparing natural cosmetics

More than 200 recipes are given in the book, some that are similar for different plants are to be used at different times of the year. Some plants can be used fresh or dried. Scented leaf plants, which include many of the herbs, will be at their most potent towards the end of summer, but they may be used fresh from early summer and dried during the rest of the year. Since the drying process is begun when the plants are at their best, their full efficacy is assured the year round.

Plants of woodland, hedgerow and field which include annuals and those perennials which come again each year after dying back in autumn and winter, are at their most potent when just coming into bloom, when the whole plant above ground, including the stems, leaves and flowers can be used. Mention is made in the recipes of the 'tops'. These are the tops of the stems, the young leaves and flowers which are most effective when used for infusions.

The plants should be used as soon as gathered or shortly after, before they lose their potent qualities by evaporation. Rinse them under a tap of cold running water and remove any dead parts, then place in a clean bowl or saucepan. This should be of ample size, to hold perhaps two large handsful of plant material and sufficient water, perhaps half a litre or more, to cover them. The water should be boiling; or the plants may be simmered over a very low flame. Most plants need gentle heat, to persuade them to release their contents more readily. It is usual to leave them 15–20 minutes to soak or simmer, (some take longer) before

straining into another bowl or into bottles. It is preferable to make up your water preparations each time they are to be used for a hair rinse or for shampoos, for water quickly loses its freshness unless kept under refrigeration. Even so, the preparations should not be allowed to become

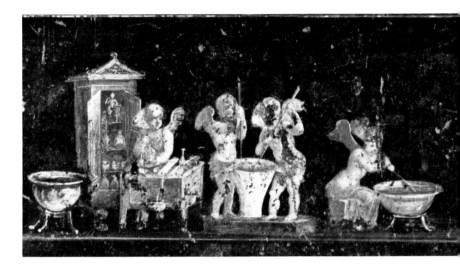

stale.

A refrigerator is a valuable asset for keeping your preparations in condition; whilst the cold temperature of fruits and lotions that have been refrigerated gives the skin a tingling sensation which stimulates the cells. That alone plays a part in the skin's rejuvenation.

Make sure that all utensils are perfectly clean before using them and that oils and fats are quite fresh and in no way rancid. A small amount of storax (styrax benzoin) added to them will prevent their becoming rancid for several months after they are made.

Take care in making up your beauty preparations for it is not easy to use milk without its curdling nor

There are natural cosmetics for all purposes, to improve the quality of the skin, nourishing it and clearing it of spots and blemishes; for the eyes, to remove tiredness and give the eyes a sparkle; for the hair, to impart a healthy gloss, for its colouring and to prevent the hair from falling, whilst correcting any dryness or excess greasiness. And there are herbal preparations to make for maintaining all parts of the body in condition and to give it a sense of well-being. Plants should be used fresh wherever possible, when all their components are at their peak of efficacy, but many plants can be saved and dried to use and will retain their quality if dried and stored with care.

Above: Roman depiction of perfume making. Wall-painting in the *House of Vettii*, Pompeii.

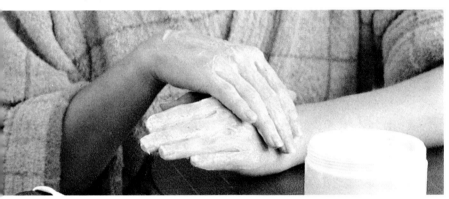

to blend water and oils in the preparation of emollients, emulsions and moisturising creams. Always add the water (which may be rose water) to the warm oil and wax (if making a cold cream), not the other way. Add it slowly, stirring all the time until the whole amount has been used up and whilst the oil is still warm. The perfume is added last, just before the mixture has become cold and at this point it is poured into the pots or jars

to set into a creamy consistency. Leave open the jars until it has set and become quite cold, then close up with the screw closures. Remove at once to a cool place.

When making up a cold cream first melt the beeswax and spermaceti which boil at low temperatures and which give the preparation a thick consistency, then add the oil, then the rose water, and very lastly the perfume. The finished product should be smooth and creamy.

When adding colouring to face powders, do so with care, for an excess will have a disastrous effect when used for one's make up. Concentrate on the more natural tints and use them sparingly.

Some preparations are more difficult to make up than others and this only comes with practice. But gathering one's own material from the countryside and translating them into preparations which are pleasing to use and enhance your beauty and well being is a most enjoyable hobby or pastime.

Except in one or two instance, all the materials mentioned are natures own and are readily obtainable. And if you do not wish to search for them in your local habitat, they may be obtained from your local shops or supermarket. Using them to make up simple beauty preparations will ensure that your skin will be free of often injurious chemicals, although your efforts will be inferior to those manufactured with a high degree of skill by established cosmetic houses.

EQUIPMENT REQUIRED

You will need the usual equipment found in kitchens everywhere – small and large cups for measuring liquids. A small tea-size cup will hold about 4 fluid ounces: a breakfast cup about twice that amount. You will require the sort of glass screw-top jars, that are used for pickles and salting beans, for pomades obtained by the maceration of flowers.

The solid mass of fat, cut up and placed in a large jar, is covered in rectified spirit to extract the essence. Large jars are also required for collecting the material from the distillation of those flowers and leaves which yield an otto or oily substance. This rises to the top and is collected and placed in a smaller jar. The

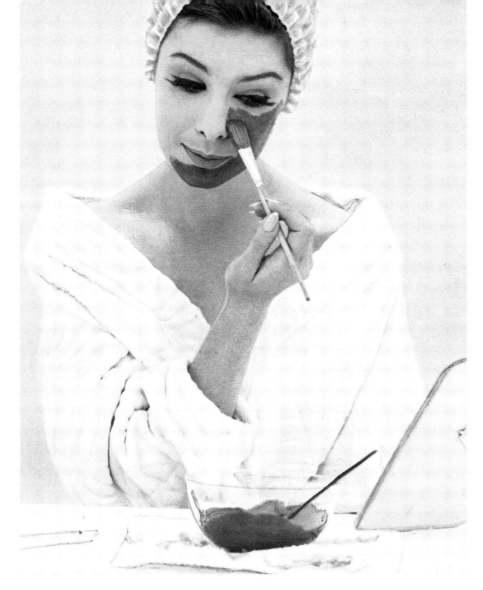

A good facial requires at least two hours, from the time of preparation to the time of removal. Different vegetables and fruit, combined with milk, are ideal ingredients for most facials, whether to treat dry, oily, or normal skin.

leaves and twigs of many plants and also their seeds yield large amounts of essential oil: flowers smaller quantities.

Exact measures of fluid ounces, pints and litres, will enable the correct amounts to be used, making for better results than estimating measurements. A pair of kitchen scales for weighing in pounds or kilos will be an advantage and they will also be used for weighing ingredients for cooking. Indeed, many of the same utensils will be used for both cooking and for making cosmetics.

A selection of wooden spoons for mixing (stirring) materials and metal spoons of various sizes for measuring dry and liquid materials will be required:

A teaspoon = 1 fluid drachm or $\frac{1}{4}$ ounce (dry)
A dessert spoon = 2 fluid drachms or $\frac{1}{2}$ ounce (dry)
A tablespoon = 4 fluid drachms or 1 ounce (dry)
Note also that: 8 fluid drachms = 1 fluid ounce = 2·8 centilitres
1 pint or 20 fluid ounces = 0·5 litres
1 oz = 28·35 grammes (30 grammes to simplify our calculations)
1 lb or 16 ounces = 0·45 kilos (0·5 kilos to simplify our calculations).

CARMELITE WATER
To make a toilet water, like that made by the nuns of the Carmelite Abbey of St Just in the 14th century:
To 16 oz (500 g) of lemon balm leaves, add 2 oz (50 g) of lemon peel, and 1 oz (25 g) each of nutmeg, cloves, coriander seed and angelica root. Place in a still with 2 pints (1 litre) of orange or elder flower water and 4 pints (2 litres) of alcohol and slowly distil, collecting the celebrated toilet water in a large jar.

Several enamel saucepans of various sizes will be a necessity and will be in constant use for infusions and for boiling waxes and fats. Several mixing bowls and basins will be required, also a strainer and a fine wire mesh sieve for face and dusting powders. A high-temperature immersion thermometer will be a valuable asset and so will an electric blender for pulping and juicing nuts, fruits and vegetables. If this is not available, a mortar and pestle will be needed to crush seeds, nuts and roots. There should be muslin or cotton wool for straining alcoholic essences and a pipette, to draw off small amounts of otto which has collected on the top of water.

Distillation will play an important part in making one's own beauty preparations and perfumes so a still will be needed. It should be of an easily manageable size to place over a burner. It should have a dome-shaped lid with a glass corkscrew shaped or gooseneck pipe through which the steam passes from the chamber which contains the flowers or leaves and water into the condenser. With the steam, the volatile oil arises and is liquified at the same time. The oil and water pass through the condenser into the separator from which the essential oil is poured into bottles. If a separator is not used, the oil must be collected from the surface of the condenser by skimming or using a pipette and placed into jars.

When placing material in the still, make it as compact as possible: it should not be loose, and it should be well covered with water so that it does not dry out during the distillation but not with more water than

necessary. As the vapour passes through the condenser as oil and water, it cools and becomes liquid when it reaches the separator. When no more oil is driven off, the operation has ended. Dry material is the best to use in a still.

After the operation has ended, dismantle the still and clean the various parts, emptying the still of its contents and placing them on the garden compost heap. It will then be ready for the next distillation.

A very simple method of distillation can be performed by filling an old large kettle with material and water and placing it over a gas burner turned very low. To the spout of the kettle fix a length of rubber tubing which leads to a glass bowl or jar into which the vapour condenses as oil and water (the tube itself must pass through a bowl of cold water to perform its task). The otto is skimmed from the bowl and placed into bottles and tightly corked. If producing cosmetics for sale, purchase bottles and jars of suitable size and shape from a specialist manufacturer and market the products with a label of good taste. If producing for your own use, save all the small bottles you can find, clean them thoroughly, rinsing them with a little alcohol and see that they have an efficient stopper. Also collect all the small pots and jars with screw-tops that one can find. They will be used for creams and pomades. Large quantities can be obtained from specialist manufacturers and should be of porcelain or plastic. Always hold on to used metal lipstick cases as well as those for eye pencils. And always make sure that all utensils and storage

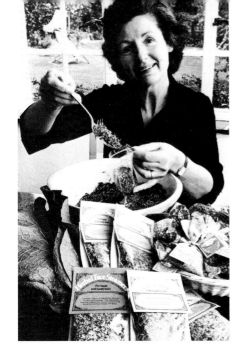

Today, a house with a scullery adjoining the kitchen is a suitable place, with the utensils and materials stored on one side. The room should be dry and cool. Materials, other than plants, which will be in constant use include beeswax, chalk, talc, spermaceti, borax, kaolin, lanolin, glycerine, honey, stearic acid and spirits of wine

To maintain the teeth in good condition, visit a dentist at least every six months. If there are fillings to be done, they can be attended to before they become bigger and tartar which coats

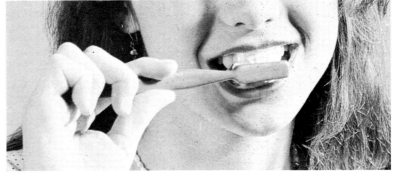

bottles and jars are clean, preferably sterilised. Cosmetic preparations put into unclean pots will not only "go off" quickly but will cause the skin to break out in blemishes and sores. It is, after all, the maintenance of the skin in as perfect a condition as possible that is the aim of all beauticians. Cleanliness is the most important aspect of cosmetics.

If a section of the refrigerator can be used to store lotions, they will last longer and will be more effective when used but make sure to keep them away from food and do not put in the refrigerator any dangerous material.

One's cosmetics should be kept in a cool place, preferably in the dark. A cupboard is a suitable place and make sure that the containers have efficient stoppers so that the creams and pomades do not lose their strength or perfume.

Materials in regular use for making cosmetics, including the utensils, should be kept in a room as near to the kitchen as possible and under lock and key.

In earlier times, most large houses had their still room where lotions and creams were compounded, a room which was used for no other purpose.

or rectified spirit (alcohol). One or two at least will appear in almost every recipe, so make certain stocks are maintained. Keep them in a cool, dry place and under lock and key. Dusting powders especially should be kept in a dry place.

Roots and leaves, however, should be kept in a warm dry place such as in a cupboard beneath the stairs or in an attic, so that they do not become mouldy.

the back of the teeth can be removed. Teeth can be made extra white by placing strawberry juice on the tooth brush and cleaning in the usual way.

DENTAL HYGIENE
Tincture of myrrh and borax is the best of all mouth washes; mastic strengthens the gums whilst ground rhatany root is included in dentifrice powders, to remove tartar from the teeth and give them a special whiteness. Mint plays a similar part in dental creams and leaves the mouth fresh and sweet.

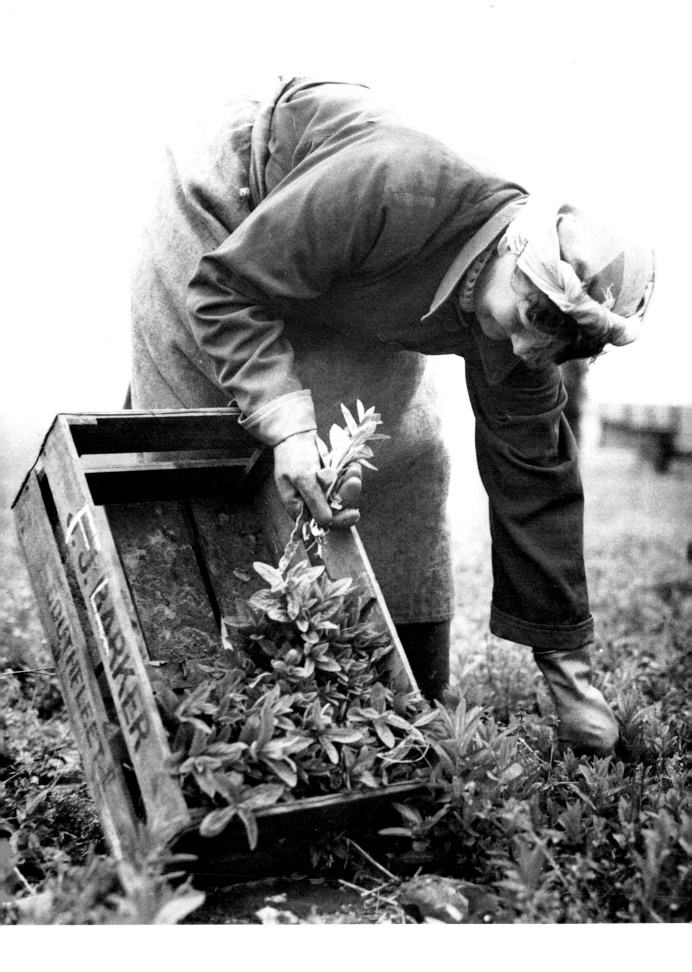

COLLECTING AND STORING MATERIALS FOR COSMETICS AND PERFUMES

Many oils and essences needed for making beauty preparations at home are obtainable from chemists and health stores who import the ingredients needed for making creams and pomades, mascaras and lipsticks from all parts of the world. It is not possible to obtain from the countryside or garden everything that is required for the home brewing of perfumes and cosmetics, but there are speciality stores catering for those needs and natural products of all types are readily available.

There are many aids to beauty and allurement which require no special knowledge in their use and which are present in abundance in hedgerows and on waste ground, or they may be grown in gardens, for not everyone has easy access to the countryside where the plants are collected each in its season. Wherever possible, plants should be used fresh when all the valuable vitamins and minerals salts that they contain are at their peak of efficacy.

Many plants can be saved and dried to use when they are not normally available and others will retain all their good qualities if dried and stored with care. The more thoroughly the work is done, the more effective the plants will be when put to their many uses. The roots of some plants can be kept almost indefinitely if dried and stored with care, amongst these being orris and rose-root, whose perfume actually increases in strength the longer they are kept. The flowers of marigolds and red roses, elder and chamomile, also increase in their fragrance and effectiveness if carefully harvested and dried, whilst the leaves of rosemary and marjoram will be as valuable when dried as when used freshly gathered. The nuts and seeds (the fruit) of a number of plants, including almonds, sesame and sunflower, can be kept in store for a considerable time without losing their strength or effectiveness, likewise the cereals, including barley and oats, which are always in demand for face packs. They can be obtained at harvest time and used throughout the year, replenishing one's stock when another year's harvesting comes round. Many plants, the most common weeds of the countryside, are available the whole year round. They spring up everywhere, not dying back in winter or only partially so, whilst some of the most useful of all herbs such as rosemary, bay laurel and balm, also retain their leaves throughout the year and so can be used at any time. Wild flowers can be collected in succession as they open and can be used fresh to make ointments and lotions which will keep for several months under refrigeration. Ointments and creams made with fats should have a few drops of oil of benjamin or oil of Tolu added, which will prevent their becoming rancid with keeping.

It must be remembered that it is the sensitive skin that is being treated and only those preparations in perfect condition must be used. Particularly when water is included in a beauty preparation the utmost cleanliness must be maintained to avoid offering a breeding ground to harmful bacteria.

In recent years, herbs and natural ingredients have made a big comeback in the world of body care. This sign from a herb farm in Kent, England is one of the many to be found throughout the English countryside.

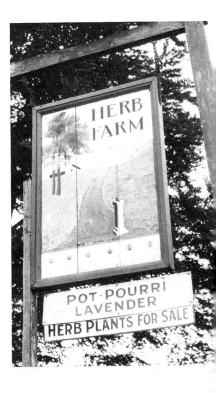

Opposite, a worker collects mint plants. The essential oil of mint is one of the most widely used in perfumery and cosmetics. To obtain the oil when it is most effective, one should harvest the plant just before it flowers, sometime in late July or early August, and preferably on a sunny day, in the late morning after the dew has evaporated.

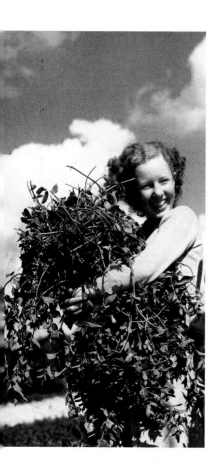

In certain regions it is the custom to gather mint and let it dry on the ground in small bundles called cocks. This happy harvester might be bringing her collection to dry somewhere in the sun or to distill it directly. The preferred method is still a matter of debate.

For this reason, lotions are best made up as required, sufficient only for a few days and keeping them under refrigeration until needed. Products that are to be kept for any length of time should be provided with suitable preservatives capable of preventing the build up of harmful bacteria. Always use sterilised equipment such as bottles and jars as containers. As most preparations usually need to be heated up at some point enamelled pans should be designated solely for that purpose so that they will not be contaminated if used for some other kitchen task.

HARVESTING AND DRYING

For purposes of drying plants for their flowers and leaves, there is a time of year when they will be at their best, when all their valuable qualities will have reached a peak. It is at this point in their growth that they should be harvested and dried. Flowers to be used either fresh or dried should be gathered when just fully open, when their cells are fully charged with essential oil. This will not be so if gathered in the half opened bud stage whilst much of the essential oil will have evaporated if the flowers have begun to die back. There is a point between the two extremes when the flowers are at their peak of perfection. Marigolds, so effective when used for face creams and lotions, and red roses for astringents, will retain their qualities long after harvesting. At one time they were kept in large wooden drums and sold by apothecaries (chemists) at so much per pound, hence the red rose (R. *gallica* or R. *rubra*) came to be called the Apothecary's Rose.

After removing the flower heads when fully open, and this is done when the sun has dried off the early morning dew, spread them out on sheets of brown paper or on wooden trays, in an airy room but away from the sun's rays. Turn the flowers daily, to dry them as quickly as possible, and after a week or ten days, remove the petals from the central disc by gently pulling them away. They should be spread out and left for another week until quite dry and, if marigolds, have turned a deep orange-brown, or, if red rose petals, have become a crimson-purple colour. They are then placed in larger paper bags (not plastic) or cardboard boxes and kept in a dark cupboard to use as required. Chamomile flowers are treated similarly and will be as effective when dry as when fresh. Lavender is dried in the same way but when fully dry (it may be hung up in bundles in an airy room or spread out on shelves), the heads are rubbed between the palms of the hands to release the tiny flowers and are then placed in paper bags or wooden containers. Do not use metal or plastic containers, for dried flowers or leaves because they sweat, causing the petals to become mildewed. Wooden drums with lids are most suitable for storing petals and leaves, for they will absorb any moisture still present, and when closed whilst their contents are stored, they will help retain the precious fragrance.

Many scented-leaf plants, such as marjoram, rosemary and sage which retain their desirable qualities for several years after drying, are treated in the same way. They should be

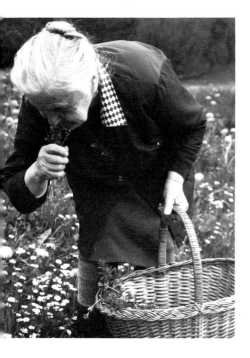

fully ripe as until then it will not have reached its maximum qualities. The capsules should be quite dry, and the seeds should rattle in the capsule when shaken. At exactly the right time, the capsules will split open longitudinally to show the seeds. The moment this occurs the capsules must be removed from the plant. Place them on a tray lined with white paper and remove to an airy room. Turn them frequently, at the same

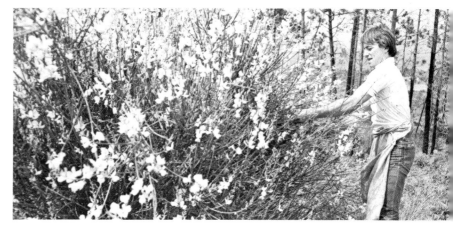

Broom, the flowering shrub whose bright yellow flowers are cultivated for many uses, takes its name from its chief use: as a device for sweeping floors. Although broom is easily cultivated from seed, its method of self-propagation makes it widely available in forests, along roadsides, and in open fields. The flowers of broom contain volatile oil and are best collected in Spring.

harvested at the end of summer when their essential oil is most potent and when the plants are dry following a period of dry weather.

Do not leave the plants too long before harvesting otherwise their essential oil will return to the base of the plant as it dies back in winter. However, it is advisable to wait for dry weather before doing so or the herbs will be difficult to dry before they become mouldy. Should this happen, they will lose their pleasant scent as well as many of their other qualities and will be of little use in perfumery or for cosmetics.

Many plants can be used fresh through summer, then dried in early autumn when they will continue to be available through winter, until the plants are ready to harvest and use fresh again. Those plants which retain their foliage in winter can be used fresh the whole year, but they will retain more of their fragrance and usefulness if carefully dried and stored.

Those plants whose seeds are to be saved must be looked over regularly, for they may have shed their seeds if harvesting is delayed. The capsules must not be removed until the seed is time pressing or shaking the seeds from the capsules. When all have left the capsules, remove unwanted material and place the seeds in small wooden or cardboard boxes. They should be stored in a dry place, such as a cupboard, and used as required. Remember to provide a different box, with a label, for each variety of seed, and remember too to avoid metal boxes which may sweat and cause the seeds to become mouldy.

When searching for material to use for your beauty preparations, set off with a number of carrier bags to place the plants in. Remove flowers and soft-stemmed plants with scissors, cutting only a few from each plant so

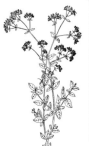
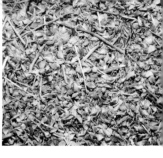

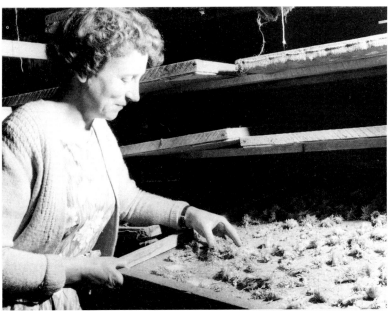

There is perhaps no better way to keep clothing free of moths in the summer and smelling sweet throughout the year than by providing in each drawer and closet a pot pourri bag of dried aromatic herbs and spices. Although the name pot pourri, connotes rottenness, the ingredients used should be carefully dried and free of mildew. Top, a woman prepares

the countryside and the rooms for drying and storing plants and for making up the various concoctions were the most important in the house. Many were prepared to the recipes of nearby monasteries where the monks were both priest and doctor.

Today, those who would make up their own beauty aids, and sweet waters to put in the bath, as well as fragrant pot pourris for the home, would do well to find a small room as in earlier times, perhaps a scullery or pantry adjoining the kitchen, where enamelled pans, bottles and jars for the purpose can be kept apart from cooking utensils. A small gas or electric ring, over which oils and resins will be heated, would be an asset and would keep the 'still room' and its activities entirely separate from the kitchen.

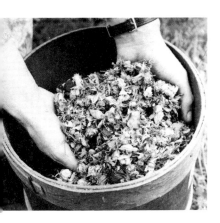

flowers for a pot pourri by spreading them out on a drying tray. Above, petals and blossoms are drying on a special round screened device made for that purpose.

as not to deplete it more than necessary. Leave on the plant some flowers which will seed themselves and so perpetuate the species. Those plants classed as weeds and which are in abundance, e.g. stinging nettles, can be cut with impunity.

Hard-wooded plants such as sage and southernwood, which, like many others mentioned can be grown in the garden, with red roses and marigolds, violets and primroses, should be cut with a pair of sharp secateurs or with a knife. Cut the stems about 3 inches (7·5 cm) above ground level. This will allow the plant to form new growth at the base and keep it free of old wood, which would die back if not removed.

After removing flowers, leaves or stems, get them to the drying room as quickly as possible and spread them out on the trays or benches. From the beginning of more enlightened times, which in Europe commenced five hundred years ago, every large house had its still-room, for the distillation of flowers and leaves was one of the chores in all households, to make sweet waters for personal cleanliness and allurement. Decoctions for some purpose or other were prepared from almost every plant of

STORING HERBS

In every house there should be a room where herbs can be dried and stored. A spare bedroom, room or attic will be most useful, or a large airy cupboard, perhaps beneath the stairs which may be a cupboard for drying clothes and fitted with wooden laths for shelves, through which warm air can circulate to complete the drying.

If a spare room is available, specially constructed trays of simple design can be made. They can be stacked one above another, in the same way that trays for macerating flowers for their perfume are used. If placed in the centre of a room, the trays will be more accessible and

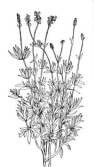
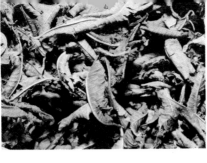
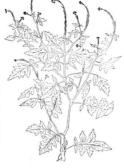
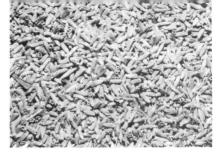

easier to attend. Each tray is made of wood, with 4 inch (10 cm) timbers for the sides and about 1 m square. Wooden slats or laths (thin strips of wood about 1 inch (2·5 cm) wide are fixed 1 inch (2·5 cm) apart to the base of each tray which are stacked to a height of about 5–6 feet (1·5 m). Over the laths, a piece of hessian (burlap, canvas or sacking) is placed. This will allow a free circulation of air to reach the plants on each tray. The trays should be stacked about 10 inches (25 cm) apart, to allow room for turning the plants, and there should be about 6 trays in each stack. They are held one above each other by pieces of timber 2 × 2 inch (5 × 5 cm) square, fixed to each corner of the trays and cut to 10 inch (25 cm) lengths to give the required height. After drying, the flowers, leaves and seeds are stored in small containers kept on shelves which may be fixed to the wall at one end of the room. In place of laths for the base, a piece of wire netting can be used, over which the canvas is placed. The trays are not heavy to move.

There should be a window to each room which can be partly opened to allow the plants to receive some fresh air which will assist with their drying. Sunlight is not required as it will scorch and dry the plants too quickly and many of their effective properties will be lost. Cover the window with sacking to keep out strong sunlight. If drying quantities of plants, you should fix an electric fan heater to one end of the room to provide a better circulation of air during warm humid weather, being careful to fix the fan where the strong current of air will not disturb the drying plants or seeds.

Another way of drying plants is to hang them in bunches from strong wire or twine fixed across a room just above head height. The plants are tied in bundles, whilst flowers for drying are placed in muslin bags and suspended from the wires. They will soon dry if given a free circulation of air.

Herbs such as sage, rosemary and thyme will be fully dry if they "crackle" when pressed in the fingers. They should break up and leave on the hands a pleasant aromatic smell, free of any mustiness. In this condition they will keep for a year or more and will be available to use at any time. They must, however, be carefully stored in a dry airy place, and are best kept in wooden drums which can be closed when the herbs are not in use.

Before placing the containers, part the leaves from the stems or, if flowers, the petals from the central boss. Place those herbs which are to be rubbed down on a table between sheets of white paper and press them with a rolling pin. Then remove the stalks, and place the leaves, which are left behind, into the containers.

DRYING AND STORING RHIZOMES

There are a number of plants whose rhizomatous roots have many uses in toiletry and particularly in the preparation of sweet-scented powders. Amongst these are the rhizomes of orris, calamus and *Cyperus longus* or galingale. Parkinson, botanist to Charles I of England, described the

The dried herbs and flowers (above) are, from left to right, oregano, verbena and lavender, all excellent ingredients in pot pourri and sachet.

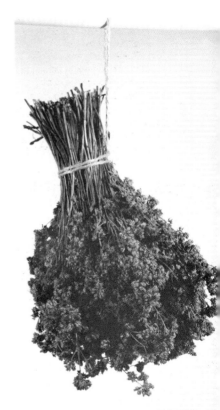

Above, a bunch of oregano is drying, blossom side down, in a cool dry place. The rafters of attics are ideally suited to hang herbs to dry.

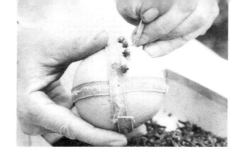

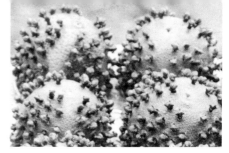

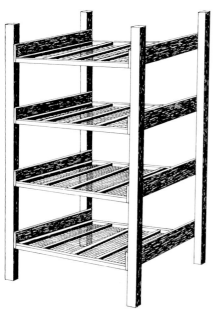

Above, a drying frame which will hold the trays containing herbs and blossoms.

last as "much used in sweet powders and to make sweet washing waters ... also in perfuming-pots, with vinegar and rose water, with a few cloves and bay leaves to perfume chambers".

The rhizomes should be lifted at the end of summer when the plant's nourishment has been returned to the roots as they die back. After lifting, spread the rhizomes out on sacks in the sun to dry and, depending upon the weather, leave out for several weeks, taking them indoors at night to protect them from heavy dew. Peel them before the drying is completed, in a warm oven if dull or wet conditions prevail outdoors. The roots of most rhizomatous plants will be mature when 2–3 years old. After you have dried them completely, store them in boxes in a warm, dry room for a year, during which time the scent will increase. The volatile oil – in the case of orris known as "orris butter" – can then be extracted or the roots can be ground down to a fine powder and mixed with starch or talc to make a violet-scented talcum powder.

Other roots have different uses. With alkanet, the red colouring matter which is used as rouge is found in the rind of the rhizome and is obtained by macerating the chopped root, after drying, in fat, or treating it with alcohol. The roots of marshmallow and horseradish are used fresh. Rose root is used for making scented waters, after drying. The bark of certain plants is used in perfumery and cosmetics, sometimes when immediately removed from the tree or after drying. With the bark of witch hazel, red elm and sassafras it is usual to include the twiggy branches in distillations. The barks of cinnamon and red elm are dried and powdered. That of red elm is so highly mucilaginous that only a pinch in a cup of water will form a thick jelly. With marshmallow and olive oil it makes a soothing face cream. These are plants of the New World, but their barks can be obtained from health stores and chemists everywhere.

Besides red elm, mucilage is obtained from quince seeds which are black, like apple "pips" and when removed from the fruit and placed in water for 10–15 minutes, form a thick mucilage which is used in skin creams and, with gum arabic, makes an effective cream mascara. Remove the seeds when making the fresh fruit into preserves, and keep them, after drying, in glass jars until required.

WAXES AND RESINS

Waxes are used in solid brilliantines, creams and lipsticks, to give strength and elasticity to cosmetics. Beeswax is used if plant wax is unobtainable. Most of the waxes are obtained from plants of the New World, carnauba being the wax palm of S America. The wax, secreted on the scales which enclose the buds, is produced in such abundance that it falls to the ground in its season and is collected and placed in vats of boiling water. It is collected from the surface, remelted and made into cakes.

The wax myrtle or candleberry is a plant of E. N. America, the berries being thickly coated in wax which is removed by immersion in boiling water. The wax collects on the surface and is skimmed off and made into wax cakes to harden. It is used to

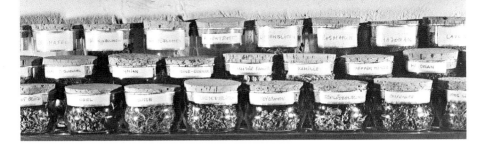

Left, jars of scented herbs for pot pourri are lined in a shop display. Below, various pomanders, from simple oranges pricked with cloves to delicate china containers suitable for hanging in closets.

solidify various cosmetics and makes an excellent lather shaving cream, for it contains an acid resembling saponin and has a refreshing balsamic scent.

The finest gums or resins, used as hair fixatives and to fix perfumes are collected from plants in the arid lands of the Near East where they grow in intense heat. In more northerly climes, valuable resins are obtained from the unopened buds of several poplar trees, that from the balsam poplar (Tacamahac) being the best. It is used in the manufacture of toilet soaps and in the less expensive perfumes, and has the smell of storax. It can be obtained by filling a bowl with the buds in spring and covering with spirits of wine. They should be left for a week, and the resin drained off into glass bottles (which should be tightly fitted with stoppers). The black poplar of Britain and North Europe also yields resin, but it is not nearly so effective.

Resin is also obtainable from the wild and garden angelica. If incisions are made in the main stem(s) early in summer when the sap begins to rise, a thick juice will exude. It is scraped off into jars containing a little spirits of wine and can be used as a fixative for home-made perfumes.

Fruits used for face packs and for the cleaning of teeth – for which purpose strawberries are highly recommended – should always be used fresh. If frozen or tinned, they will have undergone chemical changes which render them ineffective.

Refrigeration is a good method of keeping creams and lotions fresh and will enable many preparations to be made up when the flowers or fruits are in season and at their best. They can then be used as required, whilst larger quantities can be made up at one time and hence much valuable preparation time can be saved. It is also invigorating in warm weather, to use body lotions straight from the refrigerator applying them when they are ice cold. One shelf of the refrigerator should be used just for beauty preparations, to separate them from foods. Otherwise store them in as dark and cool a place as possible to prevent their losing strength or turning rancid.

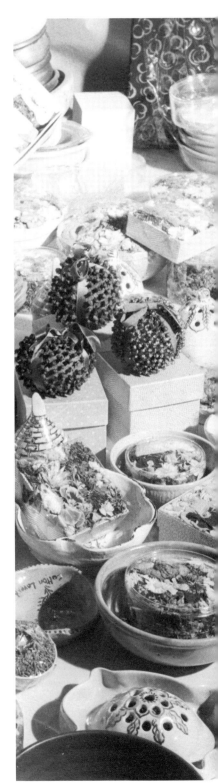

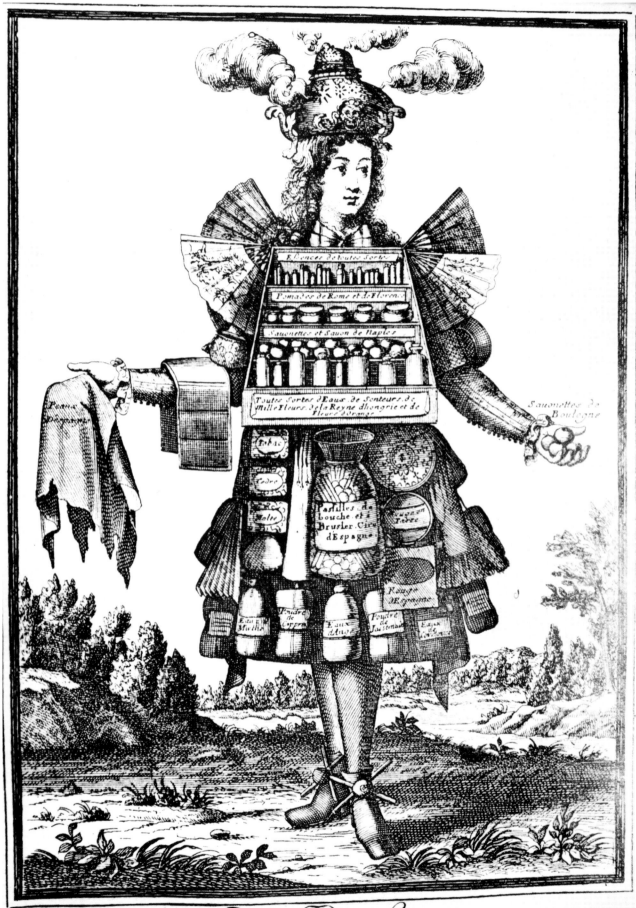

Habit de Parfumeur

The art of perfumery

A technical definition of perfume might be "a composition of scented substances whose fragrance gratifies the sense of smell and which is commonly associated with personal adornment". It is important to emphasize that perfume is not merely a pleasant scent, but a composite of many different scents. A perfume which satisfies the senses may consist of a hundred different substances, each with its separate identity, blended to produce an agreeable composition, the way the notes of a musical chord produce a single harmonic sound.

Music as a metaphor for perfume is particulary apt. Francis Bacon described the breath of flowers in the air "as it comes and goes, like the warbling of music". In *Syla Sylvarum*, he took the simile a step further, judging scent and other pleasing odours to be sweeter in the air at a distance, "for we see that in sounds likewise, they are sweeter when we cannot hear every part by itself."

When perfumes are applied to the skin, alcohol is the first substance to evaporate, for the ottos – fragrant essential oils – are fixed by a balsam, resin or oil (such as sandalwood oil) or by an animal fixative such as ambergris, civet or musk.

Without a fixative, a perfume "dies" quickly. As no two ottos are alike in their volatility, each substance used in the composition of the perfume would evaporate in turn, leaving behind others to dominate the composition and alter its character. When alcoholic solutions of various essences evaporate, they do so in direct proportion to their volatility, the most volatile being the first to

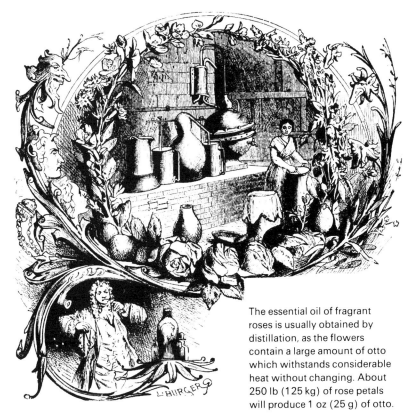

The essential oil of fragrant roses is usually obtained by distillation, as the flowers contain a large amount of otto which withstands considerable heat without changing. About 250 lb (125 kg) of rose petals will produce 1 oz (25 g) of otto.

Opposite, a French perfumer displaying his ware in a 17th century print.

evaporate, the less volatile disappearing later. That odours affect the olfactory nerves in direct proportion to their force of volatility, was observed a century ago by Dr Septimus Piesse, who called this principle "the velocity of odour". It is now an accepted law of perfumery.

Scents affect the olfactory nerves as sounds the aural nerves. As there are modes in music, so too, is there a "key" of odours in which, for example, heliotrope, vanilla and almond blend together, and a higher sharper "key" in which citron, lemon and verbena are the signature notes.

A SYMPHONY OF SCENTS

A perfumer relies on his trained sense

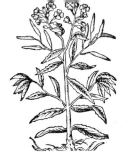
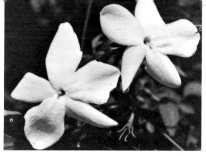
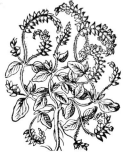

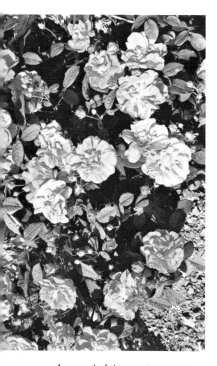

A spread of the most common flowers used in perfumery. Directly above is the *rosa gallica*, or apothecary's rose, whose otto is the *sine qua non* of perfumes from classical times to the present. Above, from left to right, are jasmine, rosemary, frangipani.

of smell to create a symphony of fragrance which may take a year to compose. His "orchestration" might use a hundred different odours until the right blend is achieved. This is known as the "chord". The "base" notes are those which have the heaviest and most lasting fragrance, whilst the "top notes", though the quickest to evaporate, have the most immediate effect upon the sense of smell. The harmony of the perfume – the right blend of top, middle and base notes – is known to the trade as layer blending. When creating a new perfume the perfumer has to adjust the balance, toning down an odour if too fierce and always remembering that one false note will completely ruin the harmony.

From the entire floral kingdom, it is estimated that there are more than 5000 substances available to the perfumer. As the concerto places emphasis on a single instrument in the orchestra, in perfumery a scent is created around a single odorous chemical substance, an otto. To arrive at the final "score", there may be as many as a hundred variations before the finished product satisfies its creator.

The "green and woody" perfumes form a bouquet of chord C and may be composed of sandalwood, cedar, vetivert, geraniol, cassie, jasmine, orange blossom and camphor. Lancôme's *Magie* with its soft flowery bouquet in which jasmine strikes the dominant "note" is representative of a "green", flowery perfume; so too is Hermès's *Calèche*, with its subtle composition of rose, gardenia, lilac and musk. Sandalwood and vetivert often strike the dominant note in perfumes of this group.

The heavier, more spicey perfumes, built around the alcohol eugenol, begin with a "green" aldehyde note, complementing carnation, tuberose, jasmine, lilac and orange blossom, followed by the "woody" notes of cedar and sandalwood, with overtones of Arabian myrrh, musk and ambergris to hold together their delicate scent.

"Bouquets" exist only as an alcoholic solution, obtained from a fatty body by way of enfleurage. These are the most delicate of perfumes, built up around white jasmine, cassie and lily of the valley. They possess a flowery lightness which has retained for them a unique popularity. They are obtained from essences, or to use the French word, *esprits*, those simple odours in alcoholic solution extracted from oils or fats in which flowers have been repeatedly infused. Mme Jeanne Lanvin's *Arpège* may be likened to an arpeggio of jasmine, rose and lily of the valley: the most difficult of all flower perfumes to reproduce. Caron's *Fleurs de Rocaille* is a blend of jasmine and rose and with undertones of the honeysuckle scent of ylang-ylang. The unique orange scent of *petit grain*, obtained from the leaves, twigs and unripe fruit of different citrus species, is also noticeable. The name *petit grain*, ("small holes"), is derived from the small globular ducts which are present in all parts of the plant. *Petit grain bigarade* is from the leaf of the Seville orange and *petit grain limon* is the distillate of lemon leaves.

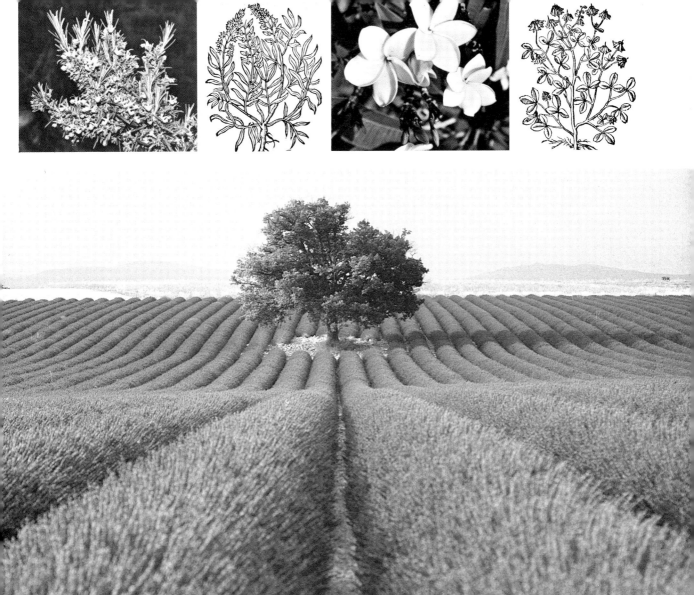

ESSENTIAL OILS

The scented substances, the essential oils, are the waste products of a plant's metabolism, first amongst the by-products of the plant's chemistry, to be thrown out as excreta. Some animal scents used in perfumery and cosmetics have a similar origin, being secreted into the cavity formed around the lanolin glands. Indol, which is present in the essential oil of many heavily scented flowers, is also one of the products of the putrefaction of animal tissue, whilst methyl indol, the active principle of civet, is a well-known excretory product. It is this "animal" quality which gives the jonquil, lily, narcissus and lilac, however fresh they may be, an unpleasant scent in a warm or badly ventilated room.

Those flowers with thick petals – e.g., jonquil, white jasmine, lily, tuberose, gardenia, magnolia, carnation, orange blossom – produce the highest quantity of essential oil, for the epidermal cells embedded in the petals contain a greater concentration of oil than in those flowers with thin

Above, a glorious field of lavender stretches out in the sunshine of Provence.
Below, a saffron crocus. Saffron flowers produce grains used to scent toilet water.

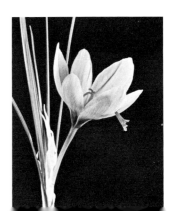

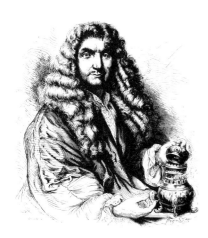

Above, a French perfumer in a late 17th century print. Below, this illustration from a late 16th century guide to the art of distillation shows a machine for the extraction of aqua vitae from herbs. Although the particular purpose of this

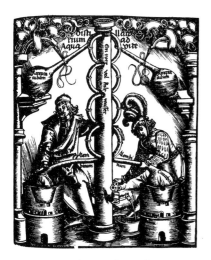

apparatus was to produce a herbal cure-all, similar distilleries were used in the increasingly industrialized world of perfumery.

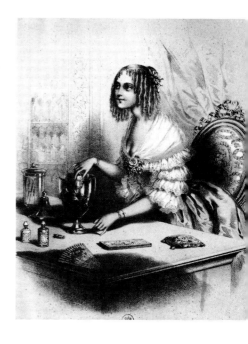

petals, and there is less rapid evaporation. White flowers (and, exceptionally, the red rose) are the most fragrant, for as pigment (colour) is bred into the flowers, the perfume vanishes. This is why many vermilion, orange, and scarlet roses, as well as the brightly coloured poppy, *lychnis chalcedonica*, and red pentstemon, are entirely devoid of perfume. Blue flowers too – whose attractiveness to bees is explained by their colour – are also in most cases scentless. Examples of scentless blue flowers are veronica, perennial scabious, gentian and campanula. White jasmine is heavily scented, the yellow is without perfume; white lilac is highly perfumed, though the dark purple lilac has little scent. The first authentic description of the essential oil of a plant (its attar or otto) was given by Arnaldo de Vilanova, a Catalan physician living at the end of the 13th century. Another hundred years were to elapse before it became known that, although essential oils are insoluble in water (otherwise rain would wash them from flowers), they will dissolve in alcohol. The alcoholic solution becomes the "essence" from which is made the "bouquets", or compounded mixture of extracts.

In leaves, the essential oil is stored in many ways. In the bay leaf, as in orange skin, it is stored in capsules which are clearly visible as pellucid dots. In the myrtle, the oil is embedded deep inside the leaf tissue and its scent is released only with pressure. With rosemary and lavender, the essential oil is stored in goblet-shaped cells which are present just below the leaf surface, and are re-

leased by the heat of the sun or by the slightest movement caused by a warm breeze. Essential oil is composed of numerous organic chemical compounds known as terpenes which contain carbon and hydrogen (hydrocarbons) and give rise to a number of oxygenated derivatives, chief of which are the alcohols and their esters, aldehydes and ketones. Alcohols occur in a number of different forms, notably geraniol in flowers, the principle substance of otto of roses; and borneol, with its camphor-like smell, which is present in a number of leaves. Another alcohol, menthol, is present in the mints, and eugenol in cloves and carnations. Eucalyptol is present in sage and rosemary.

Terpenes are present in all essential oils, especially in orange blossom and ylang-ylang, whilst benzine compounds are prominent in the ottos of heavily scented flowers. Many of the scent substances of essential oils contain in their molecules a closed ring of six carbon atoms, known as the "benzine ring". Nitrogen compounds are also present.

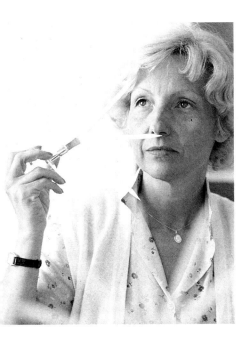

of fragrant roses is usually obtained in this way. About 250 lbs of rose petals will produce 1 oz of otto. Distillation is also used to extract the odorous principle of leaves, barks and woods.

(2) By extraction, the otto is washed from the flowers by a volatile solvent such as petroleum ether. Extraction is a gentler method than steam distillation and produces the most concentrated of essences. Cassie flowers have their essential oil extracted in this way. As the cassie flowers open in succession, extraction enables the manufacturer to make frequent changes of blossom. About 10 lbs of cassie flowers are needed to make 1 oz of otto and since

THE EXTRACTION OF PERFUME

There are several methods for obtaining essential oil: (1) distillation; (2) extraction; (3) enfleurage; (4) maceration; (5) expression.

(1) To obtain the oil by distillation calls for specialist treatment. Only stainless steel and glass vessels are now used, copper and iron for long being obsolete as they do not give the same purity of odour. Distillation is suitable only for those flowers whose otto will withstand considerable heat without suffering change. In addition, the flowers must contain a large amount of otto for the method to be profitable. The flowers are gathered without interruption, and distillation process continues throughout the night. The blooms are taken to the still which is a large tank fitted with a perforated tray. When it is almost filled, a jet of water at the base, below the tray, gushes through the perforations and through the flowers. The steam which is driven off is filled with the essential oil, which does not dissolve in water. When cooled, the oil rises to the top, the water is run off and the oil collected. The essential oil

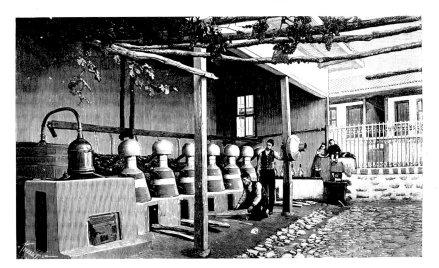

they begin to open early in January, they are the first flowers of the year which perfumers make use of.

In extraction, the flowers are placed on perforated metal trays or plates, stacked one above another, in a vat which is then hermetically sealed. At one end is a solvent tank, at the other is a vacuum still. The

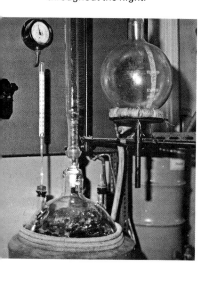

The modern process of perfume distillation has become an exceedingly technical affair, as the apparatus below attests. Because of the amount of otto needed to make the process profitable, distillation must be a round-the-clock procedure, with flowers being gathered and fed into the machine, without interruption, throughout the night.

solvent runs through the plates until charged with the scent. It is then distilled off at low pressure and returns to the tank, the otto remaining in the retort. The process is repeated again and again so that every particle of otto is extracted, the final product being solid and known as a "floral concrete". This "floral concrete" is then washed with alcohol, and the essential oil is dissolved out, the alcohol being removed by distillation to leave behind the pure essential oil known as a "floral absolute". This is the purest and most concentrated of all perfumes, the scents obtained being exactly as they are in nature. Besides cassie, and carnation, ylang-ylang, white jasmine and orange blossom will yield their essential oil by this method.

(3) Enfleurage is the preferred technique for extracting the ottos of mignonette, tuberose, white lilac, lily of the valley and white violets. Carried out entirely by hand this method is the most expensive and is only suitable for those flowers which continue to give off their essential oil long after being gathered. In enfleurage, no heat is used: it is done at ordinary room temperature, which ensures that the most delicate perfumes are in no way harmed.

The flowers are collected and spread out on sheets of glass enclosed by a wooden frame 4 in (10 cm) deep and reinforced by a wire base. This apparatus is known as a "chassis". To extract the perfume, a layer of fat about 2cm thick is spread evenly over the glass and the flowers sprinkled on top, so that they cover the entire surface. Other frames, greased on both sides and filled with flowers, are

stacked one on top of another until there are as many as twenty in the pile. They remain undisturbed for 3–4 days and nights whilst the fragrance is absorbed by the fat on both sides of the frames. The frames are then ustacked and the flowers replaced by fresh ones, though the same fat is retained. It may take up to a month before the fat is completely saturated, during which time the trays will have been changed about ten times. Because of this, the flowers used for enfleurage must bloom for about two months. After a month, the fat is scraped from the glass as a "floral concrete", and the scent is extracted by an alcoholic solution to become a "floral absolute". To prevent the fat from turning rancid during the extraction, a small quantity of oil of ben is added to it. Extract of jasmine is prepared by pouring alcohol onto the pomade (the "concrete") which has been chopped up.

(4) By maceration, heat is used to extract the scent. Melt purified lard in a porcelain pan. Put the flowers – cassie and orange respond well to maceration– in the warm fat and allow them to be digested for several

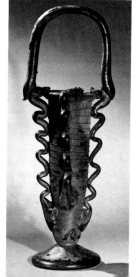
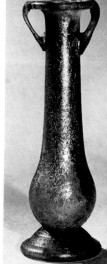

Right, two glass perfume vials of early Greek provenance.

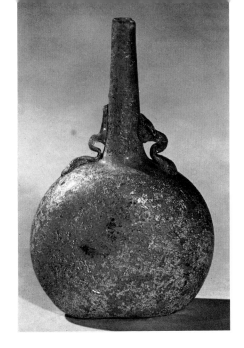

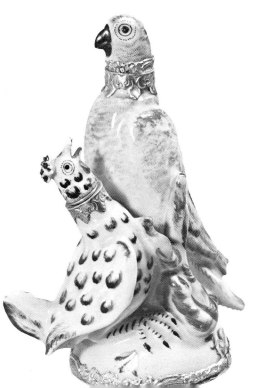

hours before removing them with a strainer. Reheat the fat and add more fresh flowers; repeat the process about 10 times until the fat has become saturated with the scent. Reheat the pomade but only sufficiently to allow impurities to settle. When cool, this becomes similar to commercial cassie or orange flower pomade. To extract the otto, you need 3 litres of rectified spirit for every 6 lbs of pomade. After a month, the essence, if cassie, will have become pale green with a violet-like perfume. The "washed"

pomatum or residue is an excellent brilliantine for the hair and still retains the cassie perfume. Cassie is one of the most "flowery" of perfumes and, with jasmine, is present in all the great floral "bouquets". It is included in François Coty's, *L'Aimant*, perfected over a period of five years, introduced in 1927 and still one of the world's great perfumes.

(5) Expression is used for obtaining essential oil under pressure, as with the skin of many types of orange. Put the peel in large muslin bags and place them in a stainless steel vat for crushing. This is done with a plate which fits inside the vessel, or by rollers. During the pressing, a water jet is sprayed onto the peel to separate the juice from the solids; the liquid being released through small holes at the bottom of the vat where the essential oil is collected with the water, from which it is separated by extraction.

THE HOME PERFUMER

Several methods can be used to make perfume at home. Though the home-made product is in no way comparable to that produced by the famous perfume houses, it will be suitable for use on handkerchiefs and clothes and as an addition to dusting powders and bath essences, soaps and shampoos. With practice you might even make a perfume that is good enough to wear.

To $\frac{3}{4}$ lb of animal fat and $\frac{1}{4}$ lb of lard, add $\frac{1}{2}$ litre of water into which has been dissolved a teaspoonful of alum. Bring to the boil, then strain through muslin and let cool. Collect

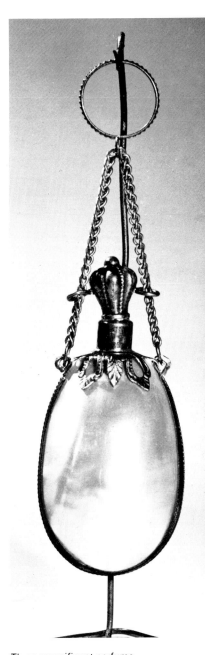

Three magnificent perfume containers – a gold-flecked glass bottle (top), Chinese ceramic birds with screw off heads, and a hanging glass bottle with its original stand.

Marie-Antoinette (right), the ill-fated wife of Louis XVI, is thought to have introduced the usage of face powder to the royal court of Versailles. Her complexion was described by one astute observer as "literally a blend of lilies and roses".

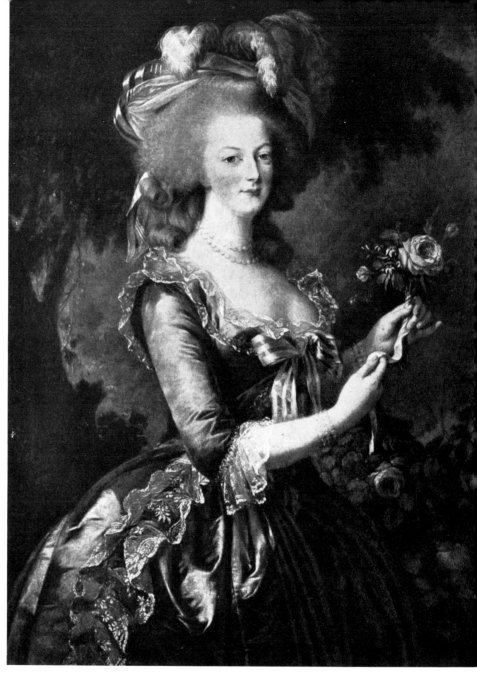

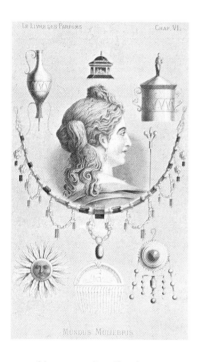

Mascara and eyeliner became increasingly in vogue in the late 19th century, and the growing cosmetic industry met the new demand for its products. Below is an advertisement for Rimmell, a mascara so renowned that throughout Europe it is still the name generically used for all mascara.

the fat on the surface and reheat it; pour it in equal amounts into two shallow dishes and let cool. Spread flowers thickly over the fat of one dish and place the inverted second dish over them, making sure the rims are in contact with each other. Leave the dishes undisturbed for 2–3 days and nights, then remove the flowers and replace them with others. Continue this process for about a month, by which time the fat will have fully absorbed the perfume. Scrape it into a wide-topped jar with a screw top and add an equal amount (by bulk) of spirits of wine. Keep the mixture in a dark place for two months and shake it up daily to extract the scent. Strain the liquid through muslin into glass bottles, to intensify the scent and, to increase its longevity, add a drop or two of sandalwood to each bottle.

Another method is to place in a large bowl ground almonds or ground sesame seeds to a depth of 1 in (2·5 cm) and to place on top the same depth of highly scented flowers which will continue to bloom for at least a month. Then add another layer of ground almonds and another of flowers and so on until the bowl is filled, topping up with the almonds. Cover with a piece of plastic and place in a warm room. Leave for 2–3 days and nights, then turn out into another bowl, with the top layer of ground almonds at the bottom. Replace the flowers with fresh ones as in the previous method. Continue for a month, then put in a muslin bag and squeeze out the oil or shake out by using spirits of wine, as described above.

Flowers can be made to yield their perfume by saturating muslin cloths in olive oil and placing them over narrow wooden laths (thin strips of wood) fixed to the base of a wooden frame 6 in (15 cm) deep. Spread out flowers over them to a depth of about 4 in (10 cm) and place another olive oil cloth over them. Every 2–3 days for about a month, change the flowers; by this time the oil will be saturated with their scent and can be squeezed from the cloths. The scent is exracted by spirits of wine as described.

CARE AND MAINTENANCE OF PERFUME

Perfumes are the ultimate in personal allurement. They should be used with discretion, and always to suit one's personality. A perfume that may be right for one person may be quite wrong for another. To find out if a perfume is right, it is necessary to "wear" it. Sniffing from a bottle is only the first step. It must then be applied to the skin, to the bosom or throat, or to the inside of the wrist where, in a few seconds, the warmth of the body will release its most subtle and intimate qualities. Only if you find the scent alluring yourself, is it the right one for your personality. If the sample you are trying elicits no reaction, take a short walk in the fresh air, then try another fragrance on the other wrist or elsewhere on the body.

Perfumes should be kept in a cool dark place. If exposed to strong light, the quality will quickly deteriorate.

Three of the great figures of the 20th century cosmetics and perfume industries. It was Coty who first exploited the enormous American market for cosmetics and perfumes, opening a New York branch in 1912. In 1922, Elizabeth Arden opened her first beauty salon on Manhattan's 5th Avenue. Today there are Elizabeth Arden beauty parlours in some forty cities throughout the world. Helena Rubinstein began her international career by importing pots of beauty cream from her native Poland to Australia.

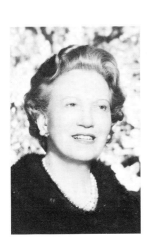

Elizabeth Arden

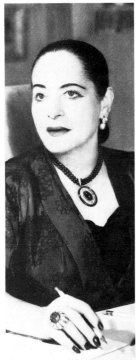

Helena Rubinstein

François Coty

Always put perfume on the body rather than on the clothes.

APPENDIX

Natural products used in perfumery and cosmetics which have no connection with plants.

BEES-WAX

A scale-like wax which is exuded by bees from between the segments on the underside of their body. At first the wax is colourless but after manipulation to make into the comb by the bees, it takes on the colour of the pollen which the bees were collecting and bringing into the hive. The bee uses the wax-like secretion to build up the walls of the honey-comb cells. After the honey is extracted, the combs are placed in hot water and the wax collected from the surface of the water. It becomes white on exposure to air. Bees-wax is used in lipsticks and mascaras and in emollient lotions.

BORAX

The white minerals colemanite and kernite were originally found on the sea-bed or after the evaporation of inland lakes. They are now mined inland and occur as prisms. Boron compounds are used for electronic tubes, for making fireproof clothing and in soaps, detergents and shampoos. Boron absorbs neutrons and so is used in atomic reactors and in solid fuels for rockets. It is also included in most eye lotions for it relieves soreness and strain. It is used as a saponifying agent in cold creams. Almost all the world's borax comes from the Western USA and W South America.

CERESIN

It is a mineral wax found in Galicia as ozokerite and becomes ceresin after treatment with sulphuric acid. It is clear yellow and used as an alternative to beeswax to raise the melting point of lipsticks.

CETYL ALCOHOL

It is produced from spermaceti and coconut oil as an odourless, wax-like powder which acts as a valuable emulsifying agent. It has an emollient effect on the skin and is used in foundation creams and in lipsticks.

COLLAGEN

The constituent parts of a white substance which, when boiled, produce gelatine.

FULLER'S EARTH

The material is the result of huge deposits of diatoms, single-celled algae, on the ocean floor millions of years ago. Where the seas have receded, thousands of tons are mined annually as diatomaceous earth, better known as Fuller's earth, for fullers have used it since earliest time to extract the natural grease from wool. It is an absorbant and being composed largely of silica, cleans without scratching. It is used in dentifrice powders and pastes and in silver polishes. It is used for mud packs or facials. Living diatoms store part of their food as oil and contribute to the earth's oil deposits.

GELATINE

Gels used for eye ointments are obtained from gelatine which is a produce of the bone cartilage of animals, after being boiled in water for a considerable time. It is transparent in thin plates, is of a yellowish-white colour, with neither smell nor taste. It is insoluble in alcohol but soluble in hot water. It has also many culinary uses.

GLYCERINE

It occurs in the fat of most animals and vegetables in combination with fatty acids. It is obtained by heating natural fat in a still with a condensing apparatus and passing steam through the melted fat, the temperature being kept below 600°F but above 550°F when the acid fats separate out in the receivers from the glycerine and water. Glycerine is a thick, colourless, inodorous syrup with a sweet taste. It mixes with water and is soluble in alcohol. It is used for preserving fruits; prevents water freezing; and is used in the making of soaps and shaving soaps which soften the skin. Used in lotions as an after shave, it prevents the skin drying.

HONEY

A product collected by bees from the nectary of plants which the honey bee swallows through its proboscis and transfers to the honey-bag. Chemical changes take place there, before the honey is transferred to the honeycomb from which it is obtained. It is used as an article of food, for sweetening and to include in hand and face creams, for it is soothing and healing. It should also be used in place of sugar for it requires no digesting to enter the blood stream.

KAOLIN

It is the purest of all forms of clay, being one of many clay minerals and has been used by man since earliest times and is still in regular use for it moulds easily and fuses at a low temperature. It is used for making pottery and china, the purest being known as china clay. It is formed by the action of rain on aluminium silicates and is distributed in Cornwall and in many European countries, also in the USA and Japan. Similar to Fuller's earth in that it is an insulator and is used in tooth and talcum powders and in face packs.

LAMPBLACK
An almost pure form of amorphous carbon obtained by the combustion of oil or resin. It is used as a black pigment in mascaras.

LANOLIN
It is the fat present in sheep's wool, many fleeces containing up to 20% fat content. It is removed by ether or by scouring with a soap solution and is yellow and inodorous with little tendency to rancidity. It is readily absorbed by the skin and leaves it soft and nourished. It is used as a base for pomades and in hair shampoos.

LARD
It is white purified pig's fat and is mostly used in enfleurage, to draw a flower's perfume and become saturated with it. To prevent rancidity, digest for an hour at 60°C with 4% gum benzoin (styrax benzoin).

LECITHIN
Egg yolks contain up to 10% and when extracted it is brown. It is also present in soya beans which are more widely used for its extraction for it is of a pleasing golden colour. It is nourishing and used in skin creams. Avocado is rich in lecithin.

PETROLEUM JELLY
A pale yellow, translucent semi-solid obtained by treating the undistilled portion of petroleum with steam and filtering it whilst hot through animal charcoal. It is insoluble in water, almost so in alcohol but dissolves in ether and benzene. It does not turn rancid on exposure to the air and so is a useful ingredient in the preparation of ointments, foundation creams and solid brilliantines.

SHELLAC
It is a resinous substance formed by the scale insect *Laccifer lacca* of S.E. Asia, the resin being collected from the stems of plants and dried. Shellac is obtained by solvent extraction as hard yellow transparent scales, 6% wax and 70% resin. It is insoluable in water but soluable in a borax solution and in alcohol. When de-waxed, it is used in hair sprays and lacquers.

SODIUM ALGINATE
It is manufactured from algae and occurs as a greyish-white powder which is mucilaginous, transparent and inodorous. The degree of mucilage is controlled by the addition of water in which borax has been dissolved. It is used in hand jellies and hair setting lotions.

SPERMACETI
An almost tasteless and inodorous fatty substance found in the head of the sperm whale and extracted by filtration and treatment by potash-ley. It is white, soft to the touch and melts between 37°–47°F. It is used in creams and ointments, usually with white wax or beeswax and almond oil. *It would be best substituted by jojoba oil to protect whales (see also cetyl alcohol)*

STEARIC ACID (STEARINE)
A constituent of fats derived from the animal and vegetable kingdom, abundant in beef and mutton suet. It is obtained by saponification with lime in the presence of steam at high temperatures, the stearate then being treated with acid and purified. It is tasteless and inodorous and used in vanishing creams. Stearyl alcohol is obtained as white flakes and is used for the control of viscosity in emulsions.

TALC It is formed by the metamorphism of magnesium (soapstone) rocks by hot vapours (steam). It is the softest of all minerals, flaking when scratched by the thumb nail. It occurs in green or white masses and has a slippery silky feel. Because of its electrical resistance, it has many uses in the electrical industry and its other commerical uses include paint and paper making, textiles, and in many food products. Talcum powders are made from ground and sifted talc, mixed with finely ground orrix root, rice starch and colouring agents. Talc is mined in the USA; Europe; and Australia.

PICTURE CREDITS

Agenzia fotografica Luisa Ricciarini, Milano: Plant lexicon: No. 128

Archivio Fratelli Fabbri Editori, Milano: 87 (Kunsthistoriches Museum, Vienna)

Ashmolean Museum, Oxford: 99 (bottom)

A-Z Botanical Collection, Dorking: 192 (top right), 193 (top, centre and right); Plant Lexicon: Nos. 15, 31, 50, 62, 103, 113, 166

Beckett Newspapers Ltd., Worthing: 187 (top)

Bibliothèque Nationale, Paris: 16 (left)

Biophotos Heather Angel, Farnham: Plant lexicon: No. 104

Bodleian Library, Oxford: 27 (left)

Botanischer Garten, Berlin-Dahlem: Plant lexicon: Nos. 20, 32

Courtesy Trustees of the British Museum, London: 90, 94 (top)

Courtesy of the British Museum (Natural History), London: Plant lexicon: Nos. 70, 80, 111

Bruce Coleman Ltd., London: 26 (R. K. Murton), 92 (right, M. Viard), 149 (top, M. Freeman), 151 (David Austen), 198 (left); Plant lexicon: Nos. 26 (WWF. H. Jungius), 35 (Erich Crichton), 36 (Sandro Prato), 74 (Hans Reinhard), 109 (Eric Crichton), 118, 142 (Peter Wilby), 146 (Michel Viard), 149 (Jan Taylor)

Bührer, Lisbeth, Lucerne: 182, 191 (left), 193 (bottom), 195 (top)

Comet-Photo, Zurich: 89 (top, Zachl)

Coray, Franz, EMB-Service, Lucerne: Artwork: 11; Plant Lexicon: Nos. 13, 14, 23, 37, 53, 136, 150, 152

De Antonis, Roma: 95 (fourth from top)

Documentation photographique de la Réunion des Musées Nationaux, Paris: 94 (top, Louvre)

Elizabeth Arden Ltd., London: 205 (left)

Egyptian Museum, Cairo: 95 (top), 98 (bottom), 99 (top left and right)

EMB Archive, Lucerne: 95 (second from the bottom)

Explorer, Basel-Paris: 191 (right), 199 (centre), 201 (bottom)

FREUNDIN-Archiv/Burda, München: 121, 122, 123, 125 (second from top and far right), 126 (middle), 128, 131, 134, 135 (top right), 136 (bottom), 144 (bottom), 145, 146, 184

Genders Roy, Worthing, Sussex: 205 (right)

Robert Harding Picture Library, London: 4 (Alistair Cowin), 8, 9, 94 (centre, left), 96, 124–125 (top), 125 (two middle, Alistair Cowin), 126 (top and centre far right, Alistair Cowin), 127 (right), 129 (Alistair Cowin), 150, 152 (M. Y. Mackenzie), 203 (bottom, coll. Mrs. Meyer Sassoon)

Hirmer Fotoarchiv, München: 92 (left), 95 (second from top), 97 (top left), 100 (top)

Institut für systematische Botanik der Universität Zürich: Photo Zuppiger: 12 (far left); Plant lexicon: No. 25

Jacana, Basel-Paris: 135 (bottom, Volot), 137 (bottom, J.-P. Champroux), 198 (top, centre, C.H. Moiton), (top, left, J.-P. Champroux; centre J. P. Hérvey; bottom, P. Darmangeat); Plant lexicon: Nos. 1 (J.-P. Champroux), 30 (R. König), 49 (R. König), 54 (Annunziata), 59 (Frédéric), 75 (M. Viard), 89 (J.-P. Champroux), 91 (Dulhoste), 93 (M. Viard), 116 (R. Volot), 120 (M. Viard), 125 (J. P. Hérvy, 140 (M. Viard), 158 (R. König), 159 (M. Viard)

KEY-Color, Zürich: 95 (bottom, ZEFA/Selitsch), 124 (bottom right, Banus), 125 (bottom, Klaus Benser), 130 (ZEFA London), 132 (B. Benjamin), 133 (G. Rettinghaus), 136 (top, J. Pfaff), 137 (top, Jonas), 144 (top, Jobron), 147 (D. Milne/ZEFA)

Kunsthistorisches Museum, Wien: 87

Mary Evans Picture Library, London: 149 (bottom), 200 (top left), 201 (bottom), 204 (left)

Museum der Bildenden Künste zu Leipzig: 88 (photo Gerhard Reinhold, Leipzig-Molkau)

Museum of Fine Arts, Boston: 96 (bottom, Robert Harding Picture Library)

Popperfoto, London: 204 (right), 205 (centre)

Photographie Giraudon, Paris: 6 (Louvre), 91, 98 (top and left)

Rauh, Prof. Dr. W., Institut für systematische Botanik und Pflanzengeographie der Universität Heidelberg: Plant lexicon: Nos. 3, 29, 38, 47, 71, 76, 105, 129

Roger-Viollet, Paris: 93, 196, 200 (top right)

British Crown Copyright. Reproduced with permission of the controller, Her (Foreign) Majesty's Stationery Office, and the Trustees, Royal Botanic Gardens, Kew 1985: Plant lexicon: Nos. 22, 58, 106, 108, 126

Silvestris Fotoservice, Kastl: 14, 124 (left), 127 (left), 128 (top and bottom, right Jogschies), 135 (top left, Jogschies/Lindenburger), 138 (left, Jogschies), 138–139 (Daily Telegraph), 139 (right, Zachl), 140 (top, Gerg; left, Jogschies), 141 (Daily Telegraph), 142 (top, Lindenburger), 143 (top, Jogschies/Lindenburger; bottom, Jogschies), 187 (right, Zachl), 202 (left, Jogschies/Lindenburger)

Harry Smith Horticultural Photographic Collection, Chelmsford: Plant lexicon: Nos. 81, 143

Smith, John Frederick, New York: 15

Storz, Wilfried, EMB-Service, Lucerne: Art work in Plant lexicon: Nos. 43, 52, 98, 119, 134, 135, 153, 171

Topham Picture Library, London: 185, 188, 189, 190, 192 (top left and bottom), 194 (top), 195 (right), 202 (bottom), 203 (top and right)

Victoria and Albert Museum, London: 148

von Matt, Leonard, Buochs: 89 (bottom), 95 (third and fifth from top), 97 (top, centre and right), 100 (left and bottom), 101, 102, 183

Published Works

Abbildungen zu Oken's allgemeiner Naturgeschichte für alle stände, Stuttgart 1843: 25

Arber, Agnes: Herbals-Their origin and evolution, Cambridge 1953: 106

Artus, Hand-Atlas, Vols. I + II: Plant lexicon: Nos. 2, 6, 21, 33, 34, 46, 48, 51, 66, 79, 83, 101, 102, 107, 115, 145, 147

Biedermann, Hans: Medicina Magica, Graz 1972: 5

Dreves, Friedrich: Botanisches Bilderbuch, Leipzig 1794: Plant lexicon: Nos. 18, 86, 96, 112, 170

Eichelberg, J. F. A.: Naturgetreue Abbildungen der merkantistischen Warenkunde, Zürich 1845: Plant lexicon: Nos. 24, 123, 157, 168

Flora Danica, Copenhagen 1770: Plant lexicon: Nos. 17, 117, 124, 127, 133, 156

Fuchs, Leonard: Kreuterbuch 1543, Reprint München 1964: 192–193 (top)

Heilmann, Karl Eugen: Kräuterbücher in Bild und Geschichte, München-Allach 1966: 2, 107, 153, 200 (bottom)

Horn, Effi: Parfum, München: 197

Künzle, Johann: Das grosse Kräuterheilbuch, Olten 1967: Plant lexicon: No. 19

Linné, Carolus A.: Abbildungen von Arzneygewächesen, Nürnberg 1784: Plant lexicon: Nos. 11, 27, 39, 42, 57, 82, 90, 99, 130, 151, 155, 164

Lonicero, Adamo: Kreuterbuch 1679, Reprint München 1962: 12–13 (top), 17

Losch, F.: Les Plantes Médicinales, Biel 1906: 27 (right); Plant lexicon: Nos. 4, 5, 40, 64, 65, 69, 72, 77, 97, 100, 122, 132, 141, 148, 154, 167, 172

Pabst, G.: Köhler's Medizinal-Pflanzen, Vols. I, II, III, Gera-Untermhaus 1887: Plant lexicon: Nos. 7, 12, 41, 44, 45, 61, 73, 84, 85, 87, 88, 102, 121, 131, 137, 138, 144, 161, 162, 163, 165

Pancony, Th.: Herbarium: 198–199 (top)

Pancovius, Herbar: 7

Schinz, Salomon: Anleitung zur Pflanzenkenntnis, Zürich 1774: Plant lexicon: Nos. 10, 139

The Complete Farmer, New York 1975: 1

Von Schuberts, Prof. Dr. G. H.: Naturgeschichte des Pflanzenreichs: Lehrbuch der Pflanzengeschichte, Esselingen 1887: 16 (top); Plant lexicon: Nos. 8, 9, 16, 28, 55, 56, 60, 63, 67, 68, 78, 92, 94, 95, 110, 114, 160, 169

Wilkomm, Dr. Moritz: Naturgeschichte des Pflanzenreichs, Esslingen s.d.: 142 (bottom)